ESSENTIALS OF
PHOTOGRAPHY

D1405079

ESSENTIALS OF PHOTOGRAPHY

PAUL W. HAYES

SCOTT M. WORTON

EDITORIAL CONSULTANT
C. GEOFFREY BERKEN
Community College
of Philadelphia

BOBBS-MERRILL
EDUCATIONAL PUBLISHING
Indianapolis, Indiana

BOBBS-MERRILL
EDUCATIONAL PUBLISHING

Indianapolis, Indiana

PAUL W. HAYES

SCOTT M. WORTON

EDITORAL CONSULTANT

C. GEOFFREY BERKEN
Community College
of Philadelphia

ESSENTIALS OF PHOTOGRAPHY

The Bobbs-Merrill Company, Inc.
4300 West 62nd Street
Indianapolis, Indiana 46206

First Edition
First Printing 1983
Design by Betty Binns
Cover design by Betty Binns

Library of Congress Cataloging in Publication Data

Hayes, Paul W., 1952–
    Essentials of photography.

    Includes index.
    1. Photography.   I. Worton, Scott M., 1949–
II. Title.
TR146.H394   1983   770   82-20755
ISBN 0-672-97492-4

CONTENTS

To Helen and Pam

Preface

We undertook this project to fill a need not met by available photography textbooks, which tend to concentrate solely on either the aesthetics of picture-taking or the scientific and technical aspects of the subject. Yet both of these areas are equally important: a good photographer blends technical competence with seasoned artistic judgment. In this book we have tried to provide the reader with a solid photographic foundation from which to expand his or her picture-taking horizons.

The reader needs no previous knowledge of photography. Anyone from the total novice to the moderately advanced amateur will find this book useful. Although the book deals primarily with black and white photography, many of the same principles can also be applied to color photography. The final two chapters are about color photography and how it works.

Wherever possible we have tried to illustrate the text with photographs taken by photography students. Seeing what can result from a little knowledge of the subject and practice may inspire those who lack confidence in their own work.

We would like to thank the various manufacturers, museums, and collections for their help and contributions. We are also grateful to our many friends, associates, and students for their comments and criticisms. Special thanks go to Helen C. Hayes and Pam Worton, who provided help and motivation throughout the project. We also wish to thank Geoff Berken, our editorial consultant, Laird Roberts, and all the people at Bobbs-Merrill for their assistance and advice.

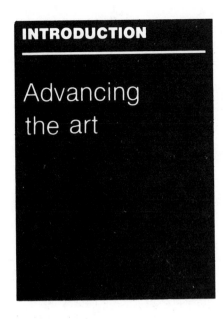

INTRODUCTION

Advancing the art

People have been keeping visual records of themselves and the things around them since prehistoric times, recording images that range from carefully drawn hieroglyphics to pictures taken on the surface of the moon. Each image—from hieroglyphic to space photography—is an attempt to communicate from one person to another the things we see.

Photography, which means "writing with light," gives us the means to record and examine our day-to-day activities. Unlike the casual glance, which often "sees" only the major elements of a scene, a photograph records the tiniest details. It then allows us time to study and understand each minute element. A photograph preserves what the memory cannot. It captures a scene with detailed accuracy, allowing us to share with others an accurate view of that same scene, even many years later. And under the unbiased scrutiny of the camera's eye, all details in that scene are accorded the same importance.

A PICTURE POSTCARD HISTORY[1]

Early study of light

The magic ability of light to transmit images was apparently first casually noted by the Egyptians some ten thousand years ago. Hiding from the fierce sun in their tents and huts, these ancients noticed that when light reflected from objects came beaming through tiny holes in the walls, the colored image of an upside-down camel or person was projected onto the tent wall. Inspired by this experience to experiment with ways to capture and preserve images, they became the first "photographers."

[1]For a more complete list of events in the history of photography, see Appendix A.

Aristotle The famous Greek philosopher first described the formation of a crude optical image in about 350 B.C. He observed that when a beam of light was allowed to enter a darkened room through a small hole, an image was formed. By holding a piece of paper six inches or so from the opening, he was able to capture the image. (Figure I-1 is an early drawing of Aristotle's concept.) Though blurred and upside-down, the image was recognizable. (See Figure I-2.)

Leonardo da Vinci Early in the sixteenth century, the Italian painter and engineer da Vinci diagrammed in his famous *Notebooks* the workings of a camera, complete with instructions on how to use it.

The camera obscura The phenomenon that Aristotle described and da Vinci illustrated became known as the *camera obscura.* This term, meaning "dark room," was introduced by the Italians, whose painters were among the first to make practical use of Aristotle's discovery. In the early 1500s, Italian painters used the camera obscura to improve proportion and perspective in their paintings.

During the next two hundred years, many improvements were made in the basic camera obscura. A glass lens that greatly sharpened the image eventually replaced the simple opening, the camera was made smaller and more portable (see Figure I-3), and mirrors were added so that the image was projected in an upright position. By the early 1700s, the basic optical equipment necessary for manufacturing a camera was available, and the camera obscura had come to look much like the basic camera of today. (See Figure I-4.) But the solution to the basic problem of preserving the camera's image continued to elude scientists. It took an additional 120 years to solve that mystery.

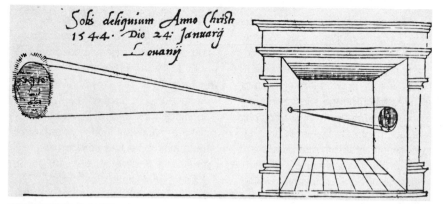

FIGURE I-1 CAMERA OBSCURA
Illustration of a camera obscura observing a solar eclipse in January 1544. The design was based on principles discussed by Aristotle many years before. (Photograph courtesy Gernsheim Collection, Humanities Research Center, University of Texas at Austin)

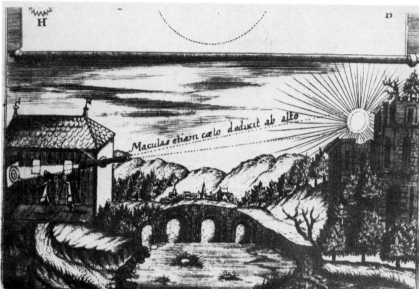

FIGURE I-2 IMAGE IN THE CAMERA OBSCURA
The image that appeared on the inner wall of the camera obscura was upside down and backward, but the proportion and perspective did not change. (Photograph courtesy Gernsheim Collection, Humanities Research Center, University of Texas at Austin)

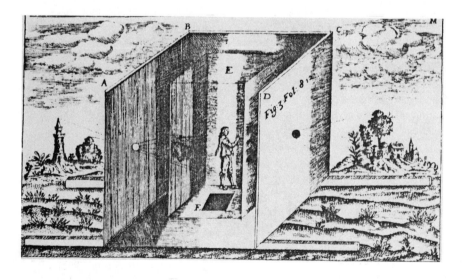

FIGURE I-3 A PORTABLE CAMERA OBSCURA
Portable camera obscura made in Germany during the 1640s. This sketch shows the camera, which was made of wood and canvas, with an inner box of paper, where the image was formed and drawn. The artist entered through a trap door in the bottom. To move the camera required four individuals—one on each corner.

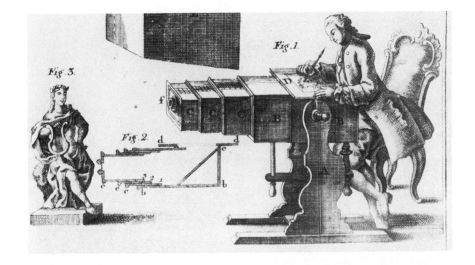

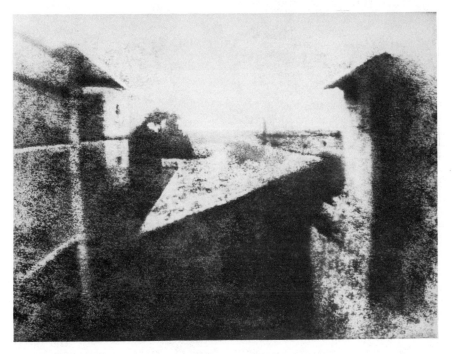

FIGURE I-4 LATE 18TH-CENTURY CAMERA OBSCURA
This table model had a glass lens to correct the image, so that it appeared upright on the screen. The lens could also be extended for close-up work. This camera was designed for use indoors and, because of its size and weight, was best used for motionless subjects. (Photograph courtesy Gernsheim Collection, Humanities Research Center, University of Texas at Austin)

FIGURE I-5 NIÉPCE'S FIRST PHOTOGRAPH
The world's first photograph, taken in 1827. The exposure time was eight hours, which is why the sun can be seen shining on both sides of the picture. (Photograph courtesy Gernsheim Collection, Humanities Research Center, University of Texas at Austin)

camera obscura to reproduce accurate drawings for his ornamental china and pottery. His son Thomas was the first to apply the idea of light-sensitive chemicals to the camera obscura. Familiar with the camera obscura because of his father's work and with Johann Schulze's discoveries about silver salts because of a lifelong interest in chemistry, Wedgwood produced silhouettes of insect wings and leaves on white leather coated with silver nitrate. However, the process was too slow to be used in the camera obscura, and there was no way to fix and preserve the silhouettes. Even Wedgwood's brilliant partner, Sir Humphry Davy, could not come up with a permanent fixing agent.

Joseph N. Niépce Partial credit for the invention of photography has also been given to Frenchman Joseph N. Niépce, who, after many disappointments, successfully produced the world's first photograph in 1827. To produce his photograph he coated a pewter plate with *bitumen of Judea,* or asphaltum, placed the plate in the camera, and made an eight-hour exposure. To develop the photograph, he rinsed the plate with lavender oil. (Figure I-5 is a copy of Niépce's original print.) Although the image was far from perfect, it was a milestone in the advancement of the art.

Making the image permanent

During the 1700s, several people were experimenting with chemicals that were sensitive to light, using as their tools combinations of different chemicals. The biggest challenge facing photographers was to find a fixing agent that would make the images permanent.

Johann Schulze A German professor of anatomy, Johann Schulze, was experimenting with the manufacture of phosphorus when he discovered that a combination of chalk, aqua regia (a mixture of nitric and hydrochloric acids), and silver nitrate turned purple when exposed to light. By the process of elimination he discovered that silver salts were the darkening agent. Unfortunately, however, he failed to make use of this discovery. The credit for applying Schulze's results goes to Thomas Wedgwood.

Thomas Wedgwood The great English potter Josiah Wedgwood used the

FIGURE I-6 DAGUERROTYPE
This picture was taken in the early 1840s. Even though the image has been carefully preserved over the years, the image is starting to deteriorate. (Courtesy Utah State Historical Society)

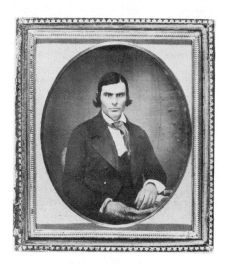

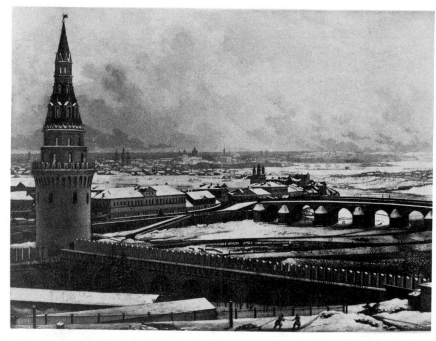

FIGURE I-7 SNOW SCENE, MOSCOW
Daguerrotypes could not be photographically reproduced. To make copies, the original had to be transferred to a wood block, from which a wood engraving was made for the printing press. The original daguerrotype was destroyed in this process. This photograph was taken by an unknown photographer *c.* 1840. (International Museum of Photography at George Eastman House)

Louis J.M. Daguerre Another Frenchman, Louis Daguerre, started his own search for the ideal fixing agent when his brief partnership with Niépce broke up. In 1837, after eight years of searching, he found what he was looking for—mercury vapor.

Daguerre patented his process as the *daguerreotype process.* The procedure involved making an exposure on silver foil that had been sensitized with iodine. Following exposure, the foil was brought into contact with mercury vapor for development. (See Figure I-6.)

Daguerreotype prints were an instant success. Studios were opened, and professional photographers began giving portrait painters stiff competition for business. Gradually, over the years, refinements were made in the lens and in the light sensitivity of the plates that were used. The popularity of daguerreotype portraits leaped

when a method was devised to soften the tones and enrich the image.

While the daguerreotype represented a fantastic advance in photography, it was far from perfect. The photographs were expensive—two dollars for a single frame. (Later modifications in the process made the prints available at two for twenty-five cents.) The images were so fragile that they had to be kept in a glass case, which made them bulky to store and awkward to look at. Also, the observer had to contend with a metallic glare. Probably the most significant disadvantage was that the daguerreotype images were positive, not negative, images, so it was difficult to manufacture reproductions. (See Figure I-7.)

William Henry Fox Talbot William Henry Fox Talbot, an English contemporary of Daguerre, made the next

major contribution to photography— production of the first negative image. Working with silver nitrate and common salt (sodium chloride), Fox Talbot produced silver chloride, a compound more sensitive to light than Daguerre's sensitized foil plates. Fox Talbot coated paper instead of glass or metal plates, to produce the first negative image in August 1835. Despite his disappointment at public indifference to his discovery, Fox Talbot made numerous experiments to perfect the process. (See Figure I-8.)

While working to improve his technique, Fox Talbot discovered the *latent image*—an invisible image formed on film after exposure but before development. Fox Talbot realized that the resulting negative would enable him to reproduce the photograph easily. (See Figure I-9.)

In 1841 Fox Talbot obtained a patent for his process, which he called the

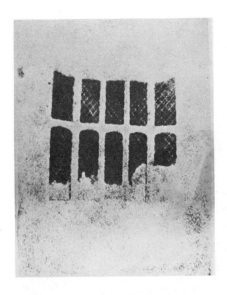

FIGURE I-8A FOX TALBOT'S FIRST NEGATIVE

The world's first paper negative was taken by Fox Talbot in 1835. It is a view of a window in his home at Lacock Abbey. (Photograph courtesy of the Fox Talbot Museum, Lacock Abbey, England)

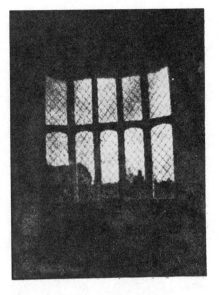

FIGURE I-8B FOX TALBOT: LATTICED WINDOW, AUGUST 1835

(Photograph courtesy of the Fox Talbot Museum, Lacock Abbey, England)

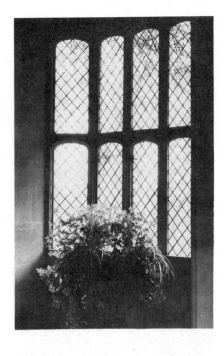

FIGURE I-8C THE LATTICED WINDOW AS IT APPEARS TODAY

(Photograph courtesy of the Fox Talbot Museum, Lacock Abbey, England)

FIGURE I-9 THE CALOTYPE PROCESS

This is a print made from the calotype process of Fox Talbot's photographic studio, the Reading Establishment, in 1845. (Photograph courtesy of the Fox Talbot Museum, Lacock Abbey, England)

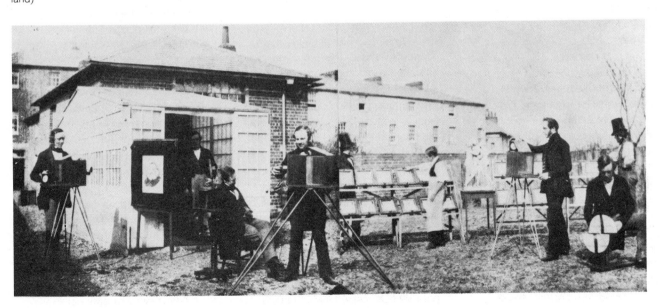

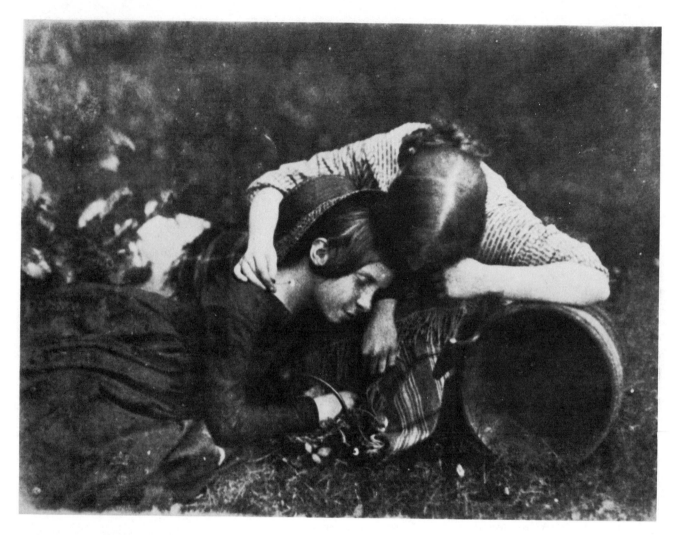

FIGURE I-10 HILL AND ADAMSON: THE MCCANDLISH CHILDREN
Calotype, c. 1845 (International Museum of Photography at George Eastman House)

calotype photographic process, derived from the Greek word calos, meaning ''beautiful.'' The beautiful thing about the calotype process was that it produced a negative, which permitted much easier reproduction of positive images that were more durable than the positive images created by the daguerreotype process.

Although Fox Talbot did not enjoy the instant success of Daguerre, his discoveries and contributions to photography were the keys that unlocked the negative–positive process, earning for him recognition as the father of modern photography.

Joseph Petzval The same year Fox Talbot patented the calotype process, a Viennese photographer, Joseph Petzval, designed the first fast portrait lens—a lens ten times faster than the landscape lenses used in the daguerreotype cameras. The daguerreotype, which was already being replaced by Fox Talbot's negative process, was further relegated to the past by Petzval's faster lens, which relieved subjects from the necessity of sitting for excruciatingly long sessions.

David Octavius Hill and Robert Adamson Using the calotype process, Scottish photographer Robert Adamson joined Scottish painter David Octavius Hill to produce some of the finest photographs of the mid-nineteenth century. Adamson was a respected portrait photographer in Edinburgh; Hill was interested in using photographs as a reference for his paintings. Although the two did photograph a number of groups, most of their photographs were of single subjects, posed outdoors in direct sunlight. The exposures were usually minutes long, and concave mirrors were used to soften the harsh shadows. (See Figure I-10.) The two worked as a team from 1842 until 1848, when Adamson died at the age of twenty-seven.

Striving for permanence, definition, and speed

By 1851, the year of Daguerre's death, photography had truly arrived. The ranks of photographers had swelled from a handful to thousands. Besides marking the end of one era, that year signalled the beginning of another, ushered in by Frederick Scott Archer's discovery of the wet collodion technique.

Frederick Scott Archer The English sculptor Frederick Scott Archer invented the *wet collodion process* while attempting to improve the calotype process he used during sculpting. Archer decided to try using collodion, a substance made by dissolving guncotton (nitrocellulose) in ether.

Archer made a mixture of the gelatin-like collodion and potassium iodide and spread it thinly over a glass plate. He then dipped the still damp plate into a solution of silver nitrate. The plate had to be exposed immediately because its light sensitivity dropped sharply as it dried. As soon as it was exposed, the plate was developed in pyrogallic acid and fixed with sodium thiosulfate. Archer's original intention was to use the collodion as a process for producing negatives, but it soon became a popular method for positive production too.

Technicians had spent years trying everything from snail slime to egg whites in an effort to achieve this result. The tough, skin-like film produced by the collodion was the ideal substance for bonding the silver nitrate salts to the glass.

Because the wet collodion glass positives looked very much like daguerreotypes, they achieved almost instant popularity in the United States. Archer's invention, which he published without restriction, was patented by Bostonian James Ambrose Cutting in 1854. The photographs were called *ambrotypes* and, like the daguerreo-

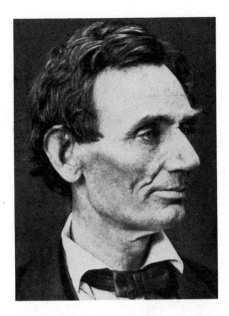

types, were usually enclosed in leather or composition cases.

By spreading the light-sensitive collodion on sheets of tin instead of glass, photographers produced the familiar *tintype*. The thin metal sheets were japanned a black or chocolate color by inventor Hamilton L. Smith, who assigned his 1856 patent to Peter Neff and Peter Neff, Jr. Manufacture of the plates was begun in 1856 under the name of *melainotypes*.

The collodion process was more technical and demanding than either the daguerreotype or the calotype process. It was especially troublesome for outdoor photographers, who had to take a complete portable darkroom into the field. But the process produced excellent results. (See Figure I-11.) With an exposure time of less than ten seconds instead of several minutes, it produced a sharp, clear, negative that could easily be reprinted.

Picture-making in the Victorian era

A strange and hotly denied partnership between painters and photographers developed during the Victorian era. The photographers labored incessantly

FIGURE I-11 HESLER: ABRAHAM LINCOLN, 1860
Wet Collodion Process (International Museum of Photography at George Eastman House)

FIGURE I-12 CAMERON: SIR JOHN HERSCHEL, 1867
(International Museum of Photography at George Eastman House)

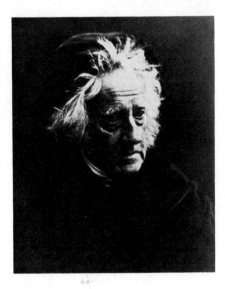

to imitate the precise and meticulous detail of the era's portrait painters. The painters, on the other hand, worked from photographs—though none would admit it. Eventually the partnership dissolved when photographers stopped trying to mimic the painters and the painters decided to leave realism to the photographers. A number of talented and brilliant photographers and artists emerged from this period of confusion.

Julia Margaret Cameron Julia Margaret Cameron, one of the most remarkable amateurs of all time, started work in the 1860s on what she considered a "divine art." In her photographs (see Figure I-12) she attempted to record "the greatness of

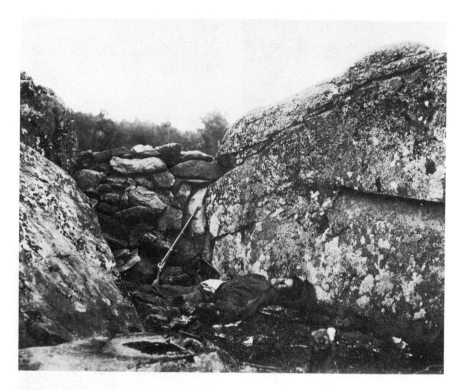

FIGURE I-13 GARDNER: "HOME OF A REBEL SHARPSHOOTER," GETTYSBURG, 1863
(International Museum of Photography at George Eastman House)

the inner as well as the features of the outer man."

She pioneered in the use of close-up techniques, large plates, and unusual lighting. She used an enormous lens and demanded that her subjects sit frozen for exposures lasting five to seven minutes. Her portrait subjects included the great, and the not so great, of the period.

Nadar A newspaperman and caricaturist, Nadar, whose real name was Gaspard Felix Tournachon, turned to photography when he realized how helpful it would be to have a photograph of the subject before him when he set to work on a caricature. His relentless pursuit of celebrities of the time won him acclaim not only as a caricaturist but also as a photographer. Eventually, he turned to full-time portraiture. His straightforward approach—a three-quarter-length view of the subject standing against a plain background under a high skylight—and his mastery of the collodion process gained him fame and brought

celebrities flocking to his studios. He photographed such notables as Baudelaire, Cézanne, Dumas, Rossini, and Wagner.

A versatile genius, Nadar built one of the world's largest balloons, *The Giant,* and snapped the first aerial photograph in 1858 while piloting the balloon. He illustrated books, wrote novels, and invented a technique called photo-interviewing.

Pioneers of reportage

Nadar's technique of photo-interviewing was refined by a group of talented photographers, who used their equipment to record snatches of history.

Roger Fenton Roger Fenton was an accomplished landscape and architectural photographer when he sailed from England in the winter of 1855. He was headed for the theatre of the Crimean War as a war photographer. Daguerreotypes of officers and men had been done during the Mexican War, but never had photographs been taken during combat. Fenton outfitted a wagon "darkroom" with five cameras, seven hundred glass plates, rations, and chemicals, and then forged to the battlefront. He was besieged from all sides. A piece of his wagon's roof was torn off by shellfire, and he was constantly bothered by requests for portraits. However, in July he returned to London with three hundred negatives, exposed by the wet collodion process. After the prints were developed, they were displayed in London and Paris. The public generally found the photographs to be dull, but they did recognize them as faithful witnesses to the situation in the Crimea, and war has since been an important subject for the photographer.

Mathew B. Brady and Alexander Gardner Mathew B. Brady's documentary photographs of the American Civil War are among the first American

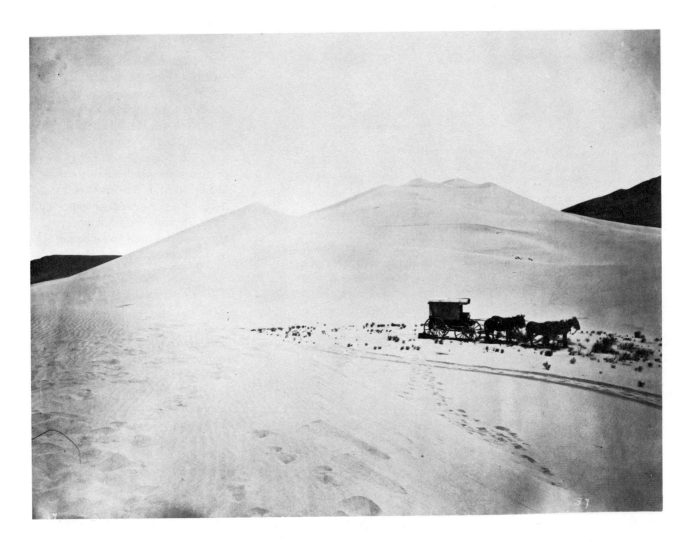

FIGURE I-14 O'SULLIVAN: SAND DUNES, NEVADA, 1867

The horses and wagon comprised a traveling darkroom. (International Museum of Photography at George Eastman House)

war photos ever recorded. Using bulky daguerreotype equipment, Brady was horribly conspicuous on the battlefield and, therefore, was constantly being shot at. His technique was exceeded only by his bravery. While Brady is renowned for his numerous high-quality photographs of the war, one of the most famous of all Civil War photographs was taken by Brady's partner, Alexander Gardner. (See Figure I-13.)

Timothy H. O'Sullivan An Irishman who worked with Brady, Timothy H. O'Sullivan had a taste for danger and excitement that inspired him to travel where even armed soldiers hesitated to go. His daring resulted in some of the most spectacular photographs of the Civil War. Then in 1867 he joined Clarence King's Geological Expedition, traveling from San Francisco to the Great Salt Lake, through the Sierra Nevadas. At Virginia City, Nevada, O'Sullivan went hundreds of feet underground to photograph the Comstock Lode mines by the light of magnesium flares—an act that could have been suicidal in a mine filled with flammable gas. Later he photographed shifting sand dunes that peaked at more than five hundred feet in height—with his only shelter a rickety ambulance "darkroom" and his only means of escape four mules. (See Figure I-14.)

William Henry Jackson The last of the great frontier photographers, Wil-

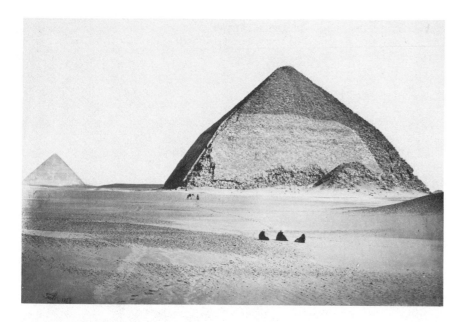

FIGURE I-15 FRANCIS FRITH: THE PYRAMIDS OF DAHSHUR, EGYPT, 1858
This print was made by the wet collodion process. (International Museum of Photography at George Eastman House)

FIGURE I-16 GEORGE EASTMAN WITH A KODAK ABOARD THE S.S. *GALLIA*, 1890
(International Museum of Photography at George Eastman House)

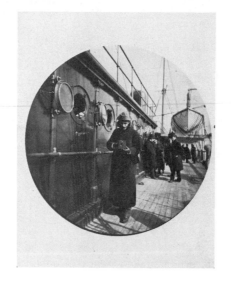

Photography for everyone

The speed of the wet collodion process revolutionized photography, but the process had drawbacks. It was messy and cumbersome. A great deal of practice was required before a photographer became skilled in the technique. So technicians sought to further decrease time needed for exposure and processing. The first step in that direction was the development of dry plates. Research produced many advancements, until finally gelatin replaced collodion as the ideal emulsifier and the era of roll film was introduced.

Eastman's simple box camera

George Eastman began as an amateur photographer in 1877. Within twenty years he controlled the largest photographic manufacturing company in the world. (See Figure I-16.)

Introduced in 1888, the Kodak No. 1, Eastman's simple box camera was the first camera to use roll film instead of plates or sheets. (See Figure I-17.) The camera appealed to the masses of amateur photographers because it was small ($6\frac{1}{2}$ inches by $3\frac{1}{2}$ inches by $3\frac{1}{2}$ inches) and simple to operate. The advertising slogan "You press the button and we do the rest" indicated that anyone who could press the button could get good pictures. Eastman chose the name "Kodak" because the word mimicked the sound the shutter made and was easily pronounced throughout the world.

The camera came loaded with enough film for one hundred pictures and cost twenty-five dollars. When the one hundred pictures had been taken, the photographer mailed the camera to the Eastman plant in Rochester, New York. The film was then processed, prints were made, the camera was reloaded with film, and the pictures and camera were returned to the owner. Total cost for the prints and new film was ten dollars.

liam Henry Jackson dragged a huge camera into the Rocky Mountains to record the spectacular scenery. The oversized camera was cumbersome, and his equipment primitive. His darkroom was a canvas tent, six feet square at the base and lined with orange calico; his developing box was a crude wooden tray. His first subject was Lake San Cristobal in Colorado; it took him three days to obtain the photograph.

Jackson's work was so stunning that when Congress saw his 1871 photographs of the Yellowstone area, that legislative body was inspired to declare it the first national park in the United States.

Francis Frith The intrepid courage of photographers of the American West was matched by photographers all over the world. Francis Frith made countless journeys from London to Egypt and the Holy Land. His travels produced a legacy of sixteen- by twenty-inch plates of Egypt's magnificent pyramids, shot under the most devilish desert conditions. (See Figure I-15.)

The rapid growth in amateur photography after 1880 created a need for mass production of photographic equipment. The Eastman Kodak Company was the first to capitalize on this opportunity to cater to an ever-increasing market, and it continues to be a primary contender today.

The age of the small camera In the 1890s, following on the heels of Kodak, a host of manufacturers attempted to compete in the vast amateur photography marketplace. The folding bellows camera, the twin-lens reflex camera, and the "nodark"—a camera that processed its own film—appealed to beginning photographers throughout the world. Small cameras became even more popular with Dr. Paul Rudolph's invention of a precision lens—the *Zeiss Tessar*.

Small precision German cameras Small, simple cameras had been developed to appeal to those novice photographers who wanted to preserve on film Ned's sixth birthday or the family's vacation on the coast. In 1925 the serious photographer was provided with a small, high-quality, hand-held camera that used 35 mm film and the Zeiss lens—the *Leica*. (See Figure I-18.) Leicas established the standards for the modern-day 35 mm cameras. The inventor of the Leica, Oscar Barnack, started work on the camera two years earlier as a means to pretest the exposure of movie film. It worked so well that on mountain hikes he substituted the smaller prototype Leica for his bulky field camera. Leicas have been in production since 1925 and have been refined and improved so that today they are still among the world's premier cameras.

The electronic flash Harold E. Edgerton's electronic flash ushered photography into an era of ultra-high speed, with shutter exposures of less than $\frac{1}{50,000}$ second. Edgerton's photo-

FIGURE I-17 THE NO. 1 KODAK ROLL FILM CAMERA
This disassembled view shows the simple internal workings of the camera. (Courtesy Eastman Kodak Company)

FIGURE I-18 THE LEICA CAMERA
This is a photograph of the Leica 1, the first production model 35 mm Leica camera. (Courtesy E. Leitz, Inc., Rockleigh, N.J.)

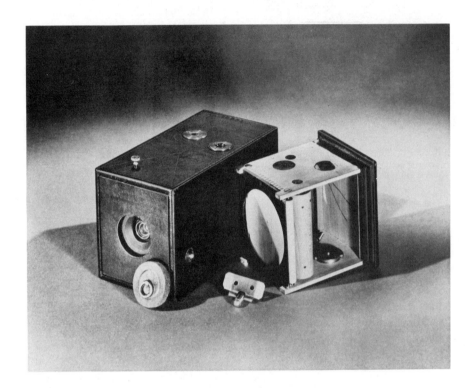

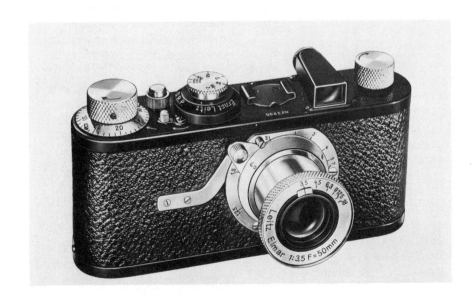

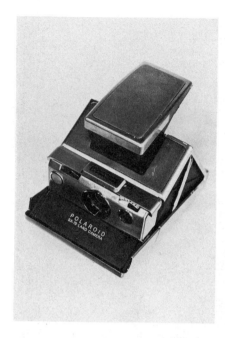

FIGURE I-19 POLAROID SX-70

graphs have shown us a drop of milk hitting a plate, a bullet passing through a light bulb, and a hummingbird resting on air.

Instant photography After World War II, amateur photography experienced another boom period. Renewed interest was in large part due to the advent of the Kodak Brownie Instamatic cameras and the 1947 invention of the Polaroid Land Camera (a camera that bore the name of its inventor, Edwin Land). The revolutionary new Polaroid produced a positive print in sixty seconds, because both the negative and the positive images were developed simultaneously. (See Figure I-19.) Despite harsh critics who said the Polaroid could not possibly last, it has endured to become a photographic mainstay among amateurs, as well as being used by many professionals.

The color breakthrough

Even the earliest photographers tried to capture color in their photographs. After all, since the camera faithfully reproduced nature, it seemed that it should be able to do so in color. Both Niépce and Daguerre made attempts, but their limited knowledge of chemistry prohibited success. Only much later were photographers able to master the complex chemical and physical balances necessary to produce color photographs.

Sir James Clerk Maxwell In what was probably the first description of modern color photography, Sir James Clerk Maxwell demonstrated in an 1861 lecture how any shade of color could be manufactured by mixing the three primary colors of light (blue, red, green) in varying proportions. He used colored glass plates to illustrate his point. The plates were combined in various ways, and a light was shone through them and projected onto a screen. His system, known as the *additive color system,* was the first theory to be applied to color photography.

Louis Ducos du Hauron French pianist Louis Ducos du Hauron described the *subtractive color system* in 1869. Colors, he said, are made of pigments that absorb all colors but their own, which they reflect. Du Hauron's and Clerk Maxwell's theories provided the basis for the introduction of color photography some sixty-five years later, with the advent of Kodachrome film.

Leopold Mannes and Leopold Godowsky In 1935 Leopold Mannes and Leopold Godowsky, working at the Eastman Kodak Laboratories, produced Kodachrome film, a film based on a dye-coupling theory. In 1941 Kodak introduced Kodacolor film, which utilized the negative—positive principle. On the color negative, the color (as well as the highlights and shadows) is reversed. A blonde woman wearing red lipstick, for example, will appear on the negative with blue hair and green lips. Any number of copies can be made using a white-base, color-sensitized paper. In 1942 Ansco brought out Ansco-Color film. Kodak followed with Ektachrome film. In 1947 Eastman Kodak produced Ektacolor film, a product that made it possible for photographers to process their own color film. Polaroid color film was developed in 1962.

PHOTOGRAPHIC STYLES OF THE TWENTIETH CENTURY

Scientists and photographers seeking to improve the art of photography have given us the rich variation in styles that characterizes twentieth-century interpretation of an art that can trace its roots back thousands of years. Incredible shutter speeds have made obsolete the stiffly posed sub-

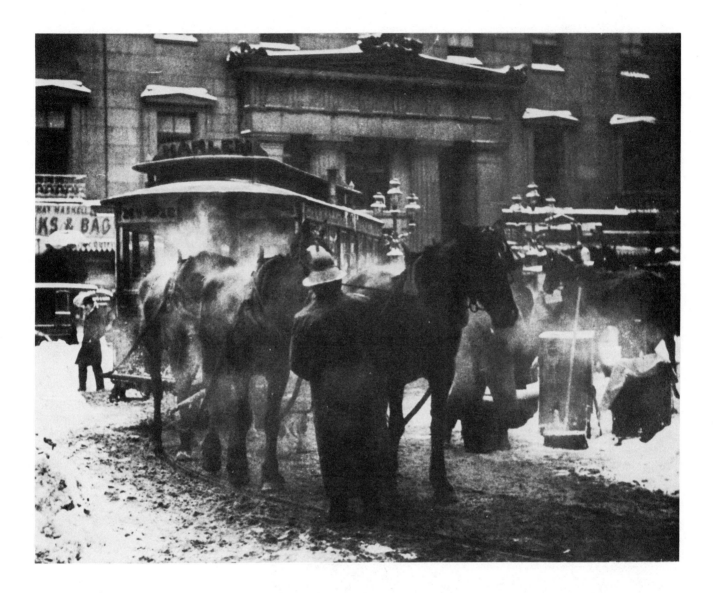

jects of the daguerreotypes. Instead, we enjoy such candid expressions as that of a baby spying a fluffy puppy. Our mastery of physics and chemistry has given us the brilliant colors of the California redwoods and the roughly hewn Grand Canyon, preserving natural wonders on film for future years.

Straight photography

Simply put, straight photography is the technique of producing a print that has not been altered in any form. A straight print is one that reproduces the original scene as faithfully as possible. Advocates of straight photogra-

phy admire its purity and its integrity with regard to its subjects.

Alfred Stieglitz One of the earliest advocates of straight photography, Alfred Stieglitz did more than any other person to establish photography as an art form. His magazine *Camera work* not only served as a vehicle for his own photography, but also exposed the work of others who became important for their photographic art. (See Figure I-20.)

Paul Strand The last two issues of *Camera Work*, dated 1916 and 1917, carried a series of photographs that

FIGURE I-20 STIEGLITZ: THE TERMINAL, 1893
From the original lantern slide (International Museum of Photography at George Eastman House)

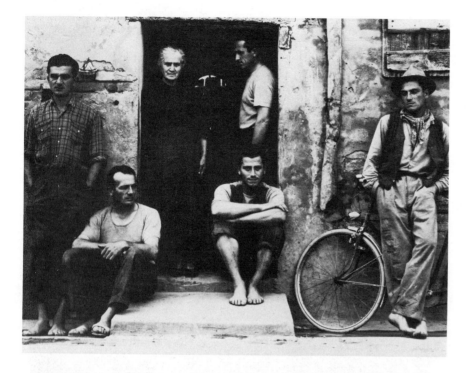

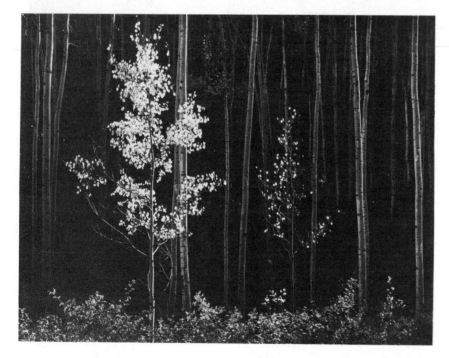

FIGURE I-21 STRAND: THE FAMILY, LUZZARA, ITALY, 1953
(International Museum of Photography at George Eastman House)

FIGURE I-22 ADAMS: ASPENS NEAR SANTA FE, NEW MEXICO, 1958
(International Museum of Photography at George Eastman House)

Stieglitz called "brutally direct, pure and devoid of trickery." This series, straight photography at its best, was by newcomer Paul Strand. Strand's landscapes, whether of Egypt or of New England, were considered lyrical. His subjects ranged from people living off the land to precision machines. (See Figure I-21.)

Ansel Adams A pianist who turned to photography, Ansel Adams began photographing West Coast landscapes in the 1920s. He eventually became an extraordinary teacher, transforming sloppy photographers into precise artisans. (See Figure I-22.)

Edward Weston An avid photographer who discovered the art at the age of sixteen, Edward Weston devoted his life to his love of cameras and all things related to them. He spent a lifetime striving for the sharpest pictures and the widest range of tones, searching for brightness and detail in every print. (See Figure I-23.) He was the first photographer to be awarded the Guggenheim Prize.

Documentary photography

In the twenties, documentary photography became a recognized form of straight photography, used to communicate, to inform, to persuade. Documentary photography tells honestly, accurately, and convincingly the story of the peasant farmer, the wounded soldier, the fragile old woman. The subject is all-important in documentary photography, and its advocates are some of the greatest storytellers of all time.

Jean Eugene Auguste Atget Virtually unknown when he died in 1927, Atget took hundreds of photographs of his beloved Paris—the iron grill work, the little people who earn their living peddling umbrellas, the ragpickers' hovels, the historic monuments. (See Figure I-24.) His technique was very

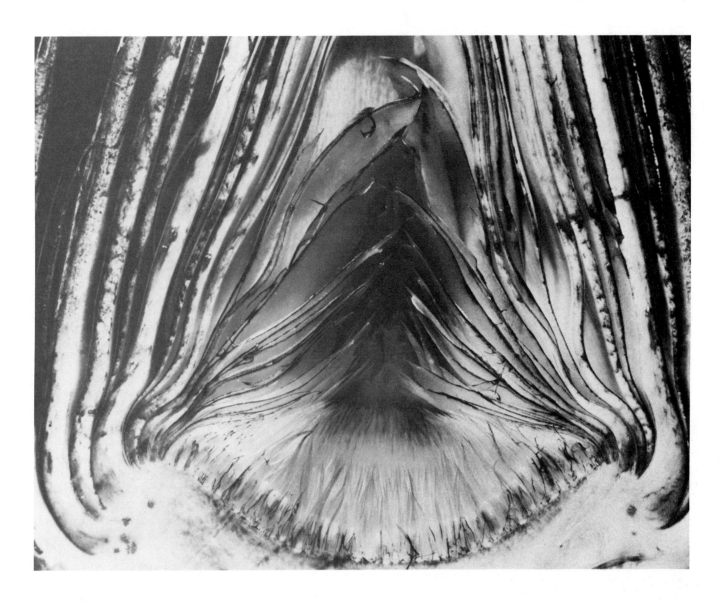

simple: he always used a view camera on a tripod. Hence the moving objects in his photographs were often blurred. He had remarkable vision and preserved on film all the poetry and lyricism of Paris as he knew it.

Dorothea Lange Devastated by what she saw in the Depression, Lange sought to bring to others the haunting sight of children in bread lines, homeless women with their tattered children, jobless men huddled along littered streets. She used her camera to help others feel what she had felt. In 1935, when the federal government realized that such photography could

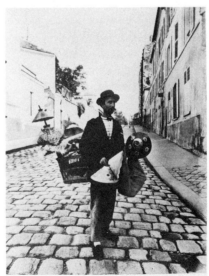

FIGURE I-23 WESTON: ARTICHOKE HALVED, 1930
(International Museum of Photography at George Eastman House)

FIGURE I-24 ATGET: LAMPSHADE PEDDLER, PARIS, C. 1910
(Collection, The Museum of Modern Art, New York. Abbott-Levy Collection. Partial Gift of Shirley C. Burden.)

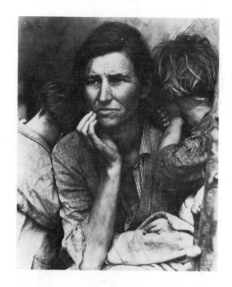

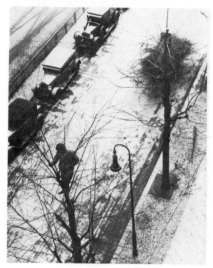

FIGURE I-25 LANGE: MIGRANT MOTHER, NIPOMO, CALIFORNIA, 1936
(International Museum of Photography at George Eastman House)

FIGURE I-26 MOHOLY-NAGY: SPRING, BERLIN, 1928
(International Museum of Photography at George Eastman House)

be an effective tool in fighting the Depression, Lange and other photographers were paid to go into stricken areas to record the sufferings of sharecroppers and other struggling Americans. The scenes Lange shot were necessarily squalid, but her interpretation was always dignified. She concentrated on the plight of migrant workers in America's farmlands. (See Figure I-25.)

Margaret Bourke-White In 1927, Margaret Bourke-White's photographic essay on Muncie, Indiana, was published in *Life* magazine. An "important American document," it was an unusually graphic cross-sectional view of an American town. It showed the rich and the poor, the mansions and the tenement dwellings. Bourke-White traveled into the intimate reaches of the city, using her camera to extract what she found for the rest of the country.

Formalistic photography

Pioneered largely by Man Ray and László Moholy-Nagy, formalistic photography seeks to isolate and organize form for its own sake, and it exploits the photographic process to accomplish this. While subject is critical to documentary photography, it may not even exist for formalistic photography; if it does, it is often not recognizable. Subjects are distorted beyond recognition; space relationships are abstracted; tones are changed; colors are reversed. (See Figure I-26.)

Metaphoric photography

Although the subject does exist in recognizable form in metaphoric photography, it is only the starting point for the vision of the photographer. Metaphoric art is rooted in the subject, and yet it extends far beyond it, taking us to a land of imagination and dreams.

Minor White Best-known of the metaphoric photographers, Minor White is a brilliant technician who uses the camera to photograph the world with great sensitivity. For White, a rock becomes an entire landscape; frost on the windowpane becomes a crashing wave spraying salty foam across the craggy coast. Contrasts are great, edges are sharp, and there is little depth. The viewer must look beyond what is obvious to what is revealed. (See Figure I-27.)

SUMMARY

What started in the seventeenth century with experiments using light-sensitive chemicals in light-tight boxes has evolved into a sophisticated art involving highly technical equipment. Generations of researchers have freed amateur and professional photographers from the kinds of scientific knowledge and technical skills that were needed by early photographers. Those who used the camera obscura could not even have imagined the advances that have resulted—such as a small built-in computer that can control all camera functions. (See Figure I-28.)

Once photography was an isolated art practiced by an eccentric few. As the photographic process became refined and improved, it grew in general popularity. Photographers opened studios to cater to increasing demand for portraits. Later, a more candid form of photography was born when a few daring souls ventured onto battlefields with their cameras. The ability of a picture to tell a story, to convey a feeling, to record history was recognized and valued by early journalistic and documentary photographers. Thanks to their art, we are able to view the past in greater detail and with more sensitivity and compassion.

Photography remained primarily in the hands of professionals until the advent of small, simple cameras.

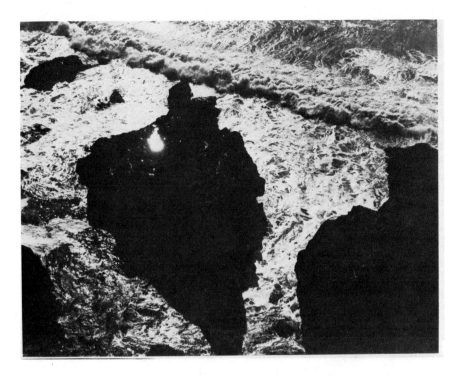

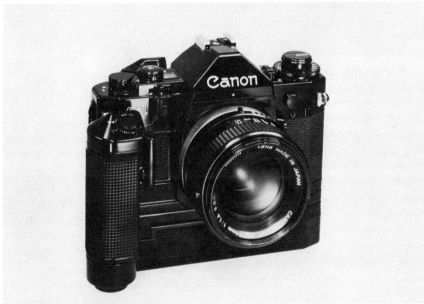

FIGURE I-27 M. WHITE: PACIFIC, 1948
(International Museum of Photography at George Eastman House)

FIGURE I-28 CANON A-1
(Courtesy Canon Camera Company)

These cameras made it possible for anyone who so desired to take pictures. The Eastman Kodak Company and scores of competitors throughout the world have made photography an economically and technically feasible hobby. The highly technological advancements in the science of photography, which have greatly enhanced the range and scope of the art, have also affected a wide spectrum of unrelated fields, such as medicine and space exploration.

Amidst the excitement of scientific discovery and development, it should not be forgotten that photography at its best remains an art form. It is one person's view of the world, interpreted through the mind's eye and the camera's lens. It is a view that can be completely realistic or completely poetic:

Of what use are lens and light
To those who lack in mind and sight?
 (Translation of Latin inscription on a 1589 Brunswick Thaler, an old German coin)

REVIEW QUESTIONS

1 Who was the first to describe the principles upon which the camera obscura was later based?

2 Who is usually given credit for producing the world's first photograph?

3 Who developed the daguerreotype process?

4 Who is called the father of modern photography and is given credit for inventing the negative–positive process?

5 In 1851 who invented the process that rapidly replaced all existing methods of photography?

6 Called one of the most remarkable amateurs of all time, who created photos characterized by qualities rare in early portraiture?

7 Who can take credit for making photography available to everyone?

8 Who developed the instant print process?

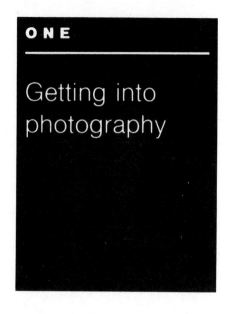

ONE

Getting into photography

Photography has the unique and almost magical ability to capture and accurately record an event as it happens. This *decisive moment,* as it is sometimes called, may last only a fraction of a second, as in the fluid motion of a hummingbird's wings in flight, or it may endure for centuries, as in the seemingly unchanging majesty of a mountain peak.

The amazing process begins in the photographer's mind and eye and ends with a photographic print. In order to produce meaningful photographic statements, the photographer must first understand each step in the photographic process and the factors that control it.

TOOLS OF THE TRADE

The following sections provide brief insights into the basics of photography. In later chapters each aspect of the photographer's skill, the parts and functions of the camera, the processes of exposure and development, and the uses of photographic materials will be discussed in greater detail.

The variety of camera equipment on the market today creates a strange paradox. Technical advances in equipment threaten to make photography so mechanized that some of the creative process may be lost—but those same technical advances have helped to make photography the recognized art medium that it is today.

Choosing camera equipment

When you purchase camera equipment, it is best to buy simple equipment of good quality. Too many people buy more tools than they need, thinking this will guarantee better photography. Instead, equipment becomes the master, and creativity suffers.

The size of film the camera uses determines the camera *format.* Cameras range in format from 110 pocket cameras (each film frame is 2.2 cm square) to cameras that use 8 × 10-inch film. Large-format cameras—once the only kind available—are used mostly by professionals today. One of the most diversified and popular formats among professional and amateur photographers alike is the 35 mm camera.

Regardless of the format and despite the amount of equipment involved, all cameras carry out only six basic functions. These depend on six basic camera parts:

a light-tight box (camera body)

a lens

a shutter

an aperture

a film transport system

a view finder.

(See Figure 1-1.) If even one of these six parts is missing or defective, the camera will not take pictures.

The camera body The body of the camera—the light-tight box—provides the supporting framework for the other parts of the camera. It also protects the film from unwanted exposure to light. The controls the photographer uses to regulate the camera functions are found on the exterior of the box.

The lens The human eye and the eye of the camera—the lens—are alike in several ways. They both concentrate and focus on the image-bearing light, and neither can focus on more than one distance at a time. You can verify this by conducting a simple experiment. Hold a pencil at arm's length. Close one eye and try to focus the open eye on the pencil and on an object about ten feet away. When you focus on the pencil, the other object looks blurry. Just as you can refocus back and forth, with an adjustable

FIGURE 1-1 BASIC CAMERA PARTS

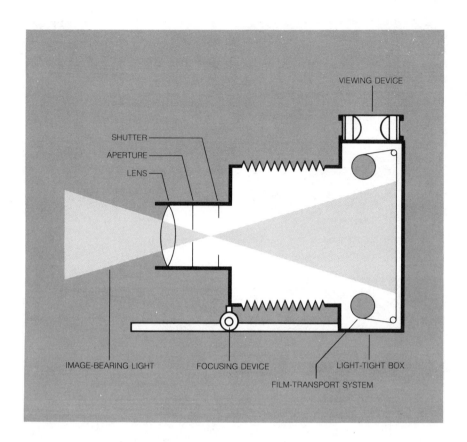

camera lens, the photographer can refocus at various distances.

Despite the similarities, there are some important differences between the human eye and the camera lens. When you look at an object, your eye sees the center of the field of vision most clearly. A camera lens, on the other hand, sees with almost identical clarity across the entire field of vision. Your eye scans the entire scene so that you can see it all; the camera lens does not. The structure of the lens, too, is very different from that of the human eye. In its simplest form, a lens is a polished circle of glass. If it is thicker at the center than at the edges, it is a simple *convex* lens. If the outer edge is thicker than the center, it is a simple *concave* lens. Simple lenses, whether convex or concave, are referred to as *lens elements*. Some cameras lenses consist of only one or two elements. Other highly complex ones have eight or ten.

The shutter The shutter controls the amount of time light is allowed to shine through the lens onto the film. The shutter is also a switch that lets the photographer choose the precise moment to turn the camera on and off.

Early shutters were simply caps that fit over the lens. The first mechanical shutters were called *drop-leaf* shutters These consisted of a metal plate with a hole that fell past the lens. The top speed was about $\frac{1}{25}$ second of exposure.

More sensitive film made more sensitive shutters necessary. The most successful designs for wide use are the *leaf* shutter and the *focal-plane* shutter. These two are capable of the high speeds demanded by today's films, reaching as high as $\frac{1}{2000}$ second.

Leaf shutters are positioned inside the lens of the camera; for this reason, they are also called interlens shutters. A leaf shutter is made up of several overlapping metal blades that open

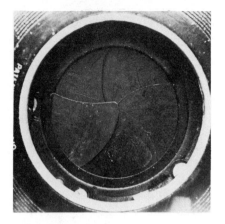

A Fully closed position

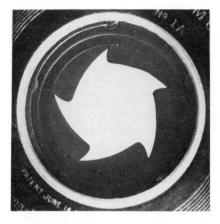

C Leaves continue to open.

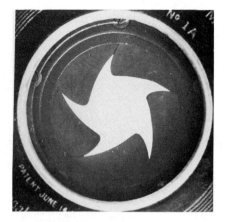

E Leaves begin to close.

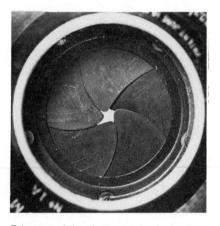

B Leaves of the shutter are beginning to open just after the shutter release has been tripped.

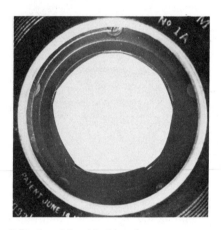

D Shutter at its widest opening

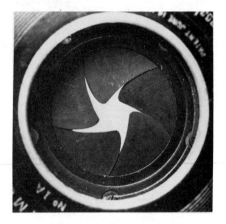

F Leaves close until the shutter is fully closed.

FIGURE 1-2A–F LEAF SHUTTER SEQUENCE

and close quickly to make the proper exposure. (See Figure 1-2.)

A leaf shutter is light and simple. It releases the tension of the shutter "primed" by a separate lever during film advance.

Focal-plane shutters are common on single lens reflex and interchangeable lens rangefinder cameras. Focal-plane shutters are located just in front of the film.

The focal-plane shutter usually consists of two fabric or metallic curtains. When the shutter is released, the primary curtain moves across the film, followed almost instantly by the secondary curtain. The two curtains are separated by a slit that exposes the film. (See Figure 1-3.) The size of the

slit and the speed it moves determine the shutter speed.

Shutter speeds are preprogrammed into the camera: you select the one you want by setting the shutter speed dial. (See Figure 1-4.) A typical shutter speed range includes B, 1, 2, 4, 8, 15, 30, 60, 125, 250, 500, and 1000. If you choose the B setting, the shutter will remain open as long as you continue to press the shutter-release button. If you choose a number on the dial, you will get a controlled time exposure. A 1 on the dial, for instance, results in a 1-second exposure; a 2 results in a $\frac{1}{2}$-second exposure; a 4 in a $\frac{1}{4}$-second exposure; a 250 in a $\frac{1}{250}$-second exposure; and so on.

Aperture The aperture—sometimes called the *iris diaphragm* or the *stop*—is another device for controlling the amount of light that passes through the lens to the film. The aperture is a small hole made by overlapping several thin metallic plates. It is located in the lens in front of or within the lens elements. By adjusting the *aperture control ring,* you change the position of the plates and therefore the size of the aperture opening. The aperture control ring is marked with a series of numbers called *f-stops,* or simply *stops,* that indicate the size of the aperture opening. A typical f-stop range for a 35 mm camera includes f/1.4, f/2, f/2.8, f/4, f/5.6, f/8, f/16, and f/22. An aperture of f/1.4 is the

FIGURE 1-3A–D HOW A FOCAL-PLANE SHUTTER WORKS
The shutter consists of two blinds, one following the other. This forms a gap that rapidly exposes the film as it passes. Gap width is controlled by the shutter speed dial.

A Shutter is cocked.

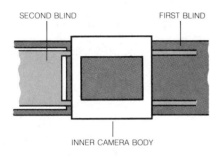

SECOND BLIND   FIRST BLIND

INNER CAMERA BODY

B First blind opens to expose the film.

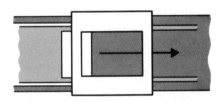

C Second blind follows. For speeds below $\frac{1}{60}$ second, the second blind is delayed and the entire frame remains uncovered for the required period.

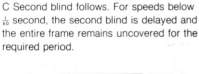

D Exposure is over. The whole frame has received the same exposure.

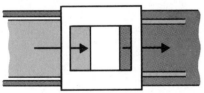

largest opening in this range, allowing the greatest amount of light to reach the film. An aperture of f/22, on the other hand, is the smallest aperture diameter and allows the least amount of light to reach the film. Reducing the aperture diameter before you shoot a picture is called *stopping down* the lens. For example, you might adjust the camera from f/4 to f/16. When you increase the diameter of the aperture opening, you are *opening up* the lens—for instance, from f/8 to f/5.6.

Film Transport System The film transport system simply replaces an exposed piece of film with an unexposed one. Usually the transport system winds the exposed film onto a take-up spool. However, some cameras use sheets of film instead of rolls. Special light-tight film carriers fit into the back of these cameras. Film is removed from the camera after each

exposure, and an unexposed piece of film is put in.

The Viewing Device All the camera parts may work together smoothly, but if you cannot see your subject, photography is impossible. When you look through the camera's viewfinder, you see essentially what the film sees. You use the viewfinder to choose what you will photograph. Viewfinders vary widely and are the basis for classifying different camera types. (This will be explained further in Chapter Two.)

THE BASIC PHOTOGRAPHIC PROCESS

Choosing the subject

The very first step in the photographic process is to choose a subject. The range of subjects is as varied as the

FIGURE 1-4 MODERN VERSION OF BASIC CAMERA PARTS

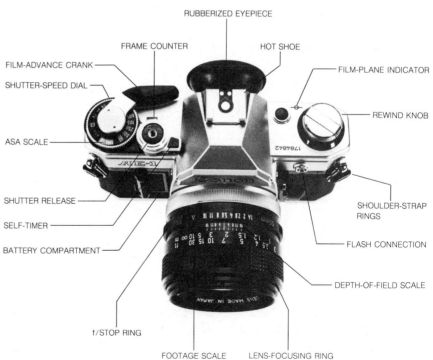

RUBBERIZED EYEPIECE
FRAME COUNTER
HOT SHOE
FILM-ADVANCE CRANK
FILM-PLANE INDICATOR
SHUTTER-SPEED DIAL
ASA SCALE
REWIND KNOB
SHUTTER RELEASE
SELF-TIMER
SHOULDER-STRAP RINGS
BATTERY COMPARTMENT
FLASH CONNECTION
DEPTH-OF-FIELD SCALE
f/STOP RING
FOOTAGE SCALE
LENS-FOCUSING RING

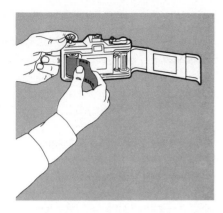

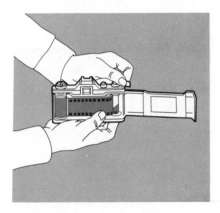

FIGURE 1-5 LOADING A CAMERA
It is always best to load film either indoors or in shade, so that sunlight cannot leak into the cassette. The emulsion—dull side of film—faces the lens. The film is advanced until both rows of holes are engaged by the sprocket teeth, and then close the back of the cassette. Make sure the cassette fits snugly into the opening.

photographer's imagination and creativity. Many beginning students attempt to photograph people, events, places, or things, without much thought for *how* these will be recorded. The experienced photographer may see these subjects quite differently and will concentrate on creating a feeling or mood so that the photograph communicates its reason for being taken, rather than just recording an image.

Visualization

Even the novice photographer knows the frustration of "seeing" the perfect picture, only to have the print turn out quite different from what was anticipated. There are a number of reasons a photograph does not look the same as the real thing. Cameras and film "see" things differently from the human eye. The untrained eye may overlook distracting elements the camera will pick up. Photographic prints have only two dimensions, so the viewer must imagine or sense depth. A black and white photograph re-creates a subject in tones of black and white and gray, and even a color photograph does not reproduce colors exactly as they appear to the eye. Finally, most photographs are either miniatures or magnifications of the real subject.

The ability to envision the final print before the picture is taken is called *visualization, previsualization,* or simply *photographic seeing.*

It is no easy task to visualize something in tones of gray when we see the world in color. Very different colors, such as red and green, are recorded by black and white film as almost identical tones of gray. A brilliantly colorful subject may be dull and uninteresting in a black and white print.

With practice you can improve your ability to visualize. Find an interesting, colorful subject, and take a black and white photograph of it. Later, compare the photograph with the original sub-

ject. Carefully note how the various colors of the subject are represented by gray tones in the print.

The ability to "see" a photograph as it will be is critical in the photographic process and is possibly the greatest asset of a successful photographer.

Taking the photograph

You load the camera with film, which will be exposed to light frame by frame as you photograph your subjects. (See Figure 1-5.) Once you have previsualized the subject, the physical part of the photographic process begins as you actually take the photograph. When the camera shutter-release button is pressed, the shutter opens, allowing light that is reflected from the subject to pass through the camera lens and form an image on the light-sensitive film.

Processing the film

After the entire roll of film has been *exposed* to light (all the pictures have been taken), then, in total darkness, the film is removed from the camera and placed in a developing tank. When the *developer solution* is poured into the tank, the negative image becomes visible on the film. After a predetermined time, the developer is poured out and an *acid stop bath* is poured into the developing tank to stop the action of the developer. A *fixer* is then used to halt further light sensitivity and preserve the negative image on the film. The film is removed from the developing tank and washed in water to remove the fixer and other chemical compounds. Finally, the developed film is hung up to dry. (See Figure 1-6.)

Making a positive print

This developed film is a strip of *negative* images. To make a positive print from a negative, you place the negative in contact with light-sensitive photographic paper. The image is formed on the light-sensitive paper by shining

FIGURE 1-6A–G PROCESSING: HOW IT WORKS

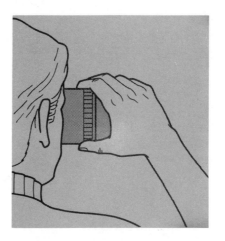

A Film is exposed in the camera.

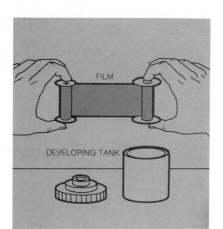

B Film is removed from the camera and loaded into the developing tank

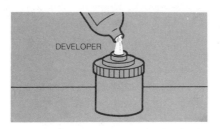

C The developer brings out the negative image on the film.

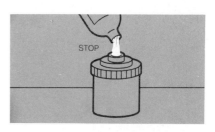

D The acid stop bath stops the development.

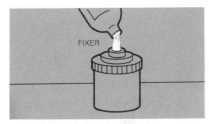

E The fixer preserves the negative image on the film.

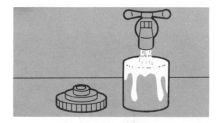

F The water wash removes the fixer and excess silver compounds.

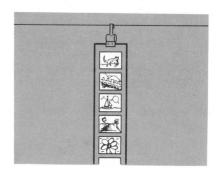

G The film is hung up to dry.

FIGURE 1-7 FROM A NEGATIVE TO A PRINT
Strip of Negatives
Negative Placed in Contact with Light-Sensitive Paper in Printing Frame
Negative in an Enlarger. Light shining through the negative forms the positive image on light-sensitive paper.

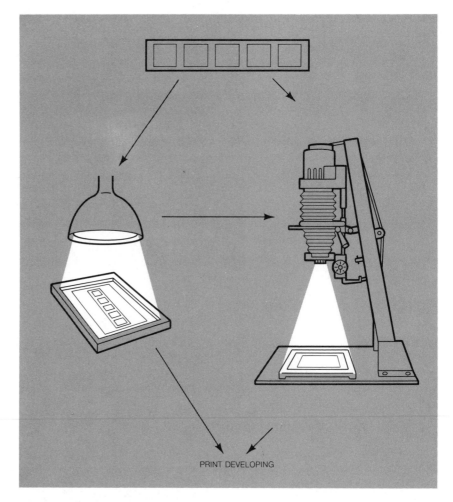

PRINT DEVELOPING

light through the negative. (See Figure 1-7.) To make an enlargement, you place the negative in an enlarger, where the same process takes place, except that the negative and the light-sensitive paper are separated. The distance of separation determines the size of the projected negative image and therefore the size of the enlargement.

Processing the paper

The steps involved in processing the light-sensitive paper are similar to those followed in producing the negative print. Developer is poured into a developing tray, and the photographic print paper is submerged in the developer until the positive image appears on the paper. An acid stop bath in a second tray stops the action of the developer, and a fixer in a third tray preserves the positive image on the paper. The positive print is then washed in water to remove the fixer and the unwanted chemicals. As the last step in the process, the print is left to dry. (See Figure 1-8.)

USING THE LIGHT

Without light, there would be no photography. Film is, in essence, light-sensitive plastic, and in order to take a photograph you must expose the film to light. As previously explained, two camera parts regulate how much light reaches the film: the aperture and the shutter.

The shutter and the aperture are two separate and distinct camera parts, but in their functions they must interrelate smoothly to produce the photograph. To better understand their relationship, imagine a gallon bottle

beneath a water tap. The tap not only turns the water on and off, but also regulates the rate of flow. If you open it wide, the bottle will fill quickly. If you open the tap only slightly, the bottle will fill slowly. In both cases, one gallon can be extracted from the tap, but if you open the tap only halfway, the bottle will need twice the time to fill. (See Figure 1-9.) Adjustments of the shutter and the aperture regulate light exposing the film in the same way adjustments of the tap regulate water passage through a pipe. Let us say that the shutter remains open for one second. The shutter controls the length of time the passage is open, and the aperture controls how large the opening is. The film will be exposed to a certain amount of light. If the aperture is adjusted to let in only half as much light, the film will receive

only half the exposure in that one second. For the exposure of the second aperture opening to equal that of the first aperture opening, the shutter would have to stay open twice as long—two seconds.

Equivalent exposure

The preceding example illustrates *equivalent exposure*—a method of using different shutter–aperture combinations to achieve identical film exposure.

Each number on the shutter speed dial has approximately half the value of the next number. For example, 250 ($\frac{1}{250}$ second) is half the value of 500 ($\frac{1}{500}$ second) and twice the value of 125 ($\frac{1}{125}$ second). A shutter speed of 250, then, is twice as fast as 125 but only half as fast as 500. (See Figure 1-10.)

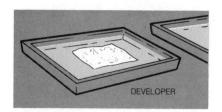

A The developer brings out the positive image on the paper.

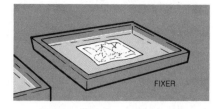

C The fixer preserves the positive image on the paper.

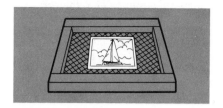

E Drying the print.

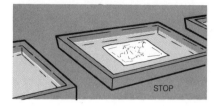

B The acid bath stops the development.

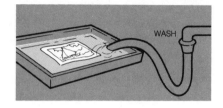

D The water wash removes the fixer and excess silver.

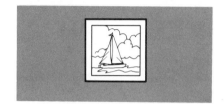

F The finished print.

FIGURE 1-8A–F PROCESSING THE PRINT: HOW IT WORKS

FIGURE 1-9 SHUTTER–APERTURE RELATIONSHIP
With tap wide open, it takes ten seconds to fill the container.
With tap only halfway open, the container is only half full after ten seconds.

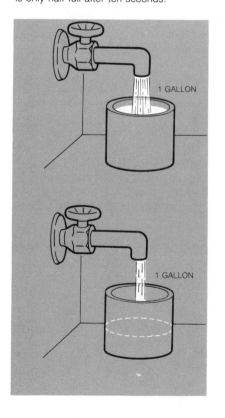

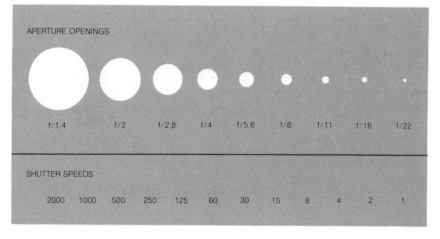

FIGURE 1-10 SHUTTER SPEED AND APERTURE SCALES
Each shutter speed is either twice or half as long as its neighbor.
All shutter speeds are expressed as fractions of a second; that is, $250 = \frac{1}{250}$ second.
The area of each aperture is either double or half its neighbor's.

FIGURE 1-11 EQUIVALENT EXPOSURE
Selected aperture is f/5.6 and the shutter speed is $\frac{1}{60}$ second. Equivalent exposures for this particular combination are given by the other aperture and shutter-speed pairs.

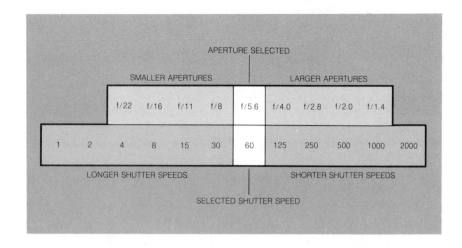

While the values of the f/stop numbers are not quite as obvious as those of the shutter speed numbers, they relate to each other in exactly the same way. An aperture diameter of f/4 lets in twice as much light as f/5.6 but only half as much as f/2.8.

By adjusting both the aperture diameter and the shutter speed, you can achieve various equivalent exposure combinations. An exposure combination of f/5.6 at 60 is equivalent to f/4 at 125. In both instances, the amount of light that reaches the film is the same because, when the lens is opened wider, the length of time the shutter is open is reduced. (See Figure 1-11.)

Equivalent exposure offers great versatility. When you want to photograph a hummingbird in flight, you need a fast shutter speed to stop the movement and prevent the image from being blurred on the film. The principle of equivalent exposure allows you to select a fast enough shutter speed to stop action and still get enough light to the film, even though the hummingbird may be hovering in the shade of a lilac bush.

Depth of field

The aperture control ring does more than just control the amount of light—it allows you to emphasize objects at certain distances within the scene. The aperture control ring regulates the depth of field. Simply speaking, depth of field is the distance in front of and beyond the lens focus distance that appears in acceptably sharp focus. For example, if a normal lens is focused at seven feet and the aperture opening is f/8, the range in acceptable focus will be from about six to nine feet. The depth of field is therefore three feet. The larger the aperture diameter, the smaller the depth of field. An f/2 aperture has a smaller depth of field than f/16, for example. Depth of field is also affected by the lens focus distance. As the lens is focused closer to the camera, the depth of field for a given f-number decreases.

Controlling the aperture opening for depth of field allows greater creativity in photography. You can choose to focus clearly on the entire panorama of a city's jutting skyline, or you can focus on a single poppy blooming in a vast, flaming meadow. (See Figure 1-12.)

Making the exposure

Much of the mystique of photography centers on the split-second timing required to properly expose film. Exposure is critical in determining what the final print will look like. When your subject is stationary—a building, for example—you can shoot pictures all day. In many cases, however, you get only one chance—to capture the look of surprise on a baby's face when a balloon explodes. Exposure is the key to getting the best possible picture in any situation.

Film speed The first step in the exposure process is choosing a film. The *film speed* identifies how sensitive the film is to light. Slow films are those least sensitive to light. Fast films, then, require less light for proper exposure than do slow films.

In the United States, film speed has in the past been denoted by an *ASA number* ("ASA" stands for *American Standards Association*—originator of the rating system). The most commonly used ASA numbers range from 25 to 400. They are usually classified into three categories: slow speed (ASA 25 to 32), medium speed (ASA 64 to 125), and high speed (ASA 160 to 400). Each has its advantages, and you should base your film selection on your subject. Fast film is best in low light, while slow film is an excellent choice for clear, sharp pictures in adequate light.

Film also carries a DIN (for *Deutsche Industrie Norm*) number.

At this writing, this somewhat perplexing system of dual numbering is

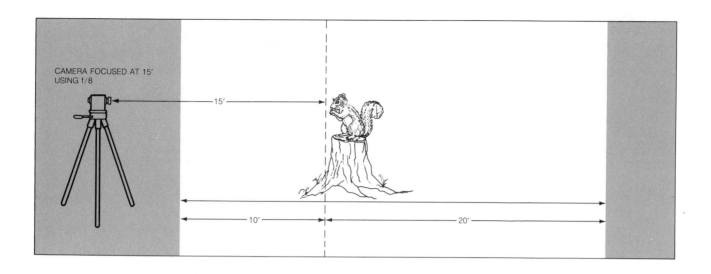

CAMERA FOCUSED AT 15'
USING f/8

15'

10'

20'

being converted to a new system: ISO, for *International Standards Organization.*

Exposure meter The light (or exposure) meter is built into most modern cameras. When you aim the camera at the subject, the light meter can be activated, and it recommends an exposure. Because light meters are so easy to use, it is tempting to let them do all the work. But there is plenty of room for error.

For one thing, the light meter determines exposure based on an average subject—one with equal areas of light and shade. If your subject is subtly shaded or brilliant with light, the meter's average reading will not be appropriate. Or the light meter may be influenced by the light in one area of the scene, while you are trying to focus on an entirely different area. If it responds to a highlighted angle of a mountain slope, for example, you will not get a proper exposure as you photograph the deeply shaded grove of pines at the base.

To best utilize your light meter, measure different parts of the scene up close whenever you can, checking the bright and dark areas separately. The correct exposure lies somewhere between these two extremes. As you measure light with the meter, make

sure that the shadow cast by the camera (or by you) does not affect the meter reading. If you are concerned about the accuracy of the meter reading, take one picture at normal exposure, then overexpose the next shot by one f/stop, and underexpose a third shot by one f/stop. This procedure is called *bracketing* the subject. For example, if you think a "normal" exposure is f/11 at 125, the overexposed bracket is f/8 at 125 and the underexposed bracket is f/16 at 125.

HOW TO HANDLE THE CAMERA

Although photography equipment may sound complicated, all you really need to practice photography is a camera and some film. Just as you would seek instruction in the best way to hold a tennis racquet, roll a bowling ball, or swing a golf club, you should know how to handle your photography equipment in order to realize the best results.

There is no single "right" way to hold a camera. Cameras come in all shapes and sizes, with the controls located at different places on each one. But there are some general guidelines to follow. An unsteady hand probably causes more spoiled pictures than any other factor. Even the slight-

FIGURE 1-12 HOW DEPTH OF FIELD WORKS
Except for close-ups, the $\frac{1}{3}$-to-$\frac{2}{3}$ rule is valid. It means that about $\frac{1}{3}$ of the focused region will be in front of the object and $\frac{2}{3}$ will be behind the object. This rule holds for any aperture, but remember: the larger the aperture, the shallower the total depth of field.

FIGURE 1-13 THE HUMAN TRIPOD
One foot is kept forward, and, if possible, a tree or building is used as a brace.

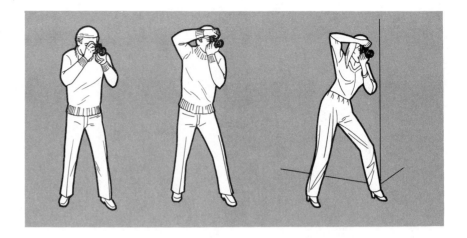

est shake or jiggle will affect image sharpness. As a rule of thumb, remember that the slowest speed you should use when hand holding a camera is 1 divided by the focal length of the lens. The focal length is the distance from the optical center of the lens to the film. For example, if the lens focal length is 50 mm, the slowest hand-held speed should be $\frac{1}{50}$ second. Since most cameras don't have a shutter speed of $\frac{1}{50}$, use $\frac{1}{60}$ or $\frac{1}{30}$ as a guide. The main goal, then, is to brace the camera so that shots as slow as $\frac{1}{30}$ second are possible without a tripod. Convert your body into a human tripod. Spread your feet comfortably apart, with one foot slightly in front of the other. Determine which arm is bearing the weight of the camera, and tuck that elbow in against your body. Use your free hand to steady the camera and operate other camera controls. (Figures 1-13 through 1-17 illustrate basic camera positions using 35 mm and 120 mm cameras.) Once you are in a proper position, inhale and exhale a few times before you shoot the picture. The moment before the picture is taken, inhale and then partially exhale. Hold your breath while you actually shoot the picture. If you are using a long lens or shooting at speeds slower than $\frac{1}{30}$ second, use a tripod or brace the camera against a solid object. (See Figure 1-18.)

COMPOSITION

The real art of photography depends on the way the picture is put together by the photographer.

The arrangement of the subject is important in any form. Arrangement—or composition—is what makes a photograph interesting to the viewer, music soothing to the listener, sculpture pleasing to the observer. Composition is not something new. Greek and Roman architecture as early as the fifth century B.C. reflects careful consideration of balance and congruity. Later, Renaissance artists used a masterful command of the art of composition to create peaceful, muted scenes. We practice good composition every day in the way we arrange furniture in our homes, the way we dress, and the way we place a simple rosebud in a fluted vase.

Photography—a visual form of communication—allows us to tell others how we feel about a scene by the manner of composition we have chosen. The better the composition, the better the communication, and the better the communication, the more meaningful the art becomes. The art works by evoking an emotional response through telling a story or making a visual statement. The photographs that communicate most effectively do not "just happen." They

require careful planning and precise composition.

The subject

The subject of every photograph should be the center of visual interest. Realizing that the actual center of interest is not what you intended it to be is a disappointment most photographers have experienced. Remember that, as a general rule, the *lightest* areas of the scene or subject will attract the eye first. To focus exactly on the subject you want, you might try holding the camera at a different angle, using a shallow depth of field, or shooting at different exposures.

Placement of the subject

Many people have a tendency to place the subject in the middle of the photograph. It might seem easiest and most natural, but in most cases "centering" should be avoided. Try placing the subject above, below, or to one side of the center of the photograph. If the subject represents movement, make sure that the movement is *into* the picture instead of out of it. Sometimes centering cannot be avoided. A large group of people, for example, will almost always be centered from side to side.

Filling the space

Everything that appears in the viewfinder will end up on your film, and the

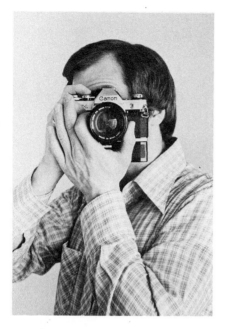

FIGURE 1-14 EYE-LEVEL CAMERA POSITION (35 MM)
Lens is held in the left hand, with the left elbow kept tightly against the body. The right hand operates the shutter release and steadies the camera.

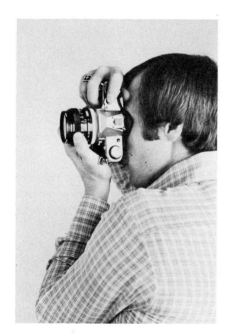

FIGURE 1-15 VERTICAL CAMERA POSITION (35 MM)
The left hand holds the lens and body of the camera. The left elbow is kept close to the body, and the right hand operates the controls. Using the right hand to support the weight of the camera in this position is very awkward.

FIGURE 1-16 EYE-LEVEL CAMERA POSITION (120)
The left hand supports the weight of the camera and is kept close to the body. The right hand, used to operate the controls, is also kept close to the body.

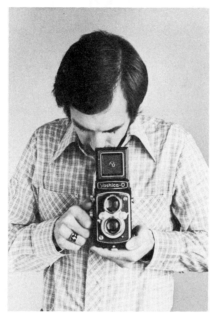

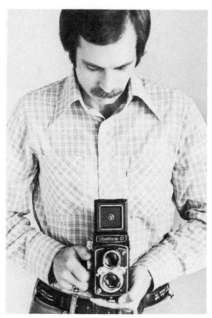

FIGURE 1-17 WAIST-LEVEL CAMERA POSITION (120)
Both arms are kept close to the body. The left hand supports the camera, and the right hand operates the controls.

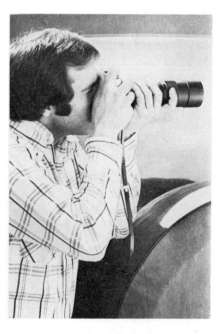

FIGURE 1-18 USING A LONG LENS
When using a telephoto or other long lens, either place the camera on a tripod or brace the lens against a stationary object.

subject usually fills only a portion of that frame. Paying special attention to the other areas as well as the subject will ensure a balanced photograph. To achieve this sense of evenness, you may need to change the angle of the camera or the shot.

Look beyond the subject

We see in three dimensions, so in reality it is easy for us to distinguish background clutter from our visual subject. But photographs have only two dimensions. Often whatever is in the background will appear to be on the same plane as the subject. Almost every novice photographer has been chagrined by a picture in which a tree or other object appears to be growing out of the subject's head. On the day the picture was taken, the subject was standing alone on an expanse of lawn, and the tree was across the yard!

To avoid this type of problem, look beyond your subject. Find out if there is anything in the background that will distract or distort. Simply narrowing the depth of field will eliminate most background problems by removing them from the viewer's eye.

SUMMARY

To the beginning photographer, the maze of equipment may seem formidable. Peering hesitantly inside a companion's camera case, the novice discovers a host of meaningless gadgets. Even the matter of selecting a camera and film is complicated by the diversity of film speeds and camera formats and styles. But understanding of all these gadgets and choices will develop as experience in photography increases. And the way to gain experience is, of course, to take pictures.

The ability to visualize is probably the successful photographer's greatest asset. For a picture to be an effective form of visual communication, it must have a meaningful subject. A good

photographer gives careful consideration to the composition of the picture— the arrangement of the subject. It must be surrounded by only those things that enhance it. There must be brilliant lights and contrasting shadows. As in all art forms, the better the composition, the better the communication.

By understanding the camera and how it works, the photographer is able to transform a mental image into a visual story that can be shared. Thus the artist blends the creative with the technical in the "magical" process of photography.

REVIEW QUESTIONS

1 What is the *decisive moment*?

2 How does a photograph differ from a view of the real thing?

3 What is the term for the ability to envision the final print before the picture is taken?

4 What is the meaning of the term "expose film"?

5 What determines a camera format?

6 How many functions does a camera accomplish?

7 Name the six essential camera parts.

8 Which two distinct camera parts regulate film exposure?

9 What is *equivalent exposure*?

10 What determines film speed?

11 List two exposure combinations that are equivalent to f/8 at 125.

12 Why is composition important?

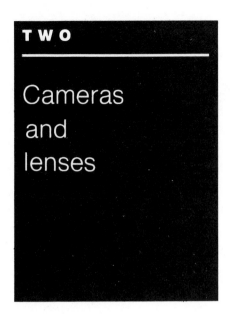

TWO

Cameras and lenses

As briefly described in the previous chapter, all cameras, from the most simple to the most complex, have six basic parts in common: a light-tight box, a lens, a shutter, an aperture, a viewfinder, and a film transport system.

Camera designs today offer a variety of formats (negative sizes), viewfinders, and body styles. The trend since the 1880s has been toward smaller, comparatively easy-to-use cameras, such as the 35 mm camera and the 126 and 110 pocket instamatic cameras.

Extensive changes since the turn of the century—interchangeable lenses, magazine backs, miniaturization, exposure automation, and instant print film—have made cameras versatile, compact instruments. Today cameras range from the ten-dollar Instamatic to the three-thousand-dollar Hasselblad. There are simple cameras small enough to tuck into a pocket, and there are others that come with cases full of accessories. However, you must remember one thing: with a ten-dollar camera, a creative photographer can achieve masterpieces that are beyond the reach of an unskilled photographer using much more expensive equipment. More sophisticated equipment will increase your options and may make it easier for you to take good pictures, but ultimately it is the photographer, not the camera, that makes the difference.

TYPES OF CAMERAS

Cameras are commonly grouped, by viewing device, into four general categories:

1 the viewfinder camera

2 the single lens reflex camera

3 the twin lens reflex camera

4 the view camera

Each is designed for a specific purpose, and each category includes cameras with a variety of different formats. See Figure 2-1 for a comparison of the most popular formats used today.

Viewfinder camera

Viewfinder cameras include simple inexpensive cameras as well as some of the finest cameras available today. Regardless of quality or cost, viewfinder cameras have three basic characteristics in common:

1 With few moving parts, they are durable and quiet to operate.

2 In formats from disk to 110 mm to 35 mm, they are lightweight and compact.

3 They are generally held at eye level while the photographer takes the picture. (See Figure 2-2.)

Viewfinder cameras have small viewing lenses, often set behind a rectangular window. (See Figure 2-3.) At first this type of viewing lens presented a difficult problem. Just as one eye has a slightly different view from the other

FIGURE 2-1 COMPARISON OF NEGATIVE SIZES

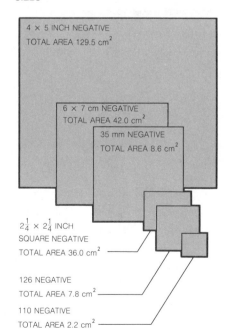

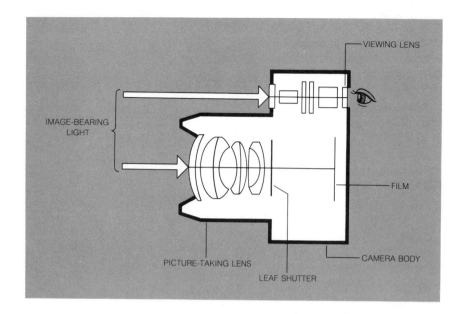

IMAGE-BEARING LIGHT

VIEWING LENS

FILM

CAMERA BODY

PICTURE-TAKING LENS

LEAF SHUTTER

FIGURE 2-2 VIEWFINDER CAMERA

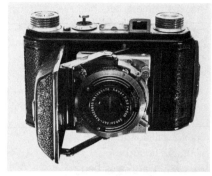

FIGURE 2-3 VIEWFINDER CAMERA

FIGURE 2-4 PARALLAX ERROR

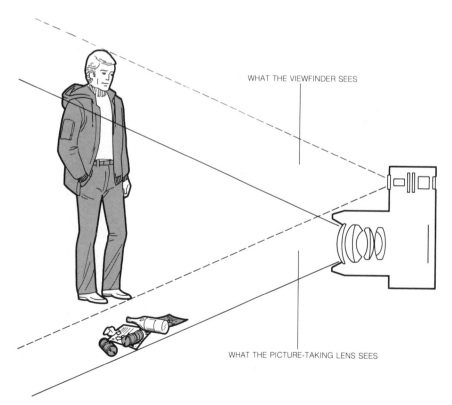

WHAT THE VIEWFINDER SEES

WHAT THE PICTURE-TAKING LENS SEES

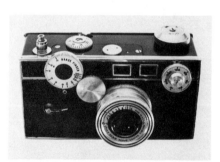

FIGURE 2-5 RANGEFINDER CAMERA

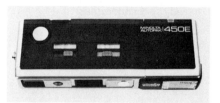

FIGURE 2-6 110 CAMERA

one, the camera lens had a slightly larger view than the viewfinder, making the area seen through the viewfinder slightly different from the area actually seen by the camera lens. (See Figure 2-4.) This fault, commonly found in early viewfinder cameras, is called *parallax error*. Parallax error made it difficult to frame and properly focus the image.

In 1932, Carl Zeiss began marketing a viewfinder camera (the Contax) with a built-in coupled *rangefinder*, a distance-measuring device that allowed for focusing. Development of the rangefinder was the first step in overcoming parallax error. The main image was seen through the viewfinder window, while the second image was transmitted from the rangefinder window to the viewfinder window by a rotating prism and an angled mirror. By turning the focusing ring on the camera lens, the photographer was able to bring the subject into focus by aligning the two images of the scene. (See Figure 2-5.)

Another way to overcome parallax error is to keep the composition within the framing lines marked on the viewfinder lens.

One of the most popular format sizes in viewfinder cameras at present is the 110 pocket Instamatic. (See Figure 2-6.) Its popularity is due to its small size and ease of operation. Its only limitation is the small size of its negative. Sold as easy-to-use cameras, most 110 and the slightly larger 126 format cameras do not have a coupled rangefinder. The 35 mm viewfinder camera, however, does incorporate a coupled rangefinder, making it a sophisticated, compact, dependable camera, chosen by many professsionals.

In February 1982, Eastman Kodak introduced its unique ultraminiature-format disk cameras. A completely electronic automatic viewfinder camera small enough to fit in a shirt pocket, it is designed to ultimately replace the 110 format cameras.

The truly unique feature is the film itself. The negatives are placed around the edge of a wafer-thin disk, $2\frac{1}{2}$ inches in diameter. There are 15 frames of the high-resolution ASA 200 Kodacolor film per disk, each measuring 8 × 10 mm. Special chemicals minimize light-scattering, and the film is coated with Estar, a heavyweight polyester used as a base for Kodak sheet film, allowing for dimensional stability.

Regardless of model, the Kodak disk cameras are small, compact, and lightweight. The camera measures 3 by $4\frac{3}{4}$ by $\frac{7}{8}$ inches and weighs $6\frac{1}{2}$ ounces. The film disk, packaged in a cassette, simply drops into the camera.

Single lens reflex camera

Currently the most popular camera among both amateur and professional photographers is the single lens reflex (SLR) camera. (See Figure 2-7.) One of the major advantages of the single lens reflex camera is that the photographer is able to see the same thing the camera lens does. A mirror positioned inside the camera at a 45-degree angle to the lens is the key to

FIGURE 2-7 SLR CAMERA

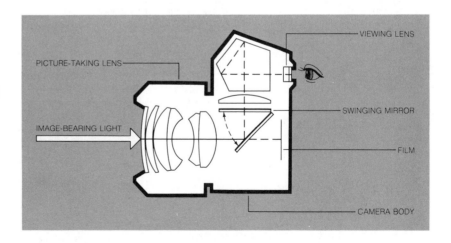

PICTURE-TAKING LENS

VIEWING LENS

IMAGE-BEARING LIGHT

SWINGING MIRROR

FILM

CAMERA BODY

FIGURE 2-8 CUTAWAY VIEW OF AN SLR CAMERA

This cutaway shot shows the various parts of an Olympus OM-2 35 mm camera and their relationship to each other. (Photo courtesy Olympus Camera Company.)

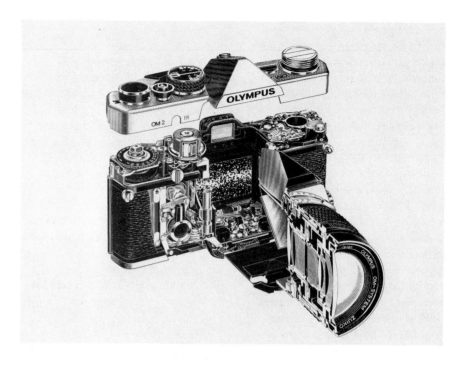

the viewing system. The mirror catches the image from the lens and reflects it up into a pentaprism in the viewfinder. The pentaprism adjusts the image so it is right side up and correct right to left. (See Figure 2-8.) This "through-the-lens viewing" eliminates parallax error, permits quick and easy focusing, increases control over composition, and allows the photographer to determine quickly which portions of the scene will be in focus.

The great flexibility of most SLR cameras is due to the availability of a variety of lenses and attachments—in some cases as many as one hundred different kinds. Some lenses allow for close-up (or *macro*) photography, while *telephoto* lenses bring a scene closer to the camera. The SLR camera, more than any other, is capable of adapting to many shooting situations.

Most SLR cameras use the 35 mm format. A standard roll of film will accommodate up to thirty-six exposures. Because of the small negative size, the 35 mm SLR camera is much less expensive to use than the larger format cameras.

The few disadvantages of the SLR cameras seem minor when compared to the advantages. The small size of the negatives—an advantage in many ways—makes reproduction of large, high-quality prints difficult. Also, the SLR cameras are not always effective at very slow shutter speeds. When the shutter is released, the mirror inside the camera must be raised out of the way quickly so that the light can expose the film. This up and down

FIGURE 2-9A–D EXPOSURE SEQUENCE FOR A 35 MM CAMERA

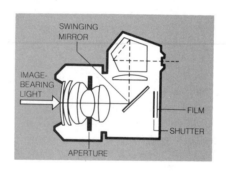

A Before the shutter-release button is pushed, the mirror is in the down position. Light enters through the lens and is reflected up through the pentaprism to the viewfinder.

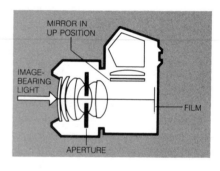

C The shutter opens, and the film is exposed.

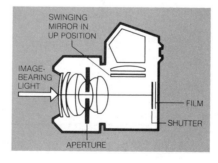

B When the shutter is released, the mirror flips up and the automatic diaphragm closes to the preset aperture.

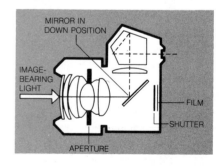

D Once the exposure is complete, the shutter closes, the aperture reopens and the mirror drops back to its original position.

movement of the mirror causes vibration. Also, since the mirror is in the raised position during exposure, the viewfinder is momentarily blocked out. Some photographers find this disturbing.

The exposure sequence of the 35 mm camera is quite complex. In order to increase image brightness in the viewfinder, 35 mm SLR cameras are focused with the aperture wide open. When the shutter release button is pressed, the mirror swings up out of the light path, allowing the light to reach the shutter but blocking it from the viewfinder. The diaphragm then automatically closes (or stops down) to the chosen aperture, and the shutter fires. When the shutter is closed, the aperture reopens and the mirror falls back into the viewing position. (See Figure 2-9.) This entire sequence happens in a fraction of a second.

Two other unique groups of cameras also fall into the single lens reflex category: the medium-format SLR and the Polaroid folding reflex instant picture camera.

Medium-format roll film single lens reflex camera Although easy to use, the medium-format roll film SLR cameras are nevertheless heavier and bulkier than their 35 mm counterparts. (See Figure 2-10.) A roll film single lens reflex camera is a versatile camera system, since there are many lenses, various film backs, and several different hoods and focusing screens available for use with it. A typical roll film SLR system is shown in Figure 2-11. The biggest advantage of the roll film SLR cameras is their larger negative size (usually $2\frac{1}{4}$ by $2\frac{1}{4}$ inches, or 6 by 7 cm). The biggest drawback is the high cost of individual components when compared to the cost of other camera systems.

Folding reflex instant picture cameras The Polaroid SX-70 is the most popular folding reflex SLR instant print camera. (See Figure 2-12 for a cuta-

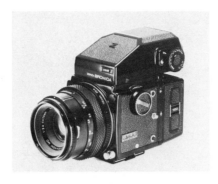

FIGURE 2-10 MEDIUM-FORMAT SLR CAMERA
(Photo Courtesy EPOI Industries, Inc.)

FIGURE 2-11 MEDIUM-FORMAT SLR SYSTEM
(Photo Courtesy Bell & Howell/Mamiya Co.)

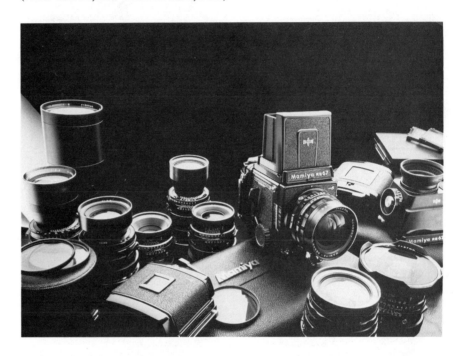

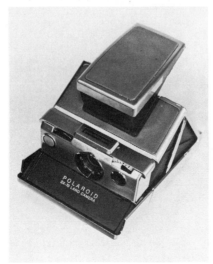

FIGURE 2-12 FOLDING REFLEX CAMERA
The Polaroid SX-70 Land Camera

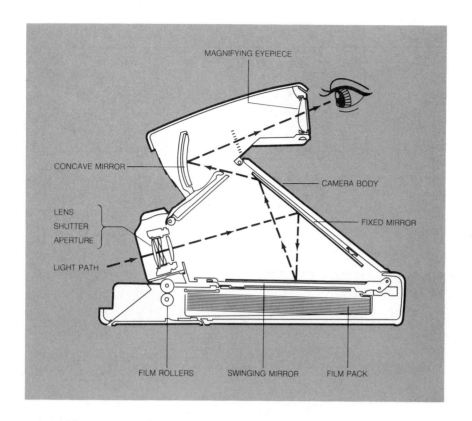

MAGNIFYING EYEPIECE

CONCAVE MIRROR

CAMERA BODY

LENS
SHUTTER
APERTURE

FIXED MIRROR

LIGHT PATH

FILM ROLLERS   SWINGING MIRROR   FILM PACK

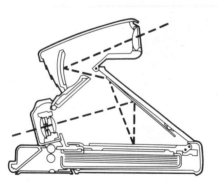

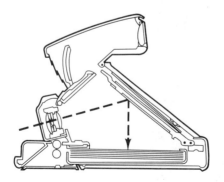

FIGURE 2-13 HOW THE FOLDING REFLEX CAMERA WORKS
Cutaway of Polaroid SX-70

FIGURE 2-14 EXPOSURE SEQUENCE FOR A FOLDING REFLEX CAMERA
To take a picture with an SX-70, first focus on an object. The swinging mirror is in the down position. As the shutter is released, the mirror swings up and the light rays from the object are reflected down onto the film.

way view, and Figures 2-13 and 2-14 for the picture-taking sequence.) This highly complex camera is electronically powered by a battery that comes in each film pack. Before exposure, light reflected from the subject enters the camera through the lens and is reflected by mirrors to the viewfinder. Additional mirrors transmit the image to the magnifying eyepiece. This image is upright and the correct way around. When the shutter release is activated, the mirrors change their positions so that the light is now reflected down onto the film. Simultaneously, a photocell measures the intensity of the incoming light and sets the proper exposure. A motor inside the camera drives the film through rollers that spread developer over the film. Finally, a framed—but blank—picture merges from the camera. In about five minutes, the colors reach full development.

Twin lens reflex camera

The twin lens camera has, in its viewing system, a ground glass plate that allows the photographer to see the composition in two dimensions, much as it will appear in the picture. Like the single lens reflex camera, the TLR camera uses a mirror to reflect the image from the lens to the photographer's eye, but the mirror of the TLR is in a fixed, rather than movable, position. As a result, there must be one lens for viewing and another for taking the picture. Both lenses are mounted on the same lens board, and both move when the focusing adjustment is used. (See Figure 2-15.)

A major advantage of the TLR system is that it uses a larger format than 35 mm. Most twin lens cameras use 120 film. The negative, which measures $2\frac{1}{4}$ inches square, has about four times the area of the 35 mm negative, thereby yielding a higher quality print when an enlargement is made. Since it has few internal moving parts, the camera is rugged, durable, and moderately priced.

The chief disadvantage of the twin lens reflex camera is parallax error. The problem is more severe in the TLR camera than in a viewfinder camera, because the lens taking the picture is below the viewing lens. (See Figure 2-16.) One can overcome parallax error by keeping the subject strictly within the framing lines. Since there is no prism in the TLR, the image in the viewfinder appears right side up but is reversed from left to right—a disadvantage that requires some adjustment, especially with fast-moving subjects.

The view camera

View cameras are medium- to large-format cameras that, because of their size and weight, are usually used on tripods or camera stands. Most view cameras use sheets of film measuring from 4 by 5 inches to 8 by 10 inches. While the large negative size allows for the highest quality enlargements, the expense of operation and the large size of the view camera limit its applications. However, the view camera is ideal for situations that do not involve action: still life, architecture, landscapes, and portraits.

The view camera uses through-the-lens viewing, but, since there is no mirror or prism, the image appears upside down and backwards on a ground glass screen at the film plane

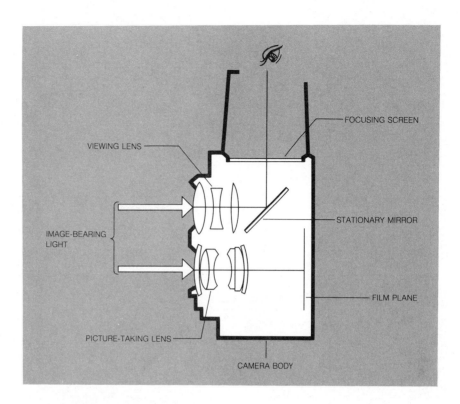

FOCUSING SCREEN

VIEWING LENS

IMAGE-BEARING LIGHT

STATIONARY MIRROR

FILM PLANE

PICTURE-TAKING LENS

CAMERA BODY

FIGURE 2-15 TWIN LENS REFLEX VIEWING SYSTEM

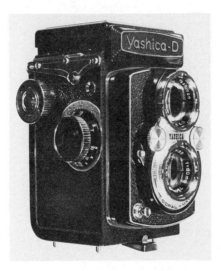

FIGURE 2-16 TLR CAMERA

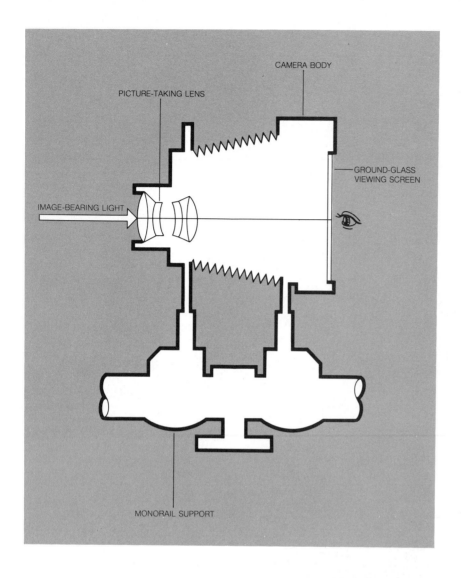

PICTURE-TAKING LENS

CAMERA BODY

GROUND-GLASS
VIEWING SCREEN

IMAGE-BEARING LIGHT

MONORAIL SUPPORT

**FIGURE 2-17 VIEW CAMERA VIEWING
SYSTEM**

**FIGURE 2-18 OMEGA 4 × 5-INCH VIEW
CAMERA**
(Photo Courtesy Berkey Marketing Companies, Inc.)

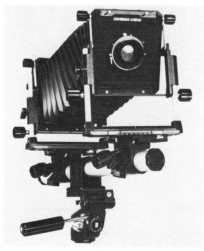

in the rear of the camera. (See Figures 2-17 and 2-18.)

CAMERA LENSES

As discussed in Chapter One, the camera lens functions in much the same way as the lens of the human eye. Both collect light rays reflected from the field of view and focus them into a sharp image. A simple camera lens with its two curved surfaces acts like a great many prisms arranged in a line. All rays of light passing through the lens are bent except those that pass directly through the center. The extent to which a lens bends the light rays is controlled by its composition and surface curvature.

In a properly designed lens, all the light rays from the same part of a subject will meet at a single point behind the lens. Thus the light-admitting hole in a camera can be quite large, since the hole is fitted with a lens that will collect light rays from the subject and cause them to converge at a certain point. A sharp image of the subject is formed where the light rays meet—the point where the film must be located if the picture is to be in sharp focus. Sophisticated lenses have made possible the short exposure times and the sharp images characteristic of today's photography.

Image formation

When reflected light from a subject passes through an optical system, the end result is an *image*. The optical system that produces the image may be as simple as a mirror or as highly complex as a modern camera lens.

One way to form an image is to use the simple tools that led to the camera obscura—a pinhole and an opaque screen. Figure 2-19 illustrates two important properties of image formation, whether it be by a pinhole or by a sophisticated optical system. First, the image is real, since it can be caught on a screen as rays that have passed through the pinhole. Second, the image must be inverted and reversed from side to side, since light rays travel in straight lines. The pinhole, of course, has limitations as a producer of images. It has poor resolution and slow speed, causing its use to be restricted to simple experiments. A lens is normally used to form an image in cameras.

The simple lens

The simple lens can be either *concave* or *convex* in design. A convex, or *positive,* lens is always thicker at the center than at the edges. A good example of a positive lens is a common magnifying glass. A concave, or *negative*, lens is thicker at the edges than at the center. Eyeglasses worn to correct nearsightedness use negative lenses. (See Figure 2-20.)

The front surface of a simple lens may be convex, concave, or planar (flat) to the incident light. The rear surface may also be convex, concave, or planar. These three designs can be combined to produce several types of simple lenses. The cross-sections of six different kinds of simple lenses are shown in Figure 2-21. One common

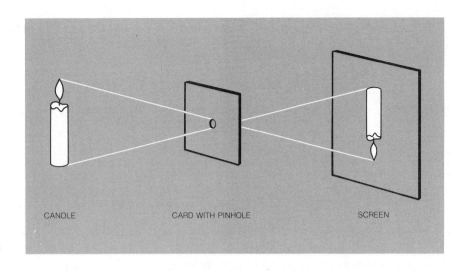

CANDLE CARD WITH PINHOLE SCREEN

FIGURE 2-19 FORMATION OF AN OPTICAL IMAGE BY A PINHOLE
The image formed by the pinhole is inverted and reversed.

FIGURE 2-20 CONCAVE AND CONVEX LENSES

SIMPLE CONVEX LENS SIMPLE CONCAVE LENS

FIGURE 2-21A SIX TYPES OF SIMPLE LENSES

FIGURE 2-21B MULTI-ELEMENT LENS, FORMED WITH SIMPLE LENSES

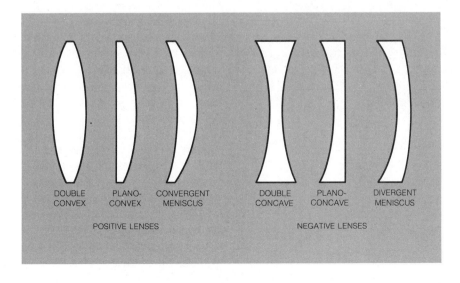

DOUBLE CONVEX PLANO-CONVEX CONVERGENT MENISCUS DOUBLE CONCAVE PLANO-CONCAVE DIVERGENT MENISCUS

POSITIVE LENSES   NEGATIVE LENSES

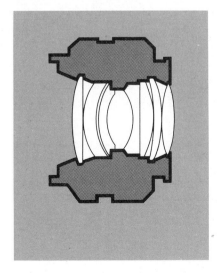

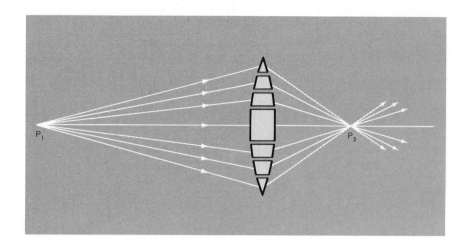

FIGURE 2-22 SIMPLE LENS WORKING LIKE A GROUP OF PRISMS
Each ''prism'' refracts light rays from point P₁ to a focus point at P₂.

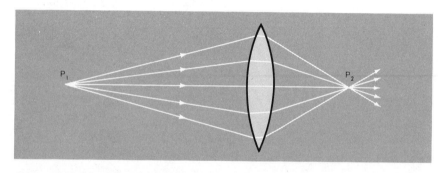

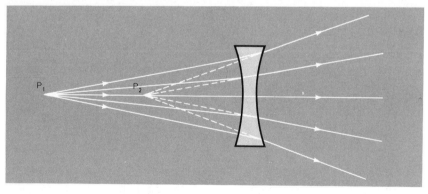

FIGURE 2-23 IMAGE FORMATION BY A POSITIVE AND NEGATIVE LENS
A positive lens concentrates the image at a point.
A negative lens expands the image, concentrating the rays at an imaginary point in front of the lens.

type of lens is a *meniscus lens,* in which the curvature of both surfaces coincides. Simple positive meniscus lenses are used as close-up lenses for many cameras.

A number of prisms form a simple lens, as shown in Figure 2-22. Light reflected from point S_1 on the subject strikes the front surface of the positive lens and is redirected by refraction to form a real image at point *I*. These reflected rays from point S_1 on the subject are said to come to a focus at point *I*. If a negative lens is used, the incident rays will be diverged even more by the refractive action of the lens. See Figure 2-23 for a comparison of the image-forming abilities of both a simple positive and a simple negative lens.

Appendix B provides a more in-depth discussion of optics and image formation.

Focal length and aperture

The common purpose of all camera lenses is to gather the reflected light rays from a subject and bring them into focus on the film plane. The basic differences in lenses are focal length and maximum aperture.

Focal length The focal length of the lens is the distance from the optical center of a lens when it is focused at infinity to the point at which it brings the image into focus. It would be extremely difficult for a photographer to figure this out, so manufacturers provide focal length information for every lens they make. The focal length is printed on either the front or the side of the lens barrel. (See Figure 2-24.)

The closest the lens can approach the film plane and still be able to focus on any subject is called the *point of principle focus.* As the lens is moved away from the film plane, there are an infinite number of other possible points of focus, depending on the distance of the subject from the lens. The closer

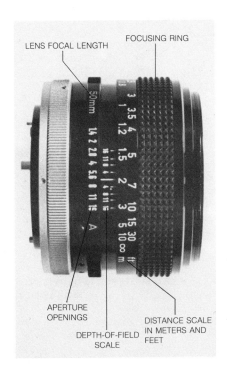

FIGURE 2-24 PARTS OF A LENS APERTURE DIAL

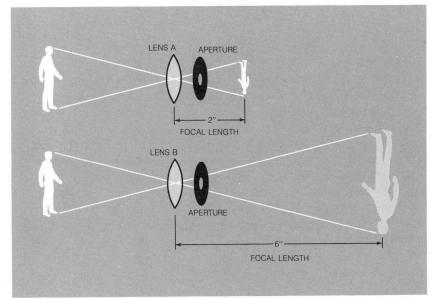

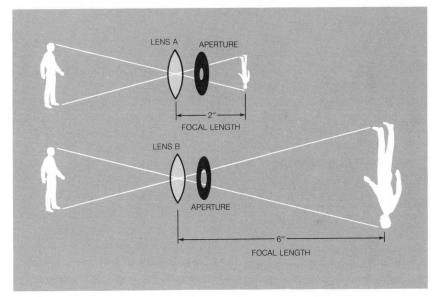

FIGURE 2-25 RELATIVE APERTURE
Two lenses with the same aperture and different focal lengths produce images with different degrees of brightness.
To make lenses interchangeable, the aperture of Lens B is changed so that the image brightness is the same for both lenses for a given f/stop.

the subject is to the lens, the more the lens must be moved away from the film plane.

Most cameras have a lens stop at infinity. When you move the lens back toward the film as far as it can go, the lens will automatically be focused at infinity. Depending on the size and construction of the camera and the focal length of the lens, infinity can be anywhere beyond about fifty feet.

The focal length of a lens determines how large an image of the subject the lens can produce and how much of the scene the lens can "see." For example, the normal lens for a 35 mm camera has a focal length of about 50 mm and a range, or angle view, of about 48 degrees. A normal lens for any format is one that "sees" about the same angle as the human eye.

Lens apertures The sizes of lens openings, or apertures, are usually expressed with f/numbers, determined by dividing the focal length of the lens by the diameter of the aperture. For

example, if the focal length of the lens is 8 inches and the aperture diameter is 2 inches, the f/number is f/4 (8 ÷ 2 = 4). A lens opening of f/4 means, then, that the aperture is only a quarter of the focal length. Similarly, f/16 means that the aperture is a sixteenth of the focal length. The smaller the f/number, the larger the lens opening. (See Figure 2-25.) Some lenses are

designed to permit the photographer to have half-f/stops between full f/stops.

Imagine two lenses, one normal and the other telephoto, focused on the same subject. If both lenses were to use the same size aperture, they would both transmit the same amount of light. Lens A, however, has a focal length of two inches; Lens B has a focal length of six inches. With Lens B the image produced on the film will be three times the size of the image produced by Lens A. The light from Lens B, with its longer focal length, is spread over an area nine times as large as the area covered by Lens A. Therefore, the image made on the film by Lens B is less bright than the image made by Lens A.

Obviously, it would be difficult to take properly exposed photographs using interchangeable lenses if the apertures on long and short focal length lenses were not equivalent. Fortunately, they are. To ensure uniformity, manufacturers make long-focal-length lenses with apertures physically larger than those of shorter-focal-length lenses. Both lenses have the same *relative* apertures, but their *physical* apertures are different sizes. In other words, if you use a lens with a normal focal length at f/8 and change to a lens with a longer focal length at f/8, the exposure will remain constant.

Effects of focal length and aperture

Image size When the distance from the lens to the subject (*u*) is very large, the corresponding image distance (*v*) is taken to be the focal length of the lens. The size of the image that will form on the negative is found by dividing the focal length by the subject distance. The size of the image, then, depends on the focal length of the lens and the distance from the lens to the subject. Consequently, using lenses with different focal lengths when photographing the same subject will produce different-sized subject images on the negatives.

Depth of field The depth of field is the area within a picture that is in acceptably sharp focus. Depth of field exists because of the difference in *resolving power* between your eyes and the camera lens. Resolving power is the ability to distinguish between objects as they decrease in size.

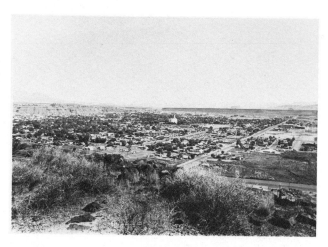

A Shot with a 28 mm lens

FIGURE 2-26A–G ANGLE OF VIEW SHOTS FOR VARIOUS FOCAL-LENGTH LENSES
Note: Camera position remained the same for all shots. As focal lengths increase, the angle of view decreases and the subject appears larger.

Angle of view The focal length of the lens also determines the angle of view—the area seen by the lens. The angle of view for any lens is calculated by dividing the diagonal of the negative by the focal length of the lens.

With one eye closed, you can normally see at an angle of about 48 degrees. Correspondingly, a normal lens should have an angle of view of approximately 48 to 58 degrees. Lenses that deviate from the standard give a different angle of view. A wide-angle lens has an angle of view of about 80 degrees; a telephoto lens has an angle of view of about 20 degrees.

Maximum angle of view is achieved only when the lens is focused on infinity. As the subject gets closer to any type of lens, the angle of view decreases. Table 2-1 shows how angle of view can change as the focal length increases; here, the object is considered to be at infinity. (See Figure 2-26.)

Under the best of conditions, our eyes can distinguish between objects about $\frac{1}{8}$ millimeter in diameter. Objects smaller than that all appear the same to the human eye.

A lens can focus perfectly on only one point at a time. As rays of light from this point pass through the lens, they are brought back to a point of sharp focus by the lens. Consequently, although the point focused on and its image formed by the lens appear sharp and clear, other points of the subject are not in sharp focus. To bring another point into perfect focus requires refocusing.

It might seem that very little of a scene would be in sharp focus. As a

TABLE 2-1 ☐ FOCAL LENGTHS AND ANGLES OF VIEW FOR NORMAL LENSES

FORMAT	NEGATIVE SIZE	DIAGONAL OF NEGATIVE	FOCAL LENGTH OF NORMAL LENS	NORMAL LENS ANGLE OF VIEW
110	14 × 17 mm	22 mm	24 mm	50°
135	24 × 36 mm	43 mm	50 mm	48°
2¼	60 × 60 mm	85 mm	80 mm	56°
4 × 5	102 × 127 mm	165 mm	150 mm	58°

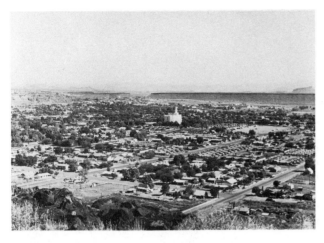

B Shot with a 50 mm lens

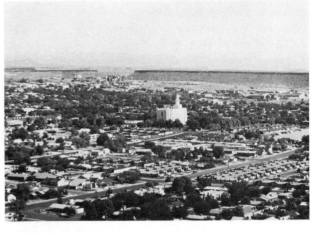

C Shot with an 85 mm lens

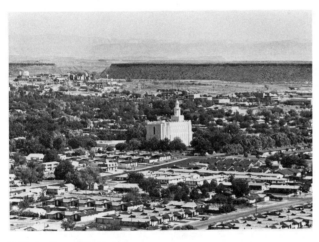

D Shot with a 135 mm lens

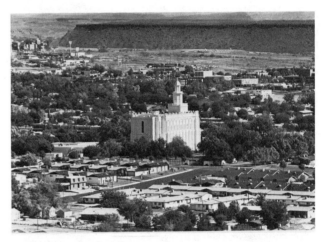

E Shot with a 200 mm lens

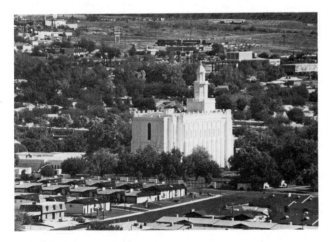

F Shot with a 300 mm lens

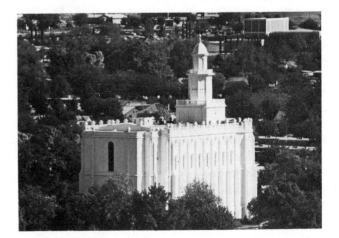

G Shot with a 500 mm lens

FIGURE 2-27 CIRCLES OF CONFUSION
The lens is focused on Point B. The aperture is wide open, resulting in large circles of confusion. The image of an object at Point A is focused in front of the film. The image of an object at Point B is focused on the film. The image of an object at Point C would be focused behind the film plane if the film were not in the way. The lens is focused on Point B. The aperture is stopped down, reducing the size of the circles of confusion.

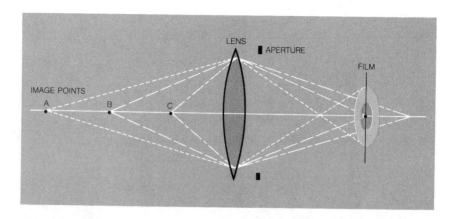

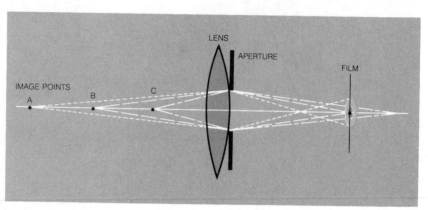

matter of fact, only the area focused on can be perfectly sharp. Objects in front of or behind this area will be out of focus to one degree or another. In practice, however, we obtain pictures that appear to have considerable depth and overall sharpness: because of the less than perfect resolving power of the eye, we can be satisfied with something less than pinpoint sharpness.

Out-of-focus points are represented at the film plane by a disc, or *circle of confusion.* These circles are cross-sections of the cones of light coming to a focus behind or in front of the surface of the film. (See Figure 2-27.) If an image point or circle of confusion is equal to or less than about ⅛ millimeter in diameter, the print will appear to be acceptably sharp in that area.

Normally, depth of field can be controlled by stopping down the lens. A large f/number, such as f/16, produces more depth of field than f/2, for example. If minimum aperture still

gives inadequate depth of field, the lens can be changed to one with a shorter focal length. The shorter the focal length of a lens, the greater the depth of field. The depth of field is also affected by the care with which the object is brought into focus and by the distance the object is from the camera. The farther away the object is, the greater the depth of field will be. For most objects, the area of sharp focus is usually divided, with one-third in front of and two-thirds in back of the object focused on.

In some applications, the photographer is concerned with the *hyperfocal distance*—the distance from the lens to the nearest object which is in acceptably sharp focus when the camera is focused on infinity. (See Figure 2-28.) The hyperfocal length varies with the depth of field—as one increases, the other decreases, and vice versa. For objects very close to the camera, the depth of field is shallow and extends about the same amount on either side

of the distance focused on.

Perspective Perspective is the apparent relationship among the shape, size, and position of three-dimensional objects captured on two-dimensional film. Sometimes called *linear* or simply *drawing perspective*, it depends on your viewpoint when you take the picture. If the viewpoint is fixed, you cannot change the perspective by using a lens of a different focal length. The only thing that will change is the apparent size of the object you focus on. Perspective will be altered, too, by changing viewpoint, moving farther away or closer, higher or lower.

No change of lens will re-create the perspective obtained from the original viewpoint. If you try to maintain object size while using lenses of longer focal lengths, for example, you will find that the distance between you and your subject will increase with increasing focal length and that the perspective will become flatter. (See Figure 2-29.)

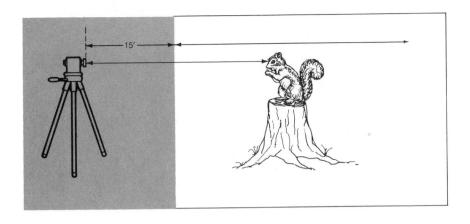

FIGURE 2-28 DEPTH OF FIELD AND HYPERFOCAL DISTANCE
By definition, the hyperfocal distance is the distance from the camera to the first point in acceptable focus when the lens is focused on infinity.

FIGURE 2-29A–F HOW PERSPECTIVE CHANGES WITH FOCAL LENGTH
The front subject was held approximately the same size in all the shots. Both subjects remained in the same positions; the camera-to-subject distance was increased with each lens change. A 35 mm camera was used.

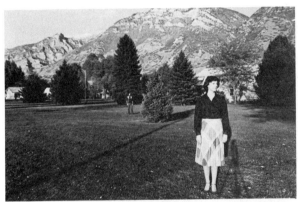

A Taken with a 28 mm lens

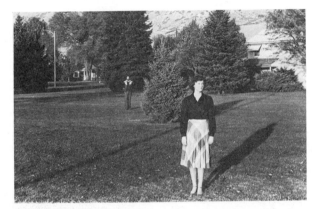

B Taken with a 50 mm lens

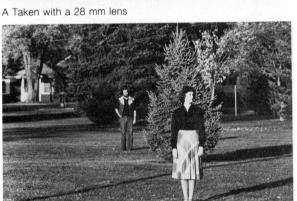

C Taken with a 135 mm lens

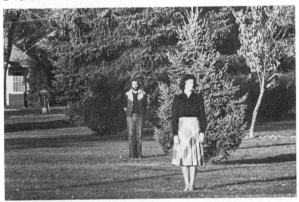

D Taken with a 200 mm lens

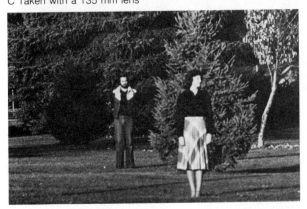

E Taken with a 300 mm lens

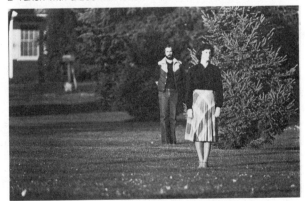

F Taken with a 500 mm lens

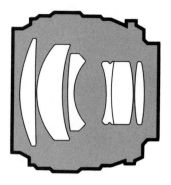

FIGURE 2-30 CROSS-SECTION OF A 50 MM LENS
A compound lens is made by placing several simple lens elements together.

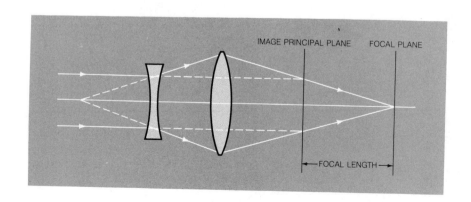

IMAGE PRINCIPAL PLANE   FOCAL PLANE

FOCAL LENGTH

FIGURE 2-31A&B OPTICS AND CONSTRUCTION OF A WIDE-ANGLE LENS
A A wide-angle lens has the negative element in front of the positive element.
B This cross-section of a modern wide-angle lens shows its various elements.

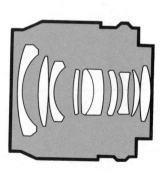

Today's camera lenses

The standard or *normal lens* offers the photographer uniform performance over its angle of view and a wide range of usable apertures. A normal lens for a particular format has a focal length that is approximately equal to the diagonal of that particular negative. A full-frame 35 mm negative is 24 by 36 mm and has a diagonal that measures 43.2 mm. The normal lens for a 35 mm camera should have a focal length between 45 and 50 mm and an angle of view of approximately 48 degrees. (See Figure 2-30.)

Standard lenses cannot meet all the requirements of every shooting situation, particularly when photographs require wide coverage in cramped surroundings or when distant, sometimes unreachable objects need to be photographed close up.

Wide-angle lenses Since the middle of the nineteenth century, wide-angle lenses have been used to capture a wide scene when the photographer could not back up. The first wide-angle lenses were no more than simple meniscus lenses; today there is a divergent or negative group in front of the lens and a convergent or positive group behind it. (See Figure 2-31.) This arrangement gives the lens a focal length that is shorter than the diagonal of the film format. Table 2-2 provides a comparison of focal lengths and angles of view for wide-angle lenses from different formats.

Wide-angle lenses can cause some distortion, but they are invaluable for capturing a wide field of view under cramped conditions—for example, when taking interior or exterior building shots where there is no room to back away.

Close-up lenses You can use a normal exposure if you use a close-up lens on your camera instead of an extension device on your lens. Close-up lenses come in various powers, such as +1, +2, +3—the higher the number, the stronger the lens and the closer you can move in to photograph the subject. You can combine two lenses to get an even more powerful total effect. For example, two +3 lenses have the effect of a +6 lens. Although you can combine two close-up lenses, you should not use more than two at once. More than two tends to cut off the corners of the image and decrease the image quality.

Since you will be photographing subjects at close distance, it is critical that you measure the distance to make sure you are focusing properly. If you are using a single lens reflex camera, you can actually see this through the viewfinder. If you are using a non-reflex camera, however, it is critical that you measure the distance down to a fraction of an inch.

Telephoto lenses The lens arrangement for the telephoto lens is the opposite of that of the wide-angle lens.

TABLE 2-2 □ FOCAL LENGTHS AND ANGLES OF VIEW FOR WIDE-ANGLE LENSES

FORMAT	NEGATIVE SIZE	DIAGONAL OF NEGATIVE	FOCAL LENGTH OF WIDE-ANGLE LENS	WIDE-ANGLE LENS ANGLE OF VIEW
110	14 × 17 mm	22 mm	18 mm	63°
135	24 × 36 mm	43 mm	28 mm	75°
2¼	60 × 60 mm	85 mm	50 mm	81°
4 × 5	102 × 127 mm	165 mm	100 mm	79°

TABLE 2-3 □ FOCAL LENGTHS AND ANGLES OF VIEW FOR TELEPHOTO LENSES

FORMAT	NEGATIVE SIZE	DIAGONAL OF NEGATIVE	FOCAL LENGTH OF TELEPHOTO LENS	TELEPHOTO LENS ANGLE OF VIEW
110	14 × 17 mm	22 mm	50 mm	25°
135	24 × 36 mm	43 mm	135 mm	19°
2¼	60 × 60 mm	85 mm	250 mm	20°
4 × 5	102 × 127 mm	165 mm	300 mm	36°

The positive or converging group is in front of the lens, and the rear group is made from negative or diverging lens elements. (See Figure 2-32.) This system yields a much greater focal length than the diagonal of the film and angles of view much smaller than those of a normal lens. Telephoto lenses also give a larger image on the film than normal lenses do.

Telephoto lenses are especially useful for:

1 Shooting a portrait without getting too close to the subject

2 Photographing dangerous subjects from a safe distance

3 Compressing space and flattening perspective

4 Shooting candid photographs without being seen or without disturbing the subject

5 Photographing sports events or other action scenes

6 Isolating detail when shooting from a fixed position

The weight of a camera fitted with a telephoto lens makes it difficult to hold the camera steady. One or more of the following will prevent blurring of the image because of camera shake: mount the camera on a tripod or other firm support; use an electronic flash; or use only high shutter speeds ($\frac{1}{250}$ to $\frac{1}{1000}$). See Table 2-3 for a comparison of various telephoto lenses and for-

FIGURE 2-32A&B OPTICS AND CONSTRUCTION OF A TELEPHOTO LENS
A In a telephoto lens, the positive element is placed in front of the negative element.
B This cross-section of modern telephoto lens shows its components.

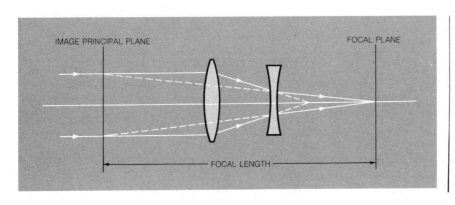

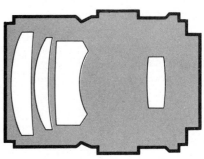

TABLE 2-4 □ VARIOUS FOCAL LENGTHS AND ANGLES OF VIEW FOR NORMAL, WIDE-ANGLE, AND TELEPHOTO LENSES

FORMAT	NEGATIVE SIZE	DIAGONAL OF NEGATIVE	FOCAL LENGTH OF NORMAL LENS	NORMAL LENS ANGLE OF VIEW	FOCAL LENGTH OF WIDE-ANGLE LENS	WIDE-ANGLE LENS ANGLE OF VIEW	FOCAL LENGTH OF TELEPHOTO LENS	TELEPHOTO LENS ANGLE OF VIEW
110	14 × 17 mm	22 mm	24 mm	50°	18 mm	63°	50 mm	25°
135	24 × 36 mm	43 mm	50 mm	48°	28 mm	75°	135 mm	19°
2¼	60 × 60 mm	85 mm	80 mm	56°	50 mm	81°	250 mm	20°
4 × 5	102 × 127 mm	165 mm	150 mm	58°	100 mm	79°	300 mm	36°

mats. Table 2-4 summarizes angle of view and focal lengths for various lenses.

Zoom lenses A zoom lens—sometimes called a variable-focus lens—allows you to change from a distant, wide-angle view of a subject to a close-up shot of the same subject without moving either the camera or the subject and without changing the lens. This is possible because a zoom lens provides an infinite number of focal lengths between the two extremes of the lens. Zoom lenses are available in a variety of focal-length ranges: from wide angle to normal, from moderately short to moderately long, and from normal to long. However, it can be difficult to maintain sharp, accurate focus over the entire range of the lens.

Lens coating

The process of coating camera lenses to improve their sharpness and speed was discovered accidentally. Early photographers wrongly assumed that the natural aging and tarnishing of the lenses' surfaces rendered them useless, so the lenses were simply thrown away when they became discolored. When it was discovered that this aging, in combination with exposure to sunlight and air, *improved* the quality and performance of the lenses, scientists began searching for a means to artificially age camera lenses. These efforts resulted in lens coating. Now almost all new lenses are precoated by the manufacturer. This coating is about four one-millionths of an inch thick. The optical interference causes greater transmission of the light—an increase of more than twenty percent in some cases.

SUMMARY

Today's photographer can choose from a tremendous selection of lenses and sophisticated cameras that allow great versatility and convenience. The avid photographer may find that no single camera or camera system will fit all the needs and situations encountered.

For fast action, it is desirable to use a 35 mm single lens reflex camera with a motor drive attachment to advance the film rapidly from one frame to the next. For landscapes, it is better to use a view camera that permits careful composition and clear, detailed enlargement. And for candid scenes, a viewfinder camera, with its quiet shutter, compact size, and light weight, is ideal.

Lenses should also be chosen according to the work planned. Those who want to photograph a wide variety of subjects will have to strike a compromise among the available lenses.

The novice will also soon realize that different camera formats and lens combinations are but one more way to realize the photographer's creativity. The first step in realizing the creative possibilities of a lens or camera is to understand how each sees the subject. The effects of wide-angle or telephoto lenses on depth of field and angle or view become extensions of the photographer's own vision—with practice and experience, these extensions will seem as familiar and ''natural'' as eyeglasses.

REVIEW QUESTIONS

1 What are the four common types of cameras?

2 Why is through-the-lens viewing so popular?

3 What is the biggest drawback to 35 mm photography?

4 What is the basic advantage of a medium-format camera?

5 What are the only disadvantages of the view camera for everyday photography?

6 What is the common purpose of all camera lenses?

7 Why are lens coatings important?

8 What is a normal lens?

9 Why is the normal lens different for various film formats?

10 How is depth of field affected as the subject gets closer to the camera?

11 How does depth of field change as the focal length increases?

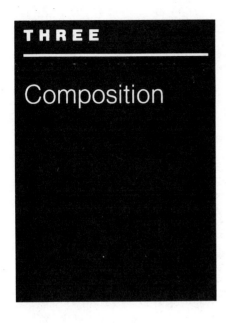

THREE

Composition

Every time a picture is taken, an image is painted with light. When light combines well with the elements of the picture, the photograph is pleasing to look at.

The basic rules of good composition have been followed at least since the times of the ancient Greeks and Romans. Later, Renaissance artists presented the world with many examples of good composition.

What exactly *is* composition? It has been defined as the pleasing arrangement of subjects or objects within a given area or as the placement of subject members to form a recognizable whole. For photographers, composition is the art of creating an understandable message by placing subject parts together so that each element adds to the overall "message." A striking photograph is one that clearly and directly transmits the photographer's message.

Although content and composition are often thought of as separate parts of a picture, neither can exist without the other. Good composition supports and clarifies picture content. A strong, clear effect is the result of a clever arrangement of content and composition.

Good composition does not usually "just happen." It requires practice. Composition skills can be broken down into two parts: learning how to "see" the composition and subject elements in your camera's viewfinder and learning how to arrange these elements effectively. Oddly enough, the harder of the two is training the eye to see all the elements in the viewfinder. Once you have mastered the basics of composition, you will naturally learn how to exercise the freedom to make your own choices when photographing a scene. This artistic license allows a photographer to break all of the rules in order to capture a special picture.

GUIDELINES FOR GOOD COMPOSITION

A novice photographer starts out taking pictures of commonplace events. As the individual grows photographically, his or her pictures show more sophistication in subject selection and arrangement. A good photographer takes each picture to make a statement, create a feeling, or communicate a mood. If the guidelines for good composition have been followed, anyone who looks at the picture will be able to understand the photographer's reason for taking it.

A talent for good composition may be inborn, but it can also be the result of planning and thought based on some general guidelines. These guidelines should help you to develop your photographic knowledge and improve the quality and impact of your photography. Use the guidelines that follow as they seem to apply, but remember that strict adherence can result in a tiresome repetition of pictoral themes. This is because understanding and imagination can *never* be replaced by memorizing a set of rules.

Center of interest

The center of interest is the subject of the photograph. A center of interest can be anything that you choose to photograph. Once you decide on the center of interest, you need to arrange the secondary parts of the scene so that they complement the subject. (See Figure 3-1.)

A common mistake often made by beginning photographers is to try to place more than one center of interest in a photograph. More than one center of interest in a single photograph is usually distracting and confusing. (See Figure 3-2.) It *is* possible to effectively use two centers of interest in a photograph if the objects or persons are

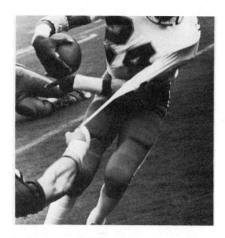

FIGURE 3-1 DYNAMIC CENTER OF INTEREST
(Nathan Pierson)

FIGURE 3-2 MULTIPLE CENTERS OF INTEREST
(Joseph T. Baiocco)

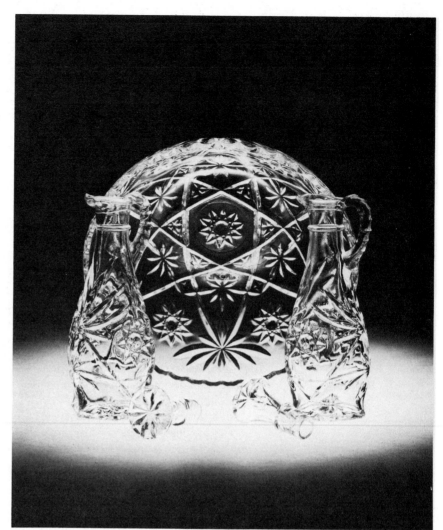

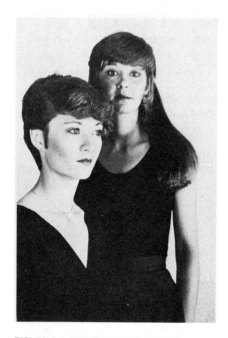

FIGURE 3-3 EFFECTIVE USE OF TWO CENTERS OF INTEREST

placed facing each other toward the center of the photograph, but extreme care must be used. (See Figure 3-3.)

Balance and proportion

Even though the center of interest is the major focus in a photograph, the area around the subject must effectively complement and strengthen it. Think of the area in the viewfinder as a sheet of paper or a canvas, then decide on the best balance and proportion to enhance the subject you are photographing.

For balance, evenly arrange large physical objects in a picture—combine light and dark areas, and use simple shapes in conjunction with complex ones. (See Figure 3-4.) Match highly detailed areas with large, empty ones, using other elements in the picture to link them to each other and to the center of interest. (See Figure 3-5.) By juggling balance and proportion you can shift the emphasis from one part of the photograph to another.

Rule of thirds

You can use the *rule of thirds* to determine ideal placement of the subject in your photograph. To get an idea of how the rule of thirds works, draw two imaginary horizontal lines across the scene you are photograph-

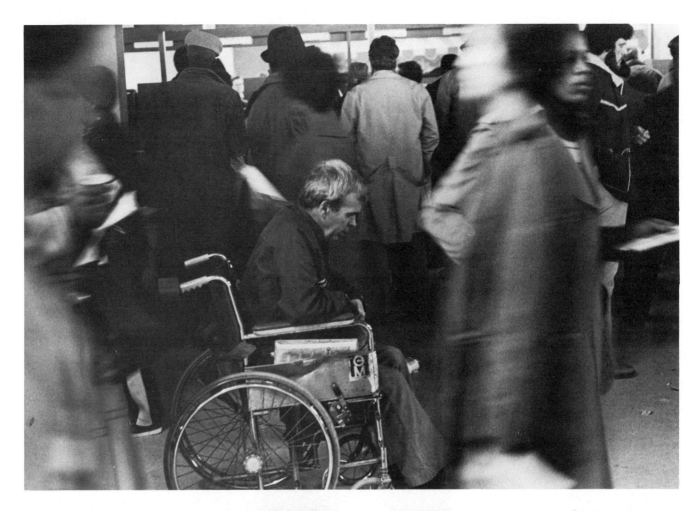

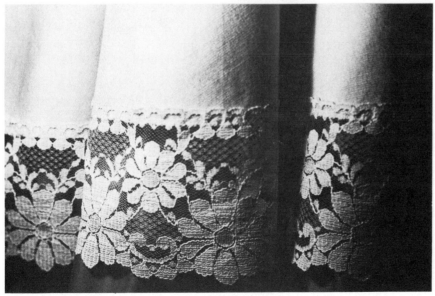

FIGURE 3-4 BALANCE OF TONES AND SHAPES
(Eileen Polsenberg)

FIGURE 3-5 HIGHLY DETAILED AREA MATCHED WITH EMPTY AREAS
(Karin F. Wheeler)

**FIGURE 3-6 SHOT WITH TWO SUBJECTS AT
OPPOSITE INTERSECTION**

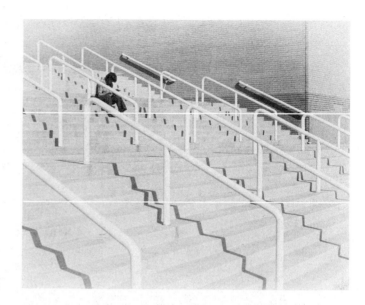

A Shot with Horizontal Lines

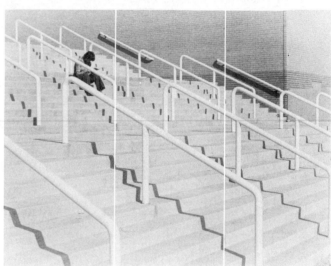

B Shot with Vertical Lines

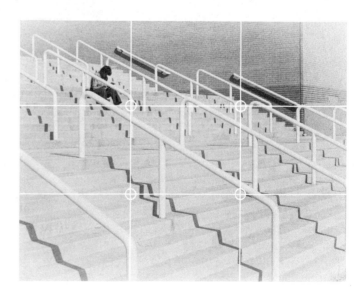

C Shot with Grid

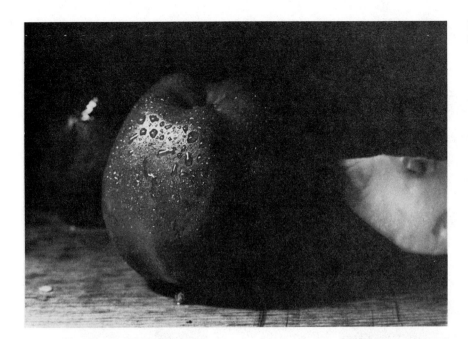

FIGURE 3-7 MOTIONLESS PRINT
(Photo Laird Roberts)

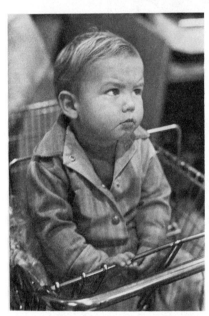

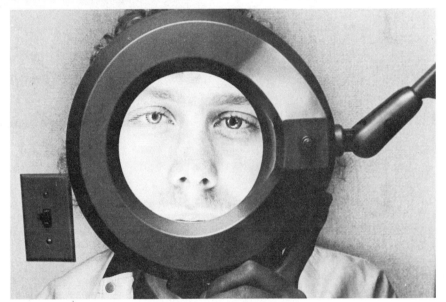

FIGURE 3-8 STRONG SUBJECT IN CENTER OF PICTURE
(Photo Laird Roberts)

FIGURE 3-9 CLOSE-UP IN CENTER OF PICTURE
(David Hering)

ing, as in Figure 3-6A. Now draw two imaginary vertical lines through the same scene as in Figure 3-6B. The subject is best placed at one of the four intersections created by your imaginary lines. (See Figure 3-6C.)

In most cases a subject in the exact center of the picture looks stiff or motionless. (See Figure 3-7.) Exceptions are a very strong subject set against a simple background, as in Figure 3-8, and a subject shot close-up, as in Figure 3-9.

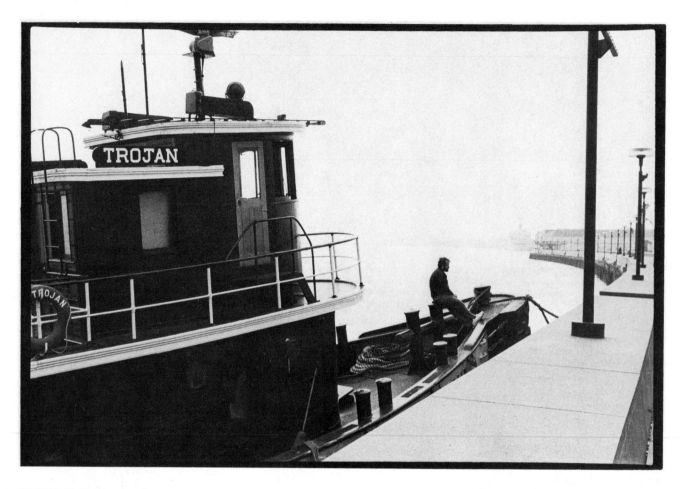

FIGURE 3-10 MOTION
(Arnold H. DiBlasi Jr.)

You should also use the rule of thirds when considering the strength or motion of the subject. The subject should be place so that its motion leads into the scene, thus creating a feeling of action. Motion should not be directed out of the picture. (See Figure 3-10.)

If you have more than one subject or center of interest in the photograph, they should be placed at opposite intersections of the imaginary grid lines.

If you are taking photographs outdoors, you may have to deal with the horizon line—the line produced where the sky meets either land or water. A horizon line that cuts across the center of a picture can make it look out of balance. (See Figure 3-11A.) The horizon line should go through the top third of the picture, emphasizing the foreground (Figure 3-11B), or through the bottom third of the picture, emphasizing the sky (Figure 3-11C). If the horizon line cuts through the center of interest, rearrange the camera's viewpoint to eliminate the problem.

Mergers

Mergers are the little devils that can ruin a good picture.

Object merger An object merger occurs when an unnecessary object in the foreground interferes with the subject. Once again, having spotted an object merger in the viewfinder, you can simply change the camera angle to eliminate it.

Foreground—background merger
The most common merger is the foreground—background merger. It occurs when an unwanted object in the background merges with the subject in the foreground. (See Figure 3-12.) Once you see it in the viewfinder, you can correct a foreground—background merger by changing the camera angle. (See Figure 3-13.)

Color merger In nature, a color merger—poor separation of hues or colors between the foreground and the background—is often a means of survival for an organism: we call this *camouflage.* It poses a great deal of difficulty for a photographer, though, both in color and in black and white photography.

In color photography, a color merger may occur when a picture is com-

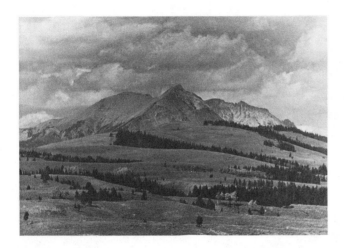

FIGURE 3-11A HORIZON LINE THROUGH CENTER OF PICTURE

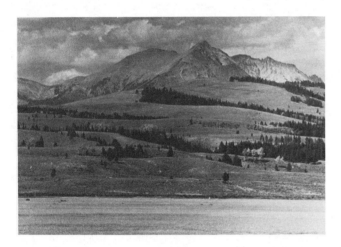

FIGURE 3-11B HORIZON LINE THROUGH TOP THIRD OF PICTURE

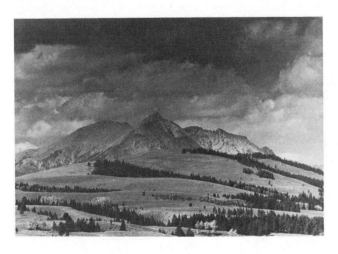

FIGURE 3-11C HORIZON LINE THROUGH BOTTOM THIRD OF PICTURE

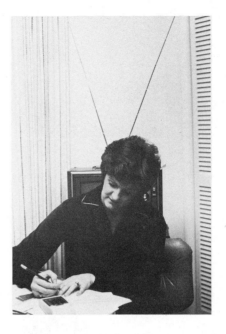

FIGURE 3-12 FOREGROUND—BACKGROUND MERGER
Note position of rabbit ears

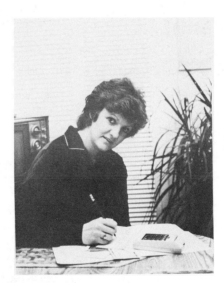

FIGURE 3-13 FOREGROUND—BACKGROUND MERGER CORRECTED
The camera position was changed.

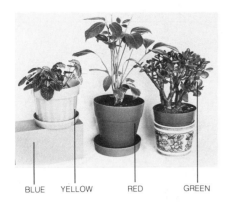

FIGURE 3-14 UNFILTERED SHOT OF SCENE CONTAINING YELLOW, RED, GREEN, AND BLUE OBJECTS

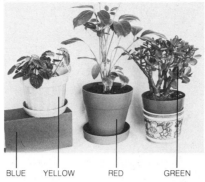

FIGURE 3-15A
Shot of Scene Using a Yellow Filter

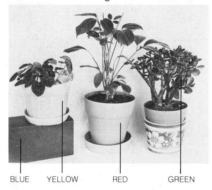

FIGURE 3-15B
Shot of Scene Using a Red Filter

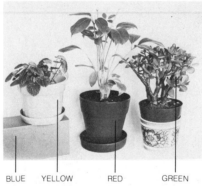

FIGURE 3-15C
Shot of Scene Using a Green Filter

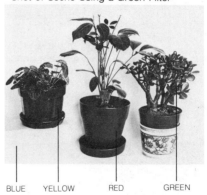

FIGURE 3-15D
Shot of Scene Using a Blue Filter

posed entirely of different shades of the same color. In black and white photography, a color merger occurs when two or more colors are recorded by the film as the same shade of gray. (See Figure 3-14.) The problem of color merger is easily corrected through use of the proper color filter. (See Figure 3-15A–D.) For a complete discussion on the use of color filters in black and white photography, see Chapter Ten.

Border merger A border merger occurs when the photographer forgets to watch the edges of the viewfinder, gets in too close, and cuts off some of the subject. Almost all amateur photographers have inadvertently left out people standing at the sides of a group or "cut off" a person's head with a border merger. To solve the problem, back off slightly. A good photographer will train his or her eye to spot potential problems in the view-finder before they end up in the print. Always remember to take a moment to look beyond the subject and analyze how *every* element in the picture relates to every other element and to the subject.

Framing

In framing, a special kind of merger, the photographer increases the feeling of depth in a picture by using objects in the foreground to complement the center of interest. Doorways, windows, limbs of trees, buildings, and so on can serve as natural frames. (See Figure 3-16.) Another way to frame the center of interest is to emphasize it by keeping either the foreground or the background out of focus. This effect can be achieved by manipulating the lens aperture, which controls the depth of field. (See Figure 3-17.)

Whether or not you use a frame will depend on the particular photographic situation. Stay on the lookout for good frames, but make sure you do not choose a frame that is so heavy it dominates the subject.

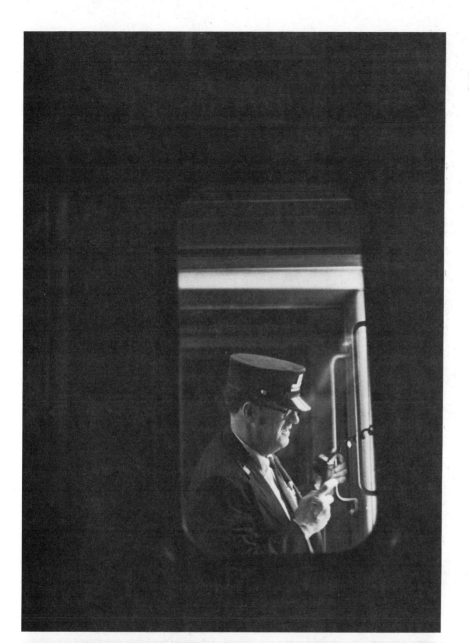

FIGURE 3-16 NATURAL FRAME PICTURE
(W.F. Mruk)

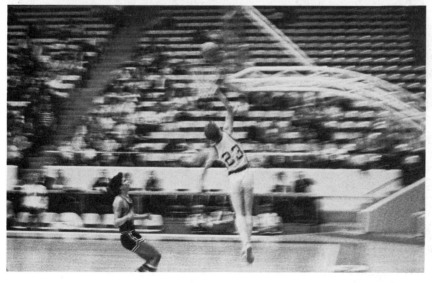

FIGURE 3-17   Selective Focus

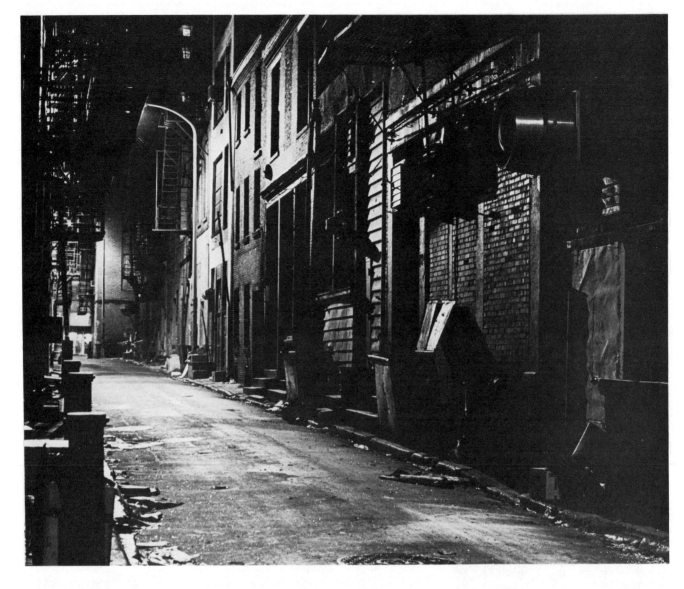

FIGURE 3-18 LEADING LINES (John J. McGurk)

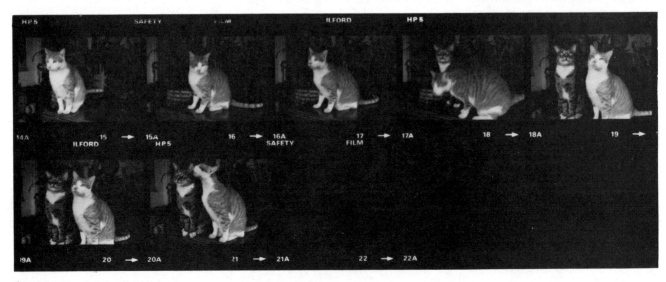

FIGURE 3-19 Judging the Moment

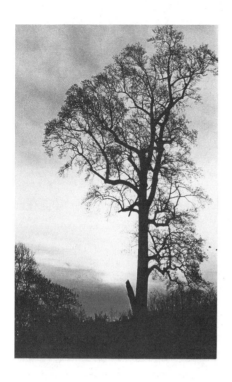

FIGURE 3-20 STRONG SHAPES AGAINST A
SIMPLE BACKGROUND
(Paul E. DeWalt)

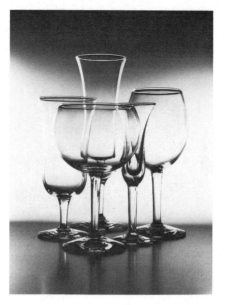

FIGURE 3-21 STRONG SHAPES WITH A FULL
RANGE OF TONES
(Patrice Williams)

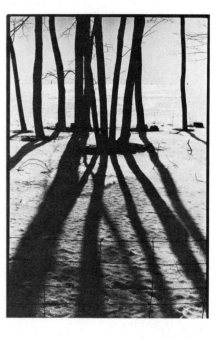

FIGURE 3-22 INTERACTION OF LINES AND
PICTURE FRAME
(Michael J. Huffert)

Leading lines

Leading lines cause the viewer's attention to be focused rapidly on the picture's center of interest. They lead the eye toward the main subject of the photograph. A leading line might be a row of trees, a river, or a fence. (See Figure 3-18.)

FORMING AN EFFECTIVE COMMUNICATION

Organizing the elements in a scene helps improve communication, but other practices can add dynamic impact to your photographs.

Judging the moment

A still life, a landscape, and other static subjects allow you the time to consider every aspect of the picture carefully. But for those scenes in which the relationships among people, objects, and settings change from one fleeting moment to the next, you need to exercise artistic license in choosing which ones to capture.

Consider the scene in Figure 3-19. This picture was present for only one brief moment. To capture this "decisive moment," you have to locate the most promising viewpoint and lighting, then roughly compose the shot within the viewfinder almost instantaneously. Carefully watch the massing and placing of shapes and forms as they interact in the viewfinder. Learn to react quickly when the right moment occurs. Above all, do not let the mechanics of photography come between you and the subject.

Using shape, pattern, and texture

Shape There are many ways of using and highlighting shape in a composition. You can emphasize the outline of a subject by contrasting it to a plain or simple background, such as sky or water. (See Figure 3-20.) Outlines and forms can be emphasized further and internal detail suppressed by using the right kind of lighting. Proper lighting is basic to photographing shapes and forms. You can convey the effect of three dimensions with a full range of tones from pure black to pure white. (See Figure 3-21.)

With very careful composition, each line of the subject's shape can be related to the other lines in the scene and to the edges of the frame. (See Figure 3-22.) The simpler the picture content, the stronger its shapes are likely to be. Decide which shapes are important, and then eliminate all unnecessary detail.

Pattern A compositional arrangement that helps strengthen a single motif, pattern can bring order to confusion.

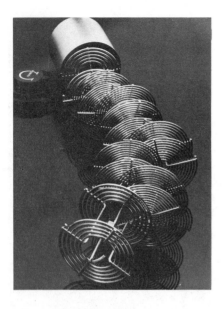

FIGURE 3-23 PATTERN
(Charles D. Hatcher)

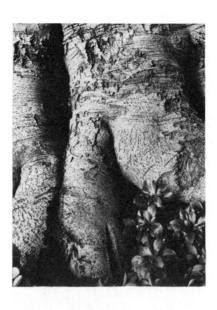

FIGURE 3-25 TEXTURE
(Randi Lyn Schor)

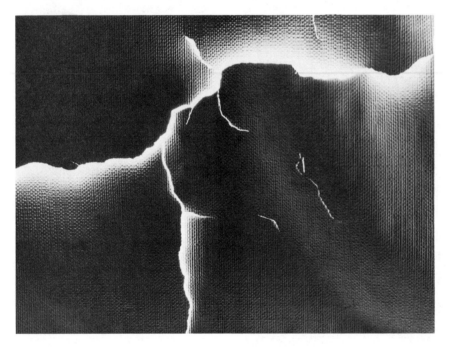

FIGURE 3-24 TEXTURE   (Lois B. Sharkey)

(See Figure 3-23.) You might discover a pattern in the simple shape of a tree or in the complex collection of buildings along a downtown parkway.

The key to working with patterns is to be selective with camera viewpoint and subject lighting. With all three-dimensional subjects, camera position determines how various elements and planes align and relate to one another. Proper lighting of the pattern will enhance its effect; improper lighting will destroy it.

Texture Texture in a photograph suggests how a surface would feel if we could touch it. Is the object rough and irregular, or is it smooth and shiny? When you want to show the depth and form of a subject, texture is a vital element. Consider the texture of a windblown landscape, an old woman's face, or a basket of ripe fruit. Texture in a photograph almost always makes the shot more interesting. (See Figure 3-24.)

As with shape and pattern, lighting is the key to good texture in photography. The best lighting direction is one almost parallel to the surface, so that the shadows produced help emphasize the texture. The kind of lighting you use will depend on the subtlety of the textures in the subject. Complex, rugged surfaces are best highlighted by soft lighting, while harsh lighting is better for smooth textures. (See Figure 3-25.)

Varying the camera viewpoint

Every camera tends to impose its own viewpoint. A single lens reflex camera encourages the photographer to shoot from eye level. A twin lens reflex camera dictates shooting from chest level. The old-fashioned box camera conditioned people to shoot from waist level. It is easy to fall into patterns of use, but you can often get more interesting, relevant composition by standing on a chair, crouching, or lying on the ground. (See Figure 3-26A–B.)

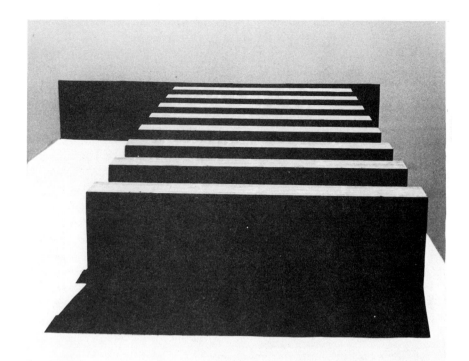

FIGURE 3-26A VERY LOW VIEWPOINT
(Kurtd Schmick)

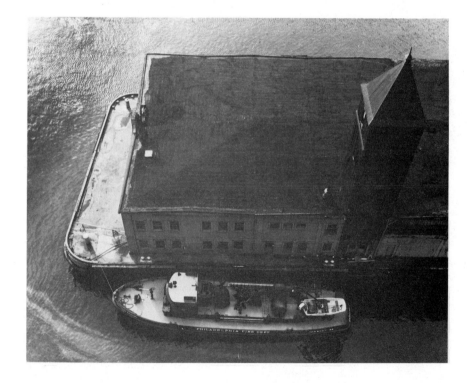

FIGURE 3-26B VERY HIGH VIEWPOINT
(Joseph T. Baiocco)

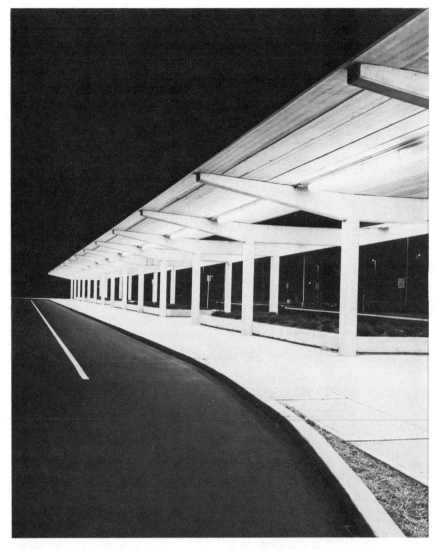

FIGURE 3-27 LINEAR PERSPECTIVE
(Robert L. Bentley)

FIGURE 3-28 AERIAL PERSPECTIVE

Before you take any picture, walk around to see how changing directions alters the scene. Carefully observe the effects of light, foreground–background relationships, lines, and shapes. When photographing a stationary subject such as a building or a landcape, try taking pictures from at least six different viewpoints, making the subject appear as different as you can in each shot.

SIMULATION OF DEPTH AND MOTION

Photographers try to compress the three-dimensional world into a two-dimensional picture. A number of tricks can help you create an illusion of depth and motion to bring a three-dimensional feeling to your photographs.

Depth

Depth in a photograph is an illusion conveyed by perspective, or the gradual changes of lines, patterns, and tones. As an example, imagine a row of telephone poles that seem to grow smaller as they march into the distance, or railroad tracks that seem to come together way off on the horizon. From experience we know that the poles are not really getting smaller, nor are the tracks getting closer together. But when you capture this sense of distance in a photograph, you have created an illusion of depth. Four techniques can help create an illusion of depth.

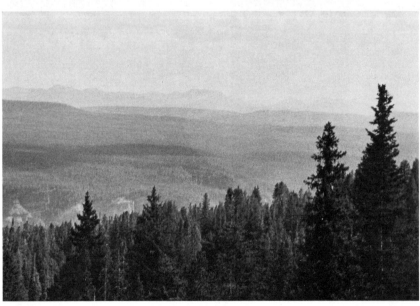

Linear perspective Linear perspective creates an illusion of depth by capturing the converging lines of an object (such as railroad tracks) or the diminishing size of similar objects (such as the row of telephone poles). When the main subject is in the middle to far distance, linear perspective offers the most effective way of giving a three-dimensional look to a photograph. With linear perspective, the viewer's eye is led into the subject area. (See Figure 3-27.)

Aerial perspective Aerial perspective is produced when atmospheric conditions separate objects at different distances with differences in tone. At dusk or dawn, mist, smoke, or haze often has a light-scattering effect. Because of this, light that travels the greatest distance through the air will produce a lighter tone. The effect of atmospheric, or aerial, perspective is most noticeable when objects are placed at distinct, well-spaced intervals. (See Figure 3-28.) The effect is enhanced if a long focus or telephoto lens is used; this makes distant images seem closer in size to those in the foreground, emphasizing the difference in tones.

Dynamic lines A dynamic form of composition makes use of various types of diagonal lines instead of horizontal or vertical lines, which tend to be much more static. Horizontal lines imply a sense of peace and calm; vertical lines add dignity and power to a scene. However, dynamic lines should not overpower or detract from the center of interest. (See Figure 3-29.)

Selective focus The technique most often used to create the illusion of depth is selective focus—throwing either the background or the foreground out of focus. By focusing on the foreground and using a wide aperture, you lose depth. On the other hand, you create a greater degree of depth by focusing on the subject and

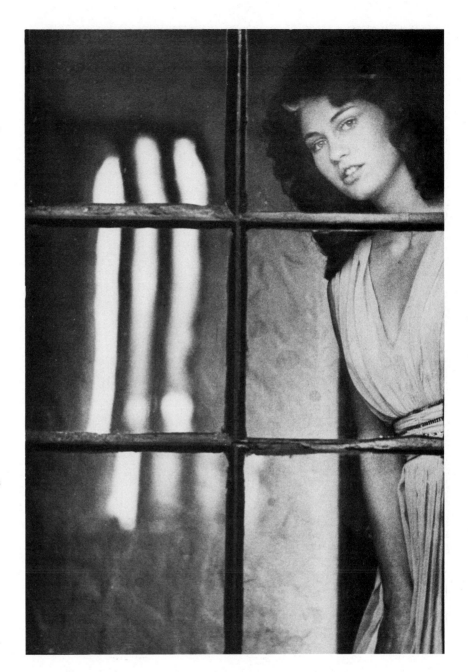

FIGURE 3-29 ALL ELEMENTS IN A VERTICAL POSITION
(Photo Laird Roberts)

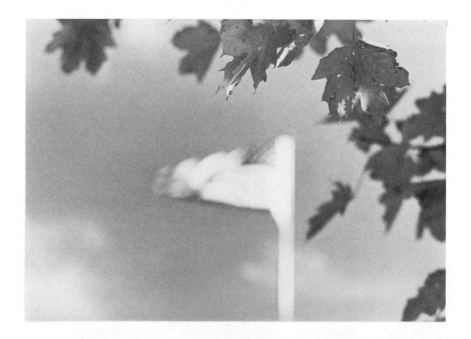

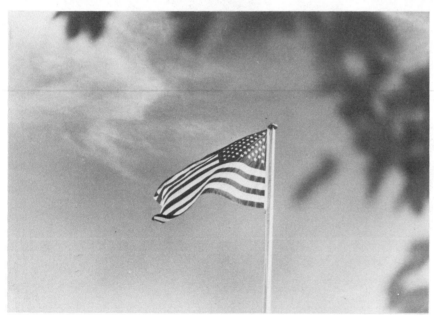

FIGURE 3-30A FOREGROUND IN FOCUS

FIGURE 3-30B FOREGROUND OUT OF FOCUS

using a small aperture. (See Figure 3-30A–B.)

The illusions of depth and form are the elements that best give a photograph three-dimensionality. However, overstressing depth in a single area of the photograph will seriously unbalance the picture.

Motion

You can imply motion in a photograph by using one of several techniques, or you can stop the action during the "decisive moment."

Shooting at low speed You can imply and capture motion by setting the shutter speed low enough to blur the action. Select a shutter speed below that necessary to stop the action: below $\frac{1}{5000}$, $\frac{1}{1000}$ for rapid motion, below $\frac{1}{250}$ to $\frac{1}{125}$ for moderate action, and around $\frac{1}{60}$ for slow movement. At speeds above $\frac{1}{60}$ second, you can safely hand-hold a camera without causing blurring. (See Figure 3-31.)

Panning The *panning* technique involves moving the camera in the same direction and at the same speed as the subject, using a moderate shutter speed. If you shoot the picture as the camera moves along with the subject, the background will be blurred and the subject in sharp focus. (See Figures 3-32 and 3-33.)

Showing obvious motion To show obvious motion, you have to stop the action at the critical point—a high diver at the top of a dive, for example, or a rodeo rider being thrown from the back of a bucking bronc. The ability to

FIGURE 3-31 INTENTIONALLY BLURRED SUBJECT

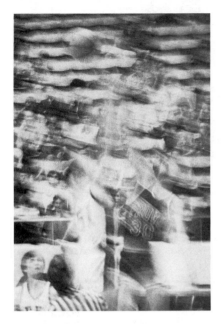

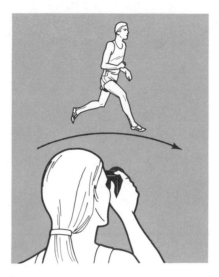

FIGURE 3-32 PANNING
You follow moving people or objects with your eyes; this action is almost unconscious, or automatic. A camera, however, does not do this automatically. You must aim the camera lens and turn with the motion, so that the subject stays in the viewfinder and the camera stays on the subject. With a slow shutter speed, the motionless background will blur, as will any part of the subject that moves in a different direction from the panning motion. For example, a runner's head and trunk will appear clear, but the arms and legs will be comparatively blurred.

FIGURE 3-33 PANNING
(Rogers C. Horsey Jr.)

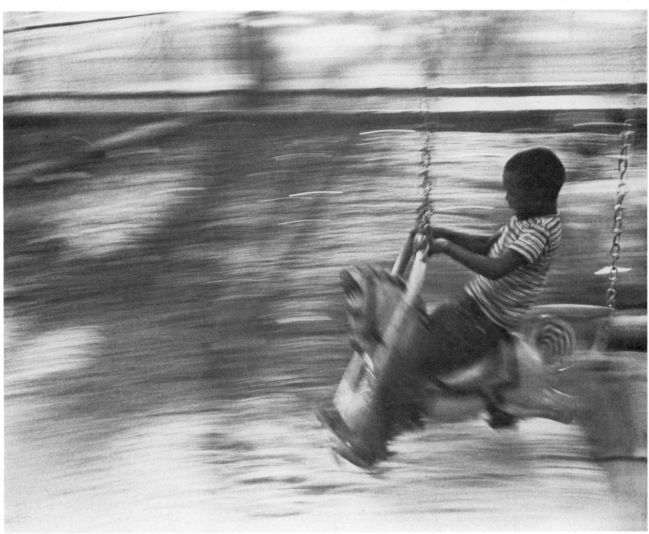

FIGURE 3-34 SHOWING OBVIOUS MOTION
(Michael Cathey)

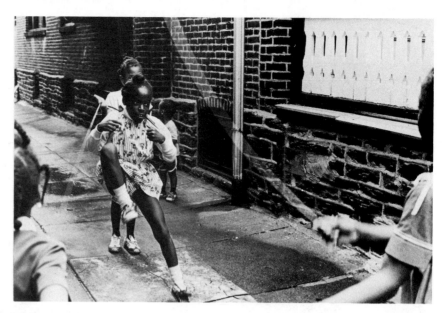

TABLE 3-1 □ MINIMUM SHUTTER SPEEDS FOR STOPPING MOTION

MOTION	SPEED (MPH)	DIRECTION IN RELATION TO CAMERA		
		SIDEWAYS	DIAGONAL	TOWARD / AWAY FROM
Walking; Hand Movement	5	$\frac{1}{250}$	$\frac{1}{125}$	$\frac{1}{60}$
Jogging; Slow Vehicle; Walking Horse	10	$\frac{1}{500}$	$\frac{1}{250}$	$\frac{1}{125}$
Dancing; Normal Traffic; Most Sports; Trotting Horse	20–30	$\frac{1}{1000}$	$\frac{1}{500}$	$\frac{1}{250}$
Fast Traffic; Speedboat; Racing Horse	40–60	$\frac{1}{2000}$	$\frac{1}{1000}$	$\frac{1}{500}$

judge the exact moment is of paramount importance. (See Figure 3-34.)

Capturing motion in the frame Use the rule of thirds when capturing motion in the frame. The motion should lead into—rather than out of—the scene. (See Table -1.)

Motion across the field of view is extremely difficult to photograph. Movement toward or away from the camera presents fewer problems. To stop the action when the object is moving across the scene, you need a faster shutter speed; when the object is approaching at an angle, one speed slower will usually work. The distance from the camera to the subject is also important: the greater the distance, the slower the speed necessary for stopping the action. See Figure 3-35A–F for a sequence of shots that illustrates this concept.

SUMMARY

A good photographer is one who can effectively recognize in the viewfinder the different elements that will combine to create the picture, can arrange and interweave these elements to produce the desired message, and can make an exposure that reproduces what appeared in the viewfinder.

Above all else, a good photographer must be successful at picture composition. Although following a set of guidelines is helpful, photographic composition is not a rule-bound art. Rather, it should be the natural expression of the photographer's sense of design, and guidelines should simply help improve that natural sense of composition.

With experience the photographer learns to recognize instinctively when one or all of these compositional guidelines can be broken to enhance the photographic purpose; this is effective use of artistic license.

REVIEW QUESTIONS

1 What is the meaning of *composition,* in the photographic sense?

2 What communicates the photographer's main reason for taking the picture?

3 What is the rule of thirds?

4 What are four common mergers?

5 What can be used to increase the feeling of depth in a picture?

6 What do leading lines do?

7 To capture that one brief, decisive moment, what must a photographer learn to do?

8 Why is an understanding of shapes necessary?

9 Texture is used to show what in a photograph?

10 A repetition of a single shape or form in a print is called what?

11 Why is it important to vary the camera viewpoint?

12 Explain linear perspective.

13 What is the term for the loss of detail and the lightening of color as objects recede into the distance?

14 What are the four basic techniques used to imply motion in a photograph?

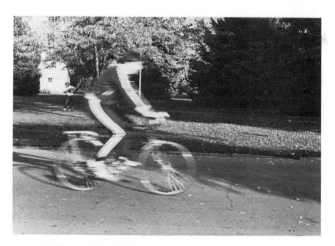

FIGURE 3-35A f/8.0 $\frac{1}{60}$ sec.

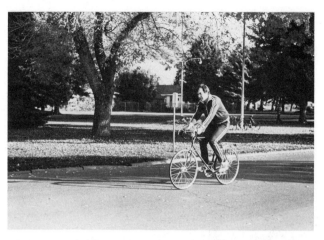

FIGURE 3-35D f/4.0 $\frac{1}{250}$ sec.

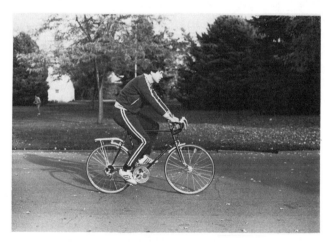

FIGURE 3-35B f/2.8 $\frac{1}{500}$ sec.

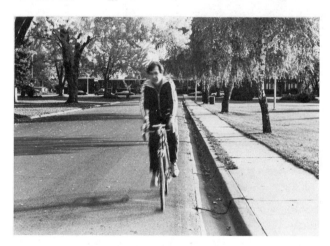

FIGURE 3-35E f/11 $\frac{1}{30}$ sec.

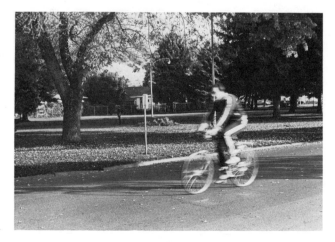

FIGURE 3-35C f/11 $\frac{1}{30}$ sec.

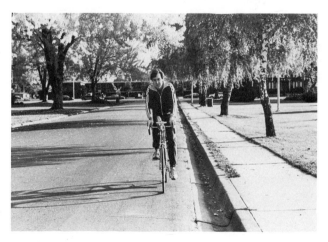

FIGURE 3-35F f/5.6 $\frac{1}{125}$ sec.

FIGURE 3-35A–F MOTION SEQUENCE
These shots illustrate motion in various directions relative to the
camera position. Blurring increases as shutter speed decreases,
but the amount varies. The biker's speed is approximately 10 mph
in all shots.

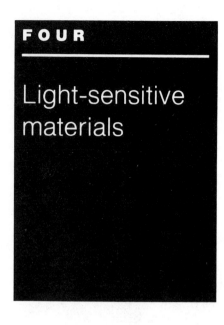

FOUR

Light-sensitive materials

Light and its reaction on photographic film provide the magic that allows us to reproduce on film almost exactly the forms and proportions that the eye sees. Modern technology has made available a variety of photographic materials that can accomplish practically any photographic task. The tremendous versatility of these materials opens up innumerable creative possibilities

LIGHT

Although scientists have developed theories to explain some of the things light does, no one really *completely* understands light. For example, the human eye is constructed to receive and see light, but unless light is striking the eye directly, light is invisible. The eye does not see objects themselves directly at all. Rather, it senses light that is emitted or reflected by objects. If an object is not emitting or reflecting light, it is invisible.

Light sources

Every visible thing in the world is a light source. Some are *primary light sources,* those that produce or emit light, like the sun; others are *secondary light sources,* those that reflect light, such as a building, a person, or a book. Whether it is primary or secondary, light and only light is the subject of photography. To begin to see how light acts and what light does, instead of just seeing the subject itself, is to begin to see photographically.

THE NATURE OF LIGHT

Scientists have developed useful theories to explain some of the things light does. None explains all of the things light is capable of, but they are useful in describing and understanding this interesting form of energy. (See Appendix C, "The Nature of Light,"

for more detail about these theories and the various properties of light.)

The particle theory

From early times up to the time of Isaac Newton, people thought of light as being composed of tiny particles, too small to distinguish individually, that were emitted by the sun and other sources of illumination. However, light seemed to lack weight and many of the other characteristics of matter. For this and other reasons, the particle theory is not a satisfactory explanation of light.

The wave theory

The wave theory described light as a form of energy, rather than matter. Rather than being matter, light was thought to be vibrations transmitted on a special kind of medium, called the ether, much as ocean waves are carried by water. One problem with this analogy is that ocean waves are also composed of water; the wave theory did not really explain *what* got transmitted, except to say that it was a form of energy. Furthermore, physicists discovered about the turn of the century that light has many characteristics that are not explained by the wave theory. Indeed, the central problem with explaining light is that it behaves like particles in some ways (it is affected by gravity, for example) and like waves in other ways (it has frequency and wavelength).

The quantum theory

The quantum theory is an attempt to resolve the contradictions between the particle and wave theories. It does not explain light completely, but it does a much better job than any previous theory.

The quantum theory describes light as packets or bundles of energy called *photons.* The quantum theory explains why light forms images. The quantum theory also explains various photo-chemical reactions, including image formation on photographic film. This theory, whose mathematical explanations are beyond the scope of this text, combines elements of the earlier theories: light is not simply a lot of particles and not simply waves, but can be thought of as packets of energy that travel in wave form.

Light is placed in the same category as cosmic rays, radio waves, microwaves, and X rays. All these are *radiant energy*, or *electromagnetic radiation*. Radiant energy wavelengths can be measured and grouped together to form the *electromagnetic spectrum*. (See Figure 4-1.) The wavelength is the distance from the peak of one wave to the peak of the next. Wavelengths of this spectrum range from a trillionth of a centimeter (cosmic rays) to several hundred miles (electrical oscillations). Visible light falls approximately in the center of this spectrum, with each color having a particular wavelength. (See Figure 4-2.)

LIGHT-SENSITIVE MATERIALS

The transformation of light energy into chemical energy is called a *photochemical reaction*. Everyday examples of it include plant photosynthesis, formation of Vitamin D by the body, and the process of sunburn. But to photographers the most interesting photochemical reaction is the one between light and film.

Early photographers made individual photographs on large, cumbersome pieces of glass. The process was complicated, and a photographer who wanted to shoot twenty pictures at the waterfront had to lug around a weighty burden. Today's lightweight strips of film allow a photographer to capture many images on a single roll and to carry many rolls in a small carrying case.

Early photographers tried many light-sensitive compounds and found that some were particularly effective for photography. Current processes, the result of a great deal of experimentation, depend on several silver compounds, known as the *silver halides*. These compounds, the result of combining metallic silver with elements known as the *halogens*, are light-sensitive. The halogens are bromine, chlorine, and iodine; the silver halides are silver bromide, silver chloride, and silver iodide.

Photographic films and papers are coated with a gelatin substance containing microscopic silver halide crystals. This light-sensitive mixture is called the *film emulsion*. The silver halide crystals, commonly referred to as *grains*, record the image formed during exposure to light.

FILM MANUFACTURE

Coating plastic or some other material with an emulsion sounds like a simple process, but modern film manufacture is actually quite complicated. A two-phase process is required to manufacture quality film.

Making the emulsion

Great progress has been made in the production of photographic emulsions.

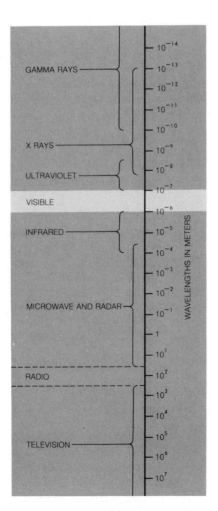

FIGURE 4-1 THE ELECTROMAGNETIC SPECTRUM

FIGURE 4-2 THE VISIBLE SPECTRUM

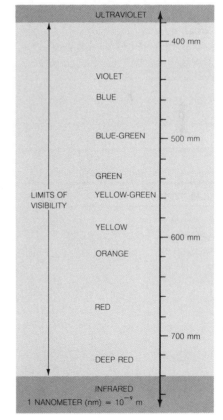

Various manufacturers have developed their own unique methods, and many guard their secrets carefully. The general principles of emulsion manufacture, however, are basic and well established. The following are the basic steps in producing black and white film:

Precipitation The first step, precipitation, brings together the silver and bromine (or other halogen) to produce the light-sensitive silver halide. At this point the gelatin is introduced to keep the material suspended.

Ripening Next, the silver halide and gelatin mixture is subjected to a heat treatment that causes the crystals of silver halide to increase in size. This is called *ripening*. The size of the crystals will determine some of the emulsion's characteristics, including how sensitive the emulsion will be to light.

Washing After the mixture is cooled, so that the gelatin sets into a jelly, it is shredded and thoroughly washed to remove any impurities.

Second ripening (chemical sensitization) The film is reheated and liquefied, then sensitizing dyes, stabilizing agents, hardeners, and wetting agents are added to give the emulsion the proper characteristics of the particular type of film it will be used for.

This step is critical because undyed silver halide is sensitive only to ultraviolet, violet, and blue light. Dyes added to the emulsion in small amounts must stick to the surfaces of the silver halide grains and sensitize them to other wavelengths. A red dye, for instance, absorbs green light energy and thus sensitizes the halide grain to green; a cyan dye absorbs red and makes the emulsion red-sensitive. If the film's emulsion is not sensitive to red, the film cannot "see" red, so any red object will appear black in the final print.

Three general black and white emulsion classifications have been developed on the basis of wavelength sensitivity. *Orthonon emulsions*, or raw emulsions, are sensitive only to blue and violet wavelengths and are often used on photographic printing paper. For this reason, it is possible to use a

"safelight" when making photographic prints—most black and white printing paper cannot "see" a yellow-amber safelight. *Orthochromatic emulsions* are sensitive to violet, blue, and green. *Panchromatic emulsions* are sensitive to all colors of the visible spectrum and are used for black and white photographic film. Table 4-1 lists some of the characteristics of common black and white panchromatic films.

Emulsion characteristics

Modern film emulsions have four general characteristics that are controlled by the manufacturing process.

Speed Film speed, a rating of the film's sensitivity to light, is directly controlled by the size of the grains in the emulsion as well as by trace amounts of sulfur present in the grains of halide. *Fast* films, which have coarse grain, are extremely sensitive to light; *slow* films, which have fine grain, are less sensitive.

Grain The size of the silver halide grain is determined by how long the emulsion grows during the first ripening phase. A short ripening will pro-

TABLE 4-1 □ BLACK AND WHITE FILM CHARACTERISTICS

FILM TYPE	FILM SPEED (ASA)	COMMENTS
Kodak Panatomic-X	32	Very fine grain, slow speed, high contrast
Ilford Pan F	50	Very fine grain, slow speed, high contrast
Agfapan 100	100	Medium speed, medium fine grain, long tonal range
Ilford FP 4	125	Fine grain, moderate speed, long tonal range. A good general-purpose film.
Kodak Plus-X	125	Fine grain, moderate speed, long tonal range. A good general-purpose film.
Kodak Verichrome Pan	125	Medium speed, fine grain, wide exposure latitude
Agfapan 400	400	Very high speed, medium course grain, wide exposure latitude; especially useful in low light
Kodak Tri-X	400	Very high speed, medium course grain, wide exposure latitude; especially useful in low light
Ilford HP 5	400	Very high speed, medium course grain, wide exposure latitude; especially useful in low light
Ilford XPI 400	400	Innovative black and white film based on color dyes rather than silver, medium grain, wide exposure latitude
Agfapan Vario-XL	Variable: 125–1600	Innovative black and white film based on color dyes rather than silver, medium grain, wide exposure latitude

duce a small, fine grain, and a longer ripening period will produce a larger, coarser grain. Fine-grain films can reproduce very fine detail. Coarse-grain films, on the other hand, produce less detailed images.

Contrast Contrast is a measure of the ratio or difference in brightness values that the film records from one portion of a scene to another. All films have a certain degree of contrast; to a large extent the quality of the contrast in a negative or print depends on the degree of exposure and on the treatment the film receives during development.

Wavelength sensitivity The sensitivity of film to various colors along the visible spectrum is dependent on dyes used during the manufacturing process.

Making the film

The final step in making film is coating the emulsion onto a suitable backing—usually paper, celluloid, plastic, or glass, depending on what the emulsion will be used for. Synthetic polymers are by far the most common type of film base used today.

A layer of liquid emulsion approximately $\frac{1}{1000}$ inch thick is fed onto the film support. The exact thickness depends on the type of film being manufactured. Sometimes another very thin layer of plain gelatin is coated over the emulsion to prevent scratches and bruises. A third layer may be applied to the back of the emulsion-support material to prevent the film from being fogged by unwanted light that is reflected back through the emulsion. This layer is called the *anti-halation backing*. (See Figure 4-3.)

REACTION OF LIGHT AND FILM

When film is in place in the camera, the silver halide crystals are ready to record the image. It is not fully under-

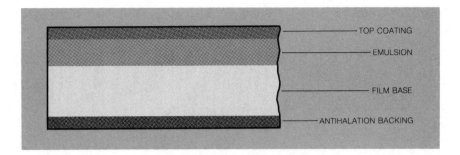

FIGURE 4-3 CROSS SECTION OF BLACK AND WHITE FILM

TOP COATING

EMULSION

FILM BASE

ANTIHALATION BACKING

stood how this image record is made. The most common theory is that when photons of light strike a silver halide crystal, part of the silver halide is changed back into metallic silver. The scale is extremely small. Perhaps only a small percentage of each crystal is changed to metallic silver as a result of this photon bombardment, but this change happens in millions of crystals simultaneously during exposure. Some crystals are affected more than others, depending on the intensity of the light striking them. After exposure, an invisible (*latent*) image exists on the film.

To make the latent image visible and permanent and to remove the unaffected crystals that are still light-sensitive, the film has to be *developed*. Developing solutions attack silver halide grains that have been partly broken down by exposure to light and further reduce them to metallic silver, which is not light-sensitive. Another step in the development process removes the silver halide grains that have not been exposed, thereby producing a permanent metallic silver image.

FILM

Achieving correct exposure is not always simply a matter of making f/stop and shutter adjustments. There are limits. For example, if the light is inadequate and using a slow shutter speed and a wide aperture still does not allow enough light to reach the

film, how can you make a proper exposure? You may be able to use a flash or choose a film with a more sensitive emulsion that better suits the situation. Good film choices can help you meet such a challenge as stopping fast action, recording minute detail, or getting that special shot in low light.

Film speed

Since the speed of a film indicates how sensitive it is to light, the correct exposure combination (f/stop and shutter speed) depends on the film that you are using. A fast film requires less light than a slow film for an exposure of the same subject under the same conditions. If the slower film exposes a subject at a camera setting of f/5.6 at a $\frac{1}{60}$ setting, the faster film may make the same exposure at f/11 and $\frac{1}{60}$ or at f/5.6 and $\frac{1}{250}$.

Rating the speed

Film speeds are determined in a standard, scientific way. In the United States, numerical film speed ratings are given by the American National Standards Institute (ANSI), previously called the American Standards Association (ASA). In Europe, the designation is *Deutsche Industrie Norm* (DIN); i.e., "German Industry Standard." Within a few years of this writing, in an effort to dispense with the sometimes confusing variation, the ratings will be given by an ISO (International Organization for Standards) number;

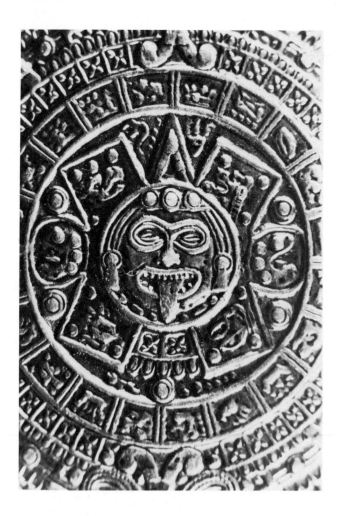 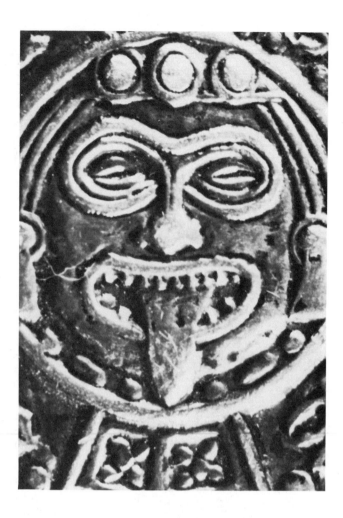

FIGURE 4-4 APPARENT GRAIN
This Aztec stone calendar was photographed with slow-speed, medium-speed, and high-speed films.

FIGURE 4-5 APPARENT GRAIN WITH A SLOW-SPEED FILM
Very moderate grain is noticable in this 100× enlargement, taken from Kodak Panatomic-X film.

many manufacturers are already including this designation on their film. The ISO rating is the same as the ASA rating. Any and all of these ratings may appear on the film package.

Choosing a film

Standard speeds for common black and white films range from ASA 32 to ASA 400; black and white Polaroid film has a speed of 3000 ASA. The best film to use depends on the way the subject is to be represented and the intent of the photographer. Black and white films generally fall into three categories.

Slow films The most obvious characteristic of a slow film is extremely fine grain. (See Figures 4-4 and 4-5.) Two commonly used slow films are

Kodak Panatomic X and Ilford Pan-F.

When an enlargement is made from a negative, everything on the negative is magnified. To make 8 × 10 prints from 35 mm negatives, one must enlarge the image on the negative approximately 100 times. Since the grain of the emulsion is enlarged by the same ratio, slow, fine-grained films are best for enlargements.

Though image quality is slightly better with slow films, shooting flexibility is at a minimum. Slow film is basically an outdoor film for use in daylight conditions; you usually need a flash when shooting indoors. Slow films are not generally the film of choice for action shooting—the fast shutter speeds required to stop action make exposing slow films difficult.

Medium-speed films Medium-speed films, with ASA ratings in the 100 to

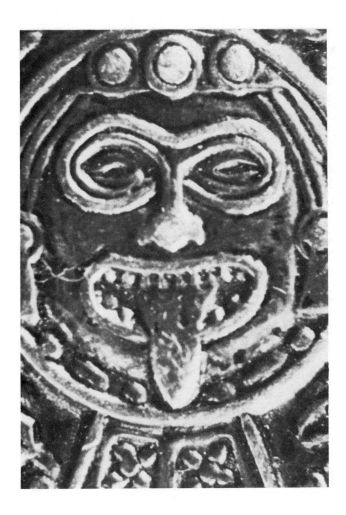

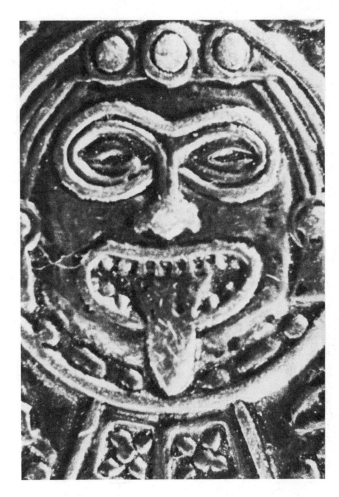

150 range, are general-use films designed to bring together some of the finer features of both slow and fast films. Medium-speed films maintain fine grain but approximately double the speed of a slow film (1 f/stop). These films work well for average shooting under average conditions. (See Figure 4-6.) Two common ones are Kodak Plus-X and Ilford FP-4, both rated at ASA 125.

Fast films Generally rated at ASA 400 or above, the fast films sacrifice grain size for greater film speed and versatility. Two films in this category are Kodak TRI-X and Ilford HP-5. Their popularity is partly due to their ability to work well in low light without a flash. Fast films also allow shutter speeds that can stop action (such as $\frac{1}{500}$ and $\frac{1}{1000}$) without sacrificing too

much depth of field. ASA 400 film is a standard among many professionals and amateurs for 35 mm photography. (See Figure 4-7.)

It is generally easier to decrease the light when the film is too fast than to find light when the film is too slow. If you have too much light and too fast a film, you can use filters to decrease the intensity of the light. But if you are working with a slow film and find there is not enough light, you may simply miss the shot.

Your choice of film speed will depend upon your style, your subject, and the way you want the final print to look.

OTHER PHOTOGRAPHIC MATERIALS

Not all photographic materials operate exactly as those discussed here. Some

FIGURE 4-6 APPARENT GRAIN WITH MEDIUM-SPEED FILM
Moderate grain is noticable in this 100× enlargement, taken from Kodak Plus-X film.

FIGURE 4-7 APPARENT GRAIN WITH HIGH-SPEED FILM
Coarse grain is noticable in this 100× enlargement, taken from Kodak Tri-X film.

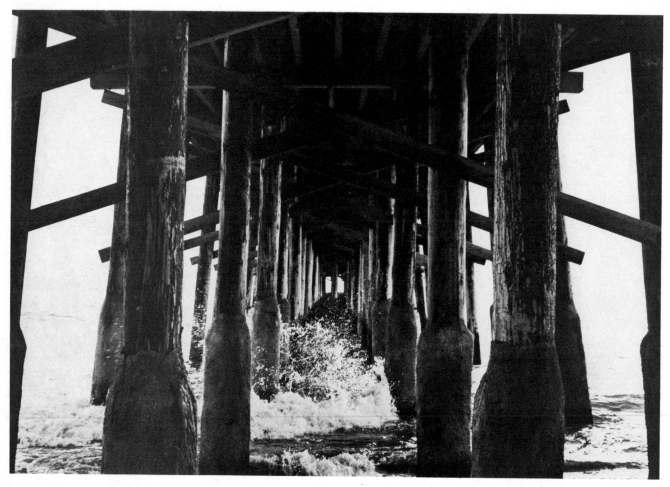

FIGURE 4-8 LATITUDE RANGE OF CHROMAGENIC FILM
(Photo: Laird Roberts)

black and white processes use silver only; some include an intermediate step in which the silver is removed entirely, so the final image is composed of dye compounds. Another process—the instant print or Polaroid process—maintains the traditional silver image, but the processing is done almost instantly after the exposure so that the camera produces a finished print.

Chromogenic black and white film

In chromogenic film, light-sensitive silver halides are used to capture the image, but the final image consists of chemical dyes rather than metallic silver. Chromogenic film has chemical dye couplers mixed with the halide crystals in the emulsion. During devel-

opment these couplers are activated and form a dye image in conjunction with the silver image on the film. The more couplers that are activated in any one area of the film, the more dense the dye image will be. Once the dye image has formed, the entire silver image is bleached from the film, leaving only dye in its place.

A big advantage of the chromogenic process is that, since the final image on the film is a dye image, the speed of the film does not need to relate to the silver grain. So while chromogenic film is fast (rated from ASA 400 to ASA 1600), the dye image it is capable of producing has a very fine grain. (See Figure 4-8.)

Instant print films

With improvements in technology, processing instant print materials has become faster and faster, enabling one to view a finished print in a matter of seconds. Instant print materials function on the same principles as other photographic processing, and the workings are really quite simple. After a film pack is loaded into the camera, a black masking paper is removed to allow the first light-sensitive sheet to face the lens. Following exposure, a tab is pulled that moves the exposed negative material into contact with a sheet of printing paper. Another tab pulls both sheets from the camera through a pair of rollers that burst a pod of developer and spread it between the sheets. Development takes place outside the camera. When development has been completed, the negative and positive materials are separated and the negative is thrown away. This kind of printmaking is called *contact printing* because the exposed negative is placed in contact with another light-sensitive sheet to form the positive print. It always produces an image the size of the image on the negative.

SUMMARY

Understanding light and how it affects film is fundamental to mastering the photographic medium. Therefore a proper film choice will make the difference between simply recording the subject and producing a dramatic interpretation of the subject.

Careful consideration of subject matter is important. For photographing scenic subjects in bright daylight, slow films will capture those important minute details and produce fine, even grain. For sporting events and other situations where fast action must be stopped and for low light where a flash cannot be used, high-speed film is a necessity.

Whatever film is used, the subject is always *light*.

REVIEW QUESTIONS

1 Match the following:

Particle theory

Wave theory

Quantum theory

A. Light is emitted in packets

B. Light is vibrations on the ether

C. Light is very small pieces of matter

2 Light belongs to what group of physical phenomena?

3 What part of the electromagnetic spectrum are we concerned with in photography?

4 What is the transformation of light energy into chemical energy called?

5 What group of chemical compounds has all four qualities necessary to be beneficial in photography?

6 What are light-sensitive silver halide suspensions called?

7 Why is gelatin so important to the photographic process?

8 What are the three general classifications of emulsions, based on their wavelength sensitivities?

9 How many steps are involved in making a photographic emulsion?

10 According to the quantum theory, the latent image is formed when grains in the film are struck by what?

11 What is the basis for all photographic processes?

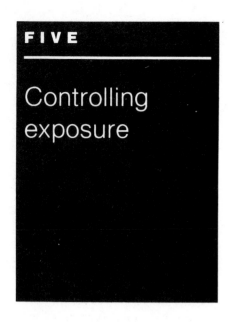

FIVE

Controlling exposure

One of the major challenges of photography is to control the light images that strike the film, transforming the vast array of tones and intensities into shades of gray that are pleasing to the eye. Achieving control of light images requires patience and a great deal of practice.

The latent image that is formed when photons of light strike some of the silver halide crystals in an emulsion depends on the amount of light that reaches the film and the length of time the light is allowed to shine on the film. This effect of light on the film is called *exposure*.

The latent image formed by this process is capable of becoming visible when the material goes through the process of normal development. Several combinations of light and time will give you an exposure, but *getting* the correct exposure is complicated in that only a particular amount of light yields an image of the desired density.

EXPOSURE CONTROLS

Two parts of the camera provide the basic tools used to control the time and the intensity of light. The shutter controls the length of the exposure, and the aperture controls the amount of light that reaches the film.

Shutter

The shutter-speed dial on most modern cameras is marked with a series of numbers. A common sequence is B, 1, 2, 4, 8, 15, 30, 60, 125, 250, 500, 1000. These numbers are the *reciprocals* of the length of time, in seconds, that the shutter is open, exposing the film to light. That is, the number 1 indicates a one-second exposure, and the rest of the numbers represent fractions of seconds: 4 represents $\frac{1}{4}$ second, 8 is $\frac{1}{8}$ second, 500 is $\frac{1}{500}$ second, and so on. Each time is approximately twice as long as the one after it and half as long as the one preceding it. If the

shutter speed is set at 250 ($\frac{1}{250}$ second), then the shutter remains open only half the time it would if it were set at 125 ($\frac{1}{125}$ second) or twice as long as if it were set at 500 ($\frac{1}{150}$ second). Many camera dials are also marked with a B (bulb) or a T (time) setting, which allows the shutter to remain open for as long as the shutter-release button is depressed. (See Figure 5-1.)

The selection of shutter speed greatly affects the way an image is recorded by the film—and it is critical in photographing moving objects. A moving subject travels a certain distance in a given amount of time; a blur results if the shutter speed is not set high enough. Even motionless objects will blur at a slow shutter speed if the camera is not immobilized to prevent vibration or shaking. Generally, a tripod should be used to stabilize the camera for any exposure at a shutter speed longer than $\frac{1}{60}$ second.

Aperture

The other half of the camera's exposure-control system is the aperture. Located in the camera lens, the aperture controls the amount of light that reaches the film. The aperture is a round hole formed by the camera diaphragm and can be adjusted to allow more or less light to pass through the lens. Various aperture settings—referred to a as *f/numbers, f/stops,* or simply *stops*—are marked on the camera lens. A typical f/stop sequence on a normal lens for a 35 mm camera is 1.4, 2, 2.8, 4, 5.6, 8, 11, and 16.

The origin of f/numbers is more complex than the simple fractions used to describe shutter speeds. The f/numbers are determined by dividing the focal length of a lens by the diameter of the aperture. Because this equation involves complex measurements, all lens manufacturers carry out the calculations and then mark the f/numbers on the lens barrel.

Aperture openings are arranged so that each opening is double or half the

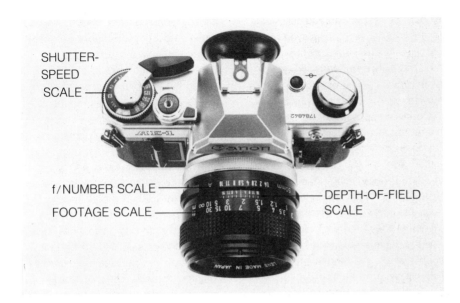

SHUTTER-
SPEED
SCALE

f/NUMBER SCALE

FOOTAGE SCALE

DEPTH-OF-FIELD
SCALE

size of the next aperture. As f/numbers become larger, aperture openings become smaller, and as f/numbers become smaller, aperture openings become larger. To illustrate, let us use the typical sequence of f/numbers listed above. An f/stop of 1.4 indicates the largest aperture opening; a maximum amount of light will reach the film when this step is used. The largest number, f/16, is the smallest aperture opening. (See Figure 5-2.)

FIGURE 5-1 SHUTTER-SPEED, F/STOP, FOOTAGE, AND DEPTH-OF-FIELD SCALES

FIGURE 5-2A–F APERTURE SEQUENCE
This shows the relationship among six of the most common apertures. Each opening has twice the area of the one before it.

EXPOSURE METERS

An essential piece of equipment for any photographer is an exposure or light meter, an instrument that uses light-sensitive cells to measure the

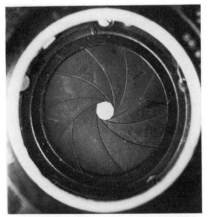

Figure 5-2A f/16

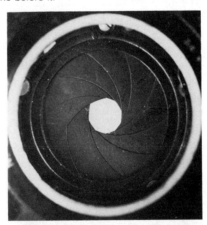

Figure 5-2C f/8

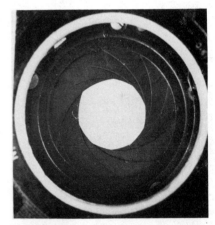

Figure 5-2E f/4

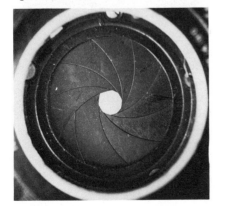

Figure 5-2B f/11

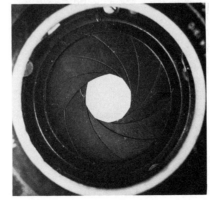

Figure 5-2D f/5.6

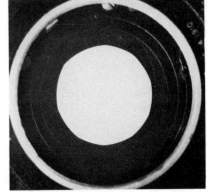

Figure 5-2F f/2.8

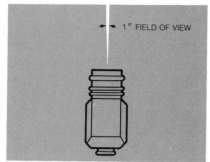

REFLECTIVE SPOT METER

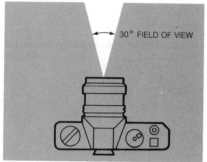

ONBOARD REFLECTIVE LIGHT METER

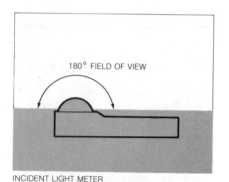

INCIDENT LIGHT METER

FIGURE 5-3 INCIDENT AND REFLECTIVE LIGHT METERS

amount of light or light intensity. This light measurement is displayed as a numerical value by the meter. The meter also incorporates a tiny computer which can be programmed with the film speed, enabling you to find the correct exposure for a particular film at the measured light intensity. (*Note*: Be sure that the exposure meter is set for the correct ASA for the film. Programming an incorrect ASA into the exposure meter will produce faulty exposure readings.)

Whether they are hand-held or built into the camera, exposure meters enable you to read the scene as the film will record it rather than as your eye sees it. Some new automatic cameras set shutter speed, aperture, or both from the reading made by a built-in meter. Depending on how they measure the light, exposure meters are divided into two types.

Incident meters Held at the subject position and aimed at the light source, an incident meter reads light that is falling on the scene. (See Figure 5-3.) An incident meter reads a wide field (180 degrees) and is often used for studio work with artificial light.

Reflective meters All built-in meters and many of today's hand-held meters are reflective. They measure the light that is reflected from the subject. Reflective meters are used from the camera position and are aimed at the subject. Most reflective meters measure an area of about 30 degrees, but some spot meters—a type of reflective meter—measure an area of only 1 degree.

RECIPROCITY LAW

One of the reasons silver halides work so well for photographic purposes is that when a certain emulsion is exposed to the same intensity of light,

the reaction is always the same. Equal amounts of light will always produce equal amounts of exposure.

Exposure is the amount of light shining on the film multiplied by the time the light is allowed to act. Mathematically, the reaction can be stated as $E = I \times T$, where E is exposure, I is the intensity, or amount of light, and T is time. This equation is called the *reciprocity law* or the *Bunsen-Roscoe law* (named for the two men who discovered it).

The reciprocity law states that as long as the product of time and the amount of light remains the same, the reaction of the film emulsion will not change. To visualize this, think of the way many combinations of two numbers multiplied together equal the number 24:

$$1 \times 24 = 24$$
$$2 \times 12 = 24$$
$$3 \times 8 = 24$$
$$4 \times 6 = 24$$

The four combinations above use different numbers, but the result is the same. In the same way, different combinations of time and amount of light result in the same exposure. In other words, if time is doubled and the amount of light is cut in half, the exposure will remain unchanged. Because of the reciprocity law, you can use a wide range of time and light combinations to produce the correct exposure.

The reciprocity law does not perform perfectly in all cases. If light intensity is very low, such as that during the late evening or in low light indoors, increasing the time to exactly correspond to $E = I \times T$ may not provide enough light for adequate exposure—a condition called *reciprocity failure*. Reciprocity failure also occurs when intensity is extremely high and time is very short. See Figure 5-4 and Table 5-1 for a guide for increasing exposure time to compensate for reciprocity failure with a particular film. Note that the guide is a sample for only one film and is not accurate for all films.

ADJUSTING EXPOSURE— EQUIVALENT EXPOSURES

The reason for using an exposure control is simple. With a light meter you can determine the correct exposure by measuring the light in a scene, programming the film speed into the light meter, and using the information it provides to select shutter speed and aperture. Once you have established what the correct exposure is, you can use the reciprocity law to decide which combinations of f/number and shutter speed will yield the correct exposure.

The step arrangements make it easy to use other combinations of shutter speeds and f/numbers to yield the same exposure as the combination recommended for correct exposure. These other combinations are called *equivalent exposures*. For example, if the shutter speed is decreased by half, the aperture must be doubled, so that the film will receive the same amount of exposure called for by the original setting.

The following analogy illustrates the reciprocity law. Four lanes of cars are waiting at a busy intersection for the light to change. The light turns green and stays green for thirty seconds, allowing a certain number of cars to pass through the intersection. If the intersection is reduced to two lanes (half) but the light stays green for sixty seconds (double the time), then the same number of cars can pass through the intersection.

Depth of field and equivalent exposures

Suppose the correct exposure for a scene can be made at f/8 for $\frac{1}{60}$ second. According to the reciprocity law, the film would react the same way if the exposure were f/5.6 at $\frac{1}{125}$, or f/4 at $\frac{1}{250}$, or f/2.8 at $\frac{1}{500}$. (See Figure 5-5.) But which one is really correct? If the subject and lighting conditions remain

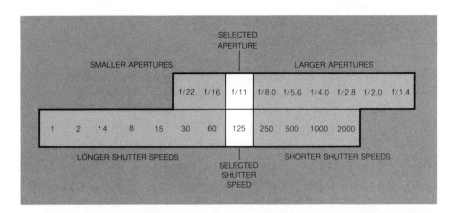

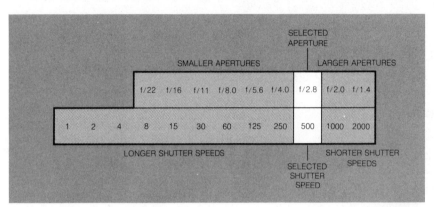

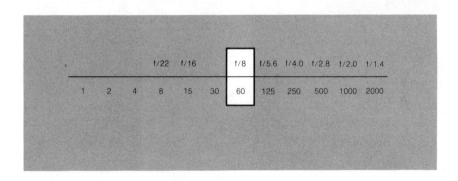

FIGURE 5-4 EQUIVALENT EXPOSURES

FIGURE 5-5 EQUIVALENT EXPOSURES FOR F/8.0 AT $\frac{1}{60}$ SECOND
All pairs are equivalent to f/8.0 at $\frac{1}{60}$ second.

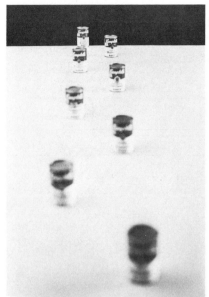

f/2   DISTANCE

1.75   2   2.5   3   3.5   4   5
16   11   8   4   2 2   4   8   11   16

DEPTH OF FIELD

Figure 5-6A Shot at f/2.0 and Focused at 3 Feet

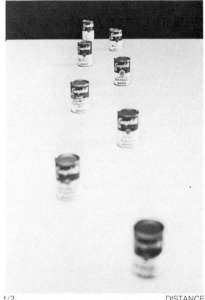

f/2   DISTANCE

3   3.5   4   5   6   7   8
16   11   8   4   2 2   4   8   11   16

DEPTH OF FIELD

Figure 5-6B Shot at f/2.0 and Focused at 5 Feet

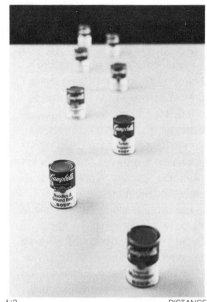

f/2   DISTANCE

4   5   6   7   8   9   10   15
16   11   8   4   2 2   4   8   11   16

DEPTH OF FIELD

Figure 5-6C Shot at f/2.0 and Focused at 8 Feet

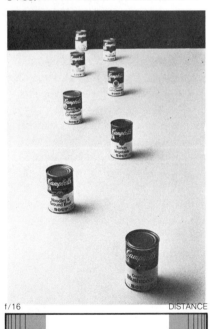

f/16   DISTANCE

1.75   2   2.5   3   3.5   4   5
16   11   8   4   2 2   4   8   11   16

DEPTH OF FIELD

Figure 5-6D Shot at f/16 and Focused at 3 Feet

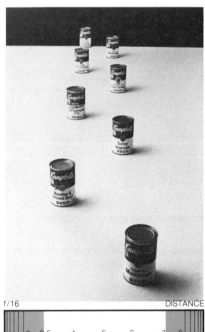

f/16   DISTANCE

3   3.5   4   5   6   7   8
16   11   8   4   2 2   4   8   11   16

DEPTH OF FIELD

Figure 5-6E Shot at f/16 and Focused at 5 Feet

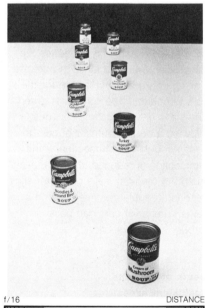

f/16   DISTANCE

4   5   6   7   8   9   10   15
16   11   8   4   2 2   4   8   11   16

DEPTH OF FIELD

Figure 5-6F Shot at f/16 and Focused at 8 Feet

FIGURE 5-6A–F DEPTH OF FIELD AND DEPTH-OF-FIELD SCALE

the same, all of the exposure combinations will produce the same reaction on the film emulsion—but the images recorded on the film will appear quite different. (See Figure 5-6A–F.)

The difference between photographs taken with different exposure combinations is a matter of *depth of field*—the distance in front of and beyond the point where the lens is focused that appears to be in focus in the picture. A wide aperture will create a shallow or narrow depth of field; a stopped-down aperture will produce an extended depth of field. The depth of field is generally divided in a $\frac{1}{3}$-to-$\frac{2}{3}$ ratio. One third of the area in focus will be in front of the point where the camera is focused, and two thirds will be behind that point of focus. The depth of field necessary for a particular shot is a critical factor that should be considered when one is selecting equivalent exposures. (See Figure 1-12.)

Motion and equivalent exposure

Freezing rapid action sometimes requires a shutter speed of $\frac{1}{500}$ or more, limiting your choices of equivalent exposures. Two different exposure combinations produce dramatically different photographs.

EXPOSING THE FILM

Light intensity and time can be varied in correct proportion to produce constant exposure, but how can you determine which combination is really right for a certain scene? You need to learn to "see" the scene before you can determine which one to use. Visualize what you want the photograph to look like, then select the exposure combination that best suits your purpose. (Chapter Twelve, where the sub-

ject of tone control is explored in depth, will further develop the topics discussed in the following sections.)

Preview the scene

Some photographers produce picture after picture of outstanding quality, while others work on the principle that, if they shoot enough pictures, the odds will allow for at least a few excellent shots. What makes the difference between the two? The photographer with the ability to "see" the picture before photographing it produces the photos of consistent quality.

An essential part of correct exposure is photographic awareness. To develop that awareness, preview each scene carefully before you start taking pictures. Notice the direction of the shadows and where the highlights are. Look carefully at the lighting condition of the main subject. Will the main subject be the center of interest, or is something else more attractive to the eye? Try to visualize the scene in black and white and various tones of gray rather than in color.

With practice, you will learn to preview a scene effectively in a brief period of time—thus mastering the first step toward the desired exposure.

Meter the scene

Exposure meters, designed to measure the available light, recommend an exposure based on the sensitivity or speed of the film being used. An "average" exposure for black and white film may be interpreted as the amount of light needed to produce a medium gray tone in the print, called *18 percent gray* because it reflects 18 percent of the light that strikes it. Many cameras feature built-in exposure meters. If yours has one, you can use the camera itself as an exposure meter. If you are shooting still life, it is more convenient to have a separate, hand-held meter, because there are a number of readings you may want to consider. (See Table 5-2.)

Average tone (gray card) readings

The average tone in a scene is most often actually a color rather than a gray, of course, but it is an object in

TABLE 5-1 □ EXAMPLES OF EXPOSURE ADJUSTMENTS TO COMPENSATE FOR RECIPROCITY EFFECTS

EXPOSURE TIME IN SECONDS	EXPOSURE ADJUSTMENT
$\frac{1}{1000}$	None
$\frac{1}{100}$	None
$\frac{1}{10}$	None
1	1 Additional Stop
10	2 Additional Stops
100	3 Additional Stops

FIGURE 5-7 18 PERCENT GRAY

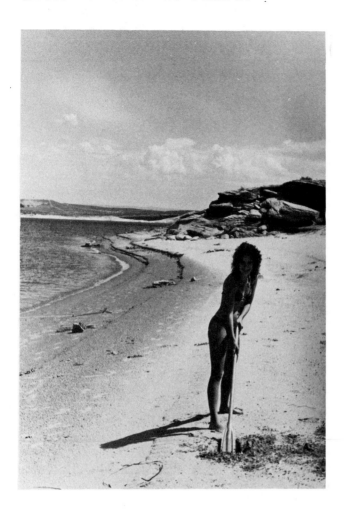

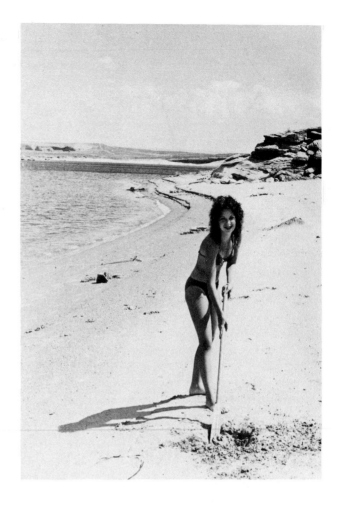

FIGURE 5-8A&B BRACKETING EXPOSURE
Figure 5-8A Underexposed Although Camera Meter Readings Were Used
Figure 5-8B Correction for Underexposure by Bracketing One Stop Either Side of Camera Meter Reading

the scene that reflects about 18 percent of the light that falls on it. Almost all photographic subjects have a tonal range that runs from light to dark, and the 18 percent gray is the middle of that range. Determine where this average tone is in your subject, and take your reading from it. If you cannot find the tone, you can meter a Kodak Gray Card, which reflects 18 percent of the light that falls on it. (See Figure 5-8.) Light meters automatically read for 18 percent gray and base exposure on that reading.

Reflectance readings To determine how much light is being reflected from your subject, you must read the subject, not the background. If you read the background instead of the subject, your subject will not be properly

exposed. If the background is lighter than the subject, the subject will be underexposed; if the background is darker, the subject will be overexposed. It is especially important that you avoid reading the sky when you are shooting outdoors. Point the meter either at the ground or close to your subject. (Often grass is the 18 percent gray in outdoor shots.) If you have trouble determining the 18 percent gray area, take readings from a dark and a light area and then average them. Make sure you choose dark shadow and bright highlight where you want detail to appear.

Incident light readings An incident light meter reads light falling on the subject rather than light reflected from it. Incident meters automatically determine the 18 percent gray, so you do not have to search for it. You simply read the light falling on the subject and shoot. Point the meter directly at the light source. There is just one important thing to remember—make sure that the light striking your subject is of the same intensity as the light striking your meter.

Bracketing the exposure If you have problems determining what your exposure should be, you can bracket the exposure when time permits. Of course, you will not be able to bracket action shots, but you have time with a still-life subject—it is not going anywhere. Take a series of photographs one stop apart; shoot one or even two underexposures, one normal exposure, and one or two overexposures. The exposures should be one stop apart, so they should progressively double. Examine the results. You may find that what you thought was a normal exposure really is an underexposure or an overexposure. On future occasions you can then adjust your exposure before you begin your photography. It is photo insurance to bracket exposures whenever possible. (See Figure 5-8.)

Select the proper exposure

The end result of all your practicing is a properly exposed piece of film. As you prepare to take each shot, you need to consider three important factors: whether you need to stop action, how much depth of field is necessary, and how much light you have. After previewing and metering, select the combination of shutter speed and f/number, and you are ready to begin photographing. Before you trip the shutter, though, take time for one last important step—visualize the composition of the scene, checking for framing, mergers, and rule of thirds. (See Table 5-3.)

TABLE 5-2 □ CONDITIONS WHERE IT PAYS TO DOUBLE-CHECK YOUR METER READING

SITUATION	PROBLEM	SOLUTION
Snow, Sand, Water	The meter will underexpose bright subjects and reduce them to average brightness.	For any brightly lighted or predominately light-colored subject, increase the exposure by one or two settings.
Fog, Rain, Other Precipitation	Moisture in the air causes a blue shift; since meters are more sensitive to blue light, the shot may be underexposed.	Increase the exposure by one setting. Bracketing will also provide insurance in bad weather.
High Subject–Background Contrast	The subject may be over- or underexposed relative to the background.	To prevent overexposing the subject, reduce exposure by one setting; to prevent underexposing, increase by one setting.
Backlighting, Sidelighting	Shadows may be darker than desired.	Use a light-colored reflector to lighten shadows.
Dim Lighting	The meter is less accurate at the low end of its scale than in the middle ranges.	Point the meter at something white or light-colored, then reduce the exposure by two or three settings.
Dark Skin	In ordinary settings, dark skin will be underexposed, except in extreme close-ups, in which the meter reads the brightness of the skin itself.	Increase exposure by one setting or meter a face close up, then shoot with that setting at the desired distance.
Dark-on-Dark	Dark subjects against a dark background can cause loss of detail.	As with night scenes, meter the scene and reduce exposure by one—perhaps two—settings.
Night	The meter will tend to overexpose the scene.	Take a close meter reading of dark areas to get detail; to lose detail in dark areas, meter the scene, then reduce the exposure by one or two settings.

TABLE 5-3 □ BASIC EXPOSURE SETTINGS FOR EXISTING LIGHT

SUBJECT/LIGHTING	EXPOSURES ASA 64–100		ASA 125–200		ASA 250–400	
Christmas Lights	$\frac{1}{4}$	f/2	$\frac{1}{4}$	f/2.8	$\frac{1}{4}$	f/4
Candlelight	$\frac{1}{4}$	f/2	$\frac{1}{8}$	f/2	$\frac{1}{8}$	f/2.8
Dim Church Lighting	$\frac{1}{8}$	f/2	$\frac{1}{8}$	f/2.8	$\frac{1}{8}$	f/4
Average Tungsten Light	$\frac{1}{8}$	f/2	$\frac{1}{8}$	f/2.8	$\frac{1}{15}$	f/2.8
Medium Firelight	$\frac{1}{8}$	f/2	$\frac{1}{8}$	f/2.8	$\frac{1}{15}$	f/2.8
Bright Tungsten Light	$\frac{1}{8}$	f/2.8	$\frac{1}{15}$	f/2.8	$\frac{1}{30}$	f/2.8
Medium-lighted Stage Shows	$\frac{1}{30}$	f/2	$\frac{1}{30}$	f/2.8	$\frac{1}{30}$	f/4
Circuses	$\frac{1}{30}$	f/2	$\frac{1}{30}$	f/2.8	$\frac{1}{60}$	f/2.8
Indoor Sporting Events	$\frac{1}{30}$	f/2	$\frac{1}{60}$	f/2	$\frac{1}{60}$	f/2.8
Brightly Lighted Stage Shows	$\frac{1}{30}$	f/4	$\frac{1}{60}$	f/4	$\frac{1}{60}$	f/5.6
Bright Fluorescent Light	$\frac{1}{60}$	f/2	$\frac{1}{60}$	f/2.8	$\frac{1}{60}$	f/4
Outdoor Night Sporting Events	$\frac{1}{60}$	f/2	$\frac{1}{60}$	f/2.8	$\frac{1}{125}$	f/2.8
Ice Shows; Hockey Matches	$\frac{1}{60}$	f/2	$\frac{1}{60}$	f/2.8	$\frac{1}{125}$	f/2.8
Bright Firelight	$\frac{1}{60}$	f/2	$\frac{1}{60}$	f/2.8	$\frac{1}{125}$	f/2.8
Spotlight	$\frac{1}{60}$	f/2.8	$\frac{1}{60}$	f/4	$\frac{1}{125}$	f/4

SUMMARY

Determining exposure can be simplified by the use of light meters and then by bracketing for insurance. Once the correct exposure has been determined, the photographer can experiment with a number of shutter speed and aperture combinations to produce the desired result.

Finding the most accurate exposure often takes some extra time. But finding the right exposure is well worth the time and effort invested in it. The reward will be crisp, eye-catching pictures that faithfully represent the tonal relationships of the original scene. With practice and patience, anyone can become the kind of photographer who turns out perfect pictures every time—not the kind who just shoots and hopes the law of averages will work in his or her favor.

REVIEW QUESTIONS

1 What is the effect of light on film called?

2 What is the reciprocity law?

3 What does the shutter control determine? What does the aperture control determine?

4 What would be an equivalent exposure for f/8 at $\frac{1}{125}$ of a second?

5 What does *depth of field* mean?

6 What is the first technique to be mastered when one is learning how to ''see'' the scene?

7 What two types of exposure meters are most commonly used in photography?

8 What is 18 percent gray?

9 What is bracketing used for?

10 At any given distance, does f/4 or f/16 produce the greater depth of field?

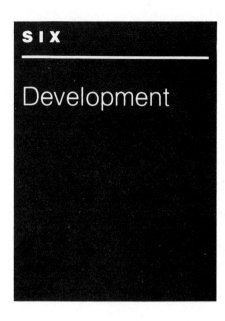

SIX

Development

A latent image is fixed on the film the moment the shutter clicks, but nothing shows on the film at this point. Not until it has been made visible by development and printing can a photograph be enjoyed.

The beauty of any print depends on how carefully the steps of developing and printing are carried out. Developing and printing your own pictures will give you almost total control over your photography.

The development of the latent image is a basic four-step process. First, the *developer,* a complex chemical solution, forms the visible image. A *stop bath* is used to halt the action of the developer. Next, *the fixer* makes the newly developed image permanent and insensitive to light. Finally, *water* is used to wash the emulsion free of processing chemicals. Careful monitoring of the developer and development yields crisp detail; careful handling of the negatives helps keep them free of dust, stains, and scratches. With special developing techniques, you can even salvage negatives with exposure problems.

THE DEVELOPMENT PROCESS

The purpose of development

Silver halides are used in photography because they are developable—the effect of light in producing an image can be amplified by a developing solution.

As explained in Chapter Four, the latent image is recorded on the film during exposure. Photons of light strike the film and activate the individual silver halide crystals, converting some of the crystalline silver halide molecules into elemental metallic silver. The developer chemically converts hundreds of thousands of other atoms of silver halide to each of the original atoms, causing a black image to appear slowly on the film. This is the

negative image, and it is exactly the reverse of the original scene—the dark areas in the negative were the bright areas of the original scene.

Film developers

Developing agents belong to a class of chemical compounds known as *reducing agents.* Only a few chemical compounds discriminate between grains that have been exposed to light and those that have not. The action of photographic reducing agents on exposed and unexposed grains is explained by *rate.* Unexposed grains eventually develop, but exposed grains develop much more quickly. With prolonged development, almost all the grains in an emulsion, both exposed and unexposed, will be converted to silver.

The amount of blackness produced as the emulsion is developed is called *density.* Negative density depends on the amount of black metallic silver that is built up in the image. The negative image is formed by varying densities of silver in the negative.

Chemical development When the photographic emulsion is placed in a developing solution, the silver halide grains are chemically attacked by the developer. Each grain that has received more than the minimum exposure is rapidly reduced to metallic silver.

Each manufacturer of developer provides a recommendation of the time necessary to reduce all the activated silver halide grains to metallic silver. In *normal development,* film is developed for the recommended time and all of the light-activated silver halide grains in the emulsion are converted. Assuming the emulsion received a normal exposure, normal development will produce a wide range of densities in the negative. Gross *overdevelopment* will cause all grains, both activated and inactivated, to be reduced to metallic silver, producing a high-density negative. *Underdevelopment* has the opposite effect—neither all the activated grains nor a majority of the inactivated grains are reduced to metallic silver, and consequently the negative has very low density.

DEVELOPING SOLUTION

Over the years, many diverse substances have been used as photographic developing agents. Not all of these agents act in the same way. The choice of an agent depends on the type of film and the exposure. Table 6-1 lists some of the qualities of each developer and the types of film recommended for use with each.

Developing agents do not work alone. A developer utilizes other chemicals that complement the actual developing agent itself to ensure that the developing solution always functions in the same way.

Developing agents

The primary task of any developing agent is to reduce the silver halide grains in the emulsion to grains of metallic silver. Three of the agents most commonly used in black and white photography are *metol, hydroquinine,* and *phenidone.*

Metol Introduced in 1891, metol is a white, crystalline powder that is easily soluble in water. Metol developers are appropriate for fast films. Because they tend to minimize grain, they are valuable when maximum shadow detail is required. Although metol can be

TABLE 6-1 □ SOME COMMON FILM DEVELOPERS

MANUFACTURER	PRODUCT	GRAIN PRODUCED	FILM SPEED TO USE WITH	COMMENTS
Agfa	Rodinal	Very fine with slow-speed films	Slow to medium	Contrast can be varied by different dilution
Acufine	Acufine	Medium to ultra-fine	High	Gives best results when used with higher-than-normal film speeds
Acufine	Diafine	Extremely fine	High	Gives best results when used with higher-than-normal film speeds
Edwal	FG-7	Fine	Most types	Compensating, general-purpose developer; has several different working dilutions
Edwal	Minicol II	Very fine	Slow to medium	Super-compensating, maximum-sharpness developer
Edwal	Super 20	Ultra-fine	Tri-X	Yields negatives that produce excellent enlargements, especially with high-speed film
Ethol	TEC	Medium to very fine	Slow	Very fine grain with slow-speed films
Ethol	UFG	Extremely fine	Medium to high	Can be used with either roll or sheet film
Ilford	Microphen	Fine	Medium to high	Effectively increases film speed up to $1\frac{1}{2}$ times normal
Ilford	Perceptol	Very fine	Medium	Especially formulated to give optimum results from high-resolution lens
Kodak	D-76	Medium fine	Most types	General-purpose film developer; can be mixed in several different dilutions
Kodak	HC 100	Moderate fine	Medium to high	General-purpose film developer; can be mixed in several different dilutions
Kodak	Microdol-X	Fine	Most types	Produces negatives with higher-than-normal contrast

used by itself with good results, it is generally combined with a second developing agent, usually hydroquinine.

Hydroquinine Noted for their ability to produce high contrast, hydroquinine developers were discovered in the 1880s. They take the form of fine white crystals that are soluble in water. By itself, hydroquinine is generally not suitable for use with a high-speed emulsion, so it is usually mixed with metol or phenidone for this purpose.

Phenidone Discovered at Ilford Photographic Laboratories in 1940, phenidone possesses most of the photographic properties of metol and some properties unique to it. Phenidone can be used alone with high-speed emulsion films, but because it produces low contrast it is generally not used by itself. Mixed with hydroquinine, phenidone produces an extremely wide range of developers.

Normal developers are designed to create an even range of gray tones. In the process, they produce good contrast and moderate grain in all parts of the negative. High-speed developers quickly build up density and graininess but have the advantage of greatly reduced developing time. High-energy developers partially compensate for underexposure by concentrating on the highlights. Fine-grain developers turn out negatives that can be enlarged into big, sharply detailed prints.

PROCESSING CHEMICALS

The developer is the first of five chemical solutions utilized in processing a roll of film. The other four are the *stop bath, fixer, washing aid,* and *drying aid.* Many of these are available on the market; experience will be the best guide as to which products suit a given situation.

Stop bath

Stop bath is two-percent solution of acetic acid that halts the action of the developer.

Fixer

The fixer removes unexposed and undeveloped silver halide grains from the emulsion. A fixing bath always contains a solvent that combines with the silver halide grains to form complexes that can be washed out with water. The solvent must not damage the gelatin base of the emulsion, nor should it attack the newly developed silver image.

Hardening, an important chemical treatment accomplished during the fixing step, has several purposes. First, the gelatin-based emulsion is hardened to prevent swelling and softening during the washing step. Second, once the emulsion is hardened, the film can be dried at higher than room temperature if necessary. Finally, a hardened emulsion is more durable and less likely to be scratched or damaged. Hardening is usually accomplished by adding a hardening agent to the fixing bath to form a *hardening fixer.*

Fixer manufacturers provide detailed fixing instructions that should be followed carefully. As a general rule, an emulsion can be considered to be fixed when it has been in the fix for twice its *clear time*—the time it takes for the fixer to remove all the unexposed silver halides. Since it is often difficult to determine the clear time, manufacturers provide this important time recommendation.

Washing aids

Washing the emulsion well with ordinary running water will remove practically all the fix and unwanted silver compounds. Thorough washing prevents the stains and discoloration that can show up months later. Unfortu-

nately, proper washing can take thirty minutes or longer and use a lot of water. Washing aids reduce the length of washing time required for the water to remove any fix and silver compounds, from thirty minutes to about five.

Drying aids

Wetting agents, or *emulsifiers,* are compounds that reduce the surface tension of water. It may seem paradoxical that wetting agents are drying aids. In fact, wetting agents minimize the chance of water spots on film, helping the film to dry more uniformly.

HOW TO PROCESS A ROLL OF FILM

Five main steps are involved in processing a roll of film:

1 Assemble all the materials needed for processing.

2 Load the film into the developing tank.

3 Add the chemicals needed to produce the negative image.

4 Wash and dry the negatives.

5 Place the negative in a protective envelope for storage.

The secret to good development lies in being careful and consistent. Familiarize yourself with the process so that you carry out each step the same way time after time.

Materials

Most of the items necessary for developing roll film are inexpensive, but make certain you do not over-economize on the *developing tank*—you will need one constructed of good-quality plastic or metal. You will also need a *timer* that shows seconds and an accurate *thermometer.* You can use any kind of *dark bottles* for storing your solutions, so long as the bottles are clean and have tight-fitting lids. Other useful items include *scis-*

FIGURE 6-1 MATERIALS NEEDED TO DEVELOP A ROLL OF FILM
A Timer
B Film-Washing Tank
C Chemical Bottles
D Stirring Rod
E Scissors
F Can Opener
G Film-Developing Tank and Reel
H Roll of Film
I Thermometer
J Funnel
K Beaker
L Film Clips

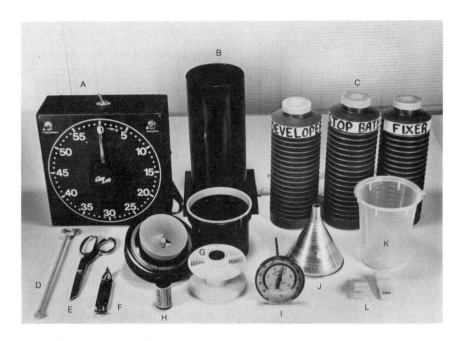

sors, a bottle opener, a stirring rod, a funnel, a beaker, and film clips. The basic equipment necessary to process a roll of film is shown in Figure 6-1.

Arrange your equipment in an orderly fashion. Once you start the developing process, things will move too quickly for you to spend precious seconds hunting around for equipment.

Loading the tank Each of the two types of tanks and reels—stainless steel and plastic—has its advantages and disadvantages. Many photographers find the plastic walk-on reel easier to load than the metal reel, but both produce excellent results. Here we show how to process a roll of 35 mm film using a plastic reel and tank.

All the equipment necessary to load the tank should be placed in a light-tight change bag or should be arranged in a darkroom.

Trimming the film A leader is placed at the beginning of a roll of 35 mm film to make the film easier to load into the camera. You need to trim the leader so the film will fit onto the developing reel more easily. You can

trim the leader in the dark after the cassette is opened, or you can trim it by not winding all of the leader back into the film cassette after the roll is exposed—a method that allows you to trim the leader in room light. (See Figure 6-2.) This is the only step for which you have an option; the remaining steps must be carried out in complete darkness.

Opening the cassette With a can opener in one hand and the film cassette in the other, pry off the end of the cassette. (See Figure 6-3.) Slide the film out and hold it gently in one hand while you secure the reel with the other hand. Hold the film by the edges, making sure that you do not touch the surface of the film.

Loading the reel Align the reel guides and insert the trimmed edge of the film. Once the film has caught, rotate one side of the reel until the roll of film has been "walked on." (See Figure 6-4.) The tail end of the film is taped to the film spool. Cut or tear the tape, and finish winding the film onto the reel. If you tear the tape rather than cut it, you may see a bluish-white

flash of static electricity. Don't worry; this will not expose the film.

Assembling the tank If the tank you are using has a center core, then after the film has been loaded onto the reel, insert the center core and place the retaining clip on the opposite end of the core. Do not forget to use the center core—it forms a light-tight seal when the lid is put on the tank. Put the reel assembly into the tank, and replace the lid tightly. (See Figure 6-5.) You may then turn on the room lights or remove the tank from the change bag, and so complete the rest of the processing steps in room light.

USING THE CHEMISTRY

Developing begins in total darkness, and once started, it moves briskly. Make sure all the needed chemicals are ready even before you arrange the essential equipment.

Dilutions

Photographic chemicals are packaged by the manufacturer as liquids or powders. Most are in concentrated form and must be mixed with water. Once the total amount of concentrate

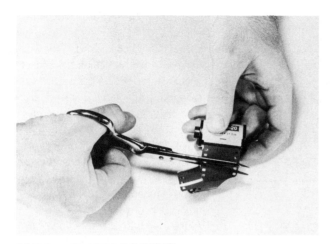

FIGURE 6-2 TRIMMING THE LEADER

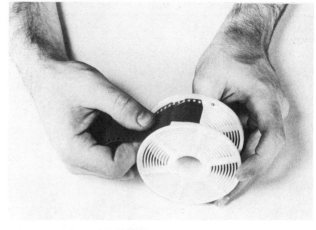

FIGURE 6-4 LOADING THE REEL

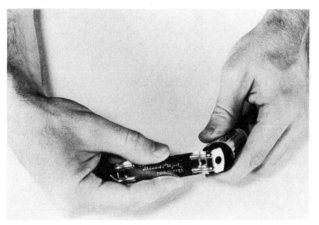

FIGURE 6-3 OPENING THE CASSETTE

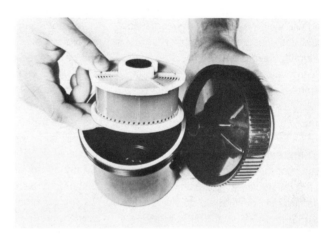

FIGURE 6-5 ASSEMBLING THE TANK

has been mixed with water according to the instructions on the package, the solution is called a *stock solution.* (Even if the chemical is in the form of a water solution, it may require further dilution before you can use it.)

Chemicals are generally stored in a stock solution. A powdered developer should be mixed into a stock solution when you first open the package. For example, you might add a package of powdered developer to a gallon of water to produce a gallon of stock solution. It is much easier to get accurate results if you use stock solutions instead of trying to mix a highly concentrated substance in small quantities.

Once a stock solution has been prepared, it is best to make up a *working*

dilution—the mixture that you will actually use. The relationship between working dilutions and stock solutions is always expressed in a ratio. For example, a working dilution of developer is a 1:1 dilution—one part stock solution and one part water. With some developers, several different working dilutions may be produced from one stock solution. Each of these working dilutions has different characteristics that affect the way the developer works. Stock solutions should be made from developers, stop bath, and fixer. Make sure you mix and dilute all chemicals carefully. Check to make sure the solution is the correct one *before* it goes into the developing tank or tray. Always follow manufacturer's recommendations.

Time, temperature, and agitation

Three variables—time, temperature, and agitation—affect the amount of development that occurs in the emulsion. All chemical processes are sensitive to both time and temperature, so it is critical that you exercise careful control over both the time and the temperature during processing. For good results you need just the right amount of time at just the right temperature.

Time The length of time that the film is left in contact with the developing solution is crucial. Obviously, the development process is not instantaneous. If you remove the film from the

TABLE 6-2 □ TIME–TEMPERATURE DEVELOPMENT CHART

FILM	ASA	65°	68°	70°	72°	75°
Pan-X	32	8 min.	7 min.	6½ min.	6 min.	5 min.
Plus-X	125	8 min.	7 min.	6½ min.	6 min.	5 min.
Tri-X	400	11 min.	10 min.	9½ min.	9 min.	8 min.
Verichrome	125	11 min.	9 min.	8 min.	7 min.	6 min.
FP-4	125		9 min.			
HP-5	400		12 min.			

KODAK D-76, diluted 1:1 (one part stock developer to one part water).

developer too soon, the process may be incomplete; if you leave it in the developer too long, the film may become overdeveloped. Underdeveloping will yield negatives with decreased contrast—less dense or thinner than normally developed negatives. Overdeveloping film tends to increase contrast and produce dense, grainy negatives, even from normally exposed film.

Temperature Heat speeds up chemical processes; cold slows them down. If the chemical developer is too hot, the film may develop so quickly that you cannot remove it from the developer fast enough to avoid overdeveloping. If it is too cold, it may take much longer to develop the film properly. If one solution is hot and the other cold, the sudden change in temperature can damage the film severely—the gelatin will crack just as a heated glass will crack when plunged into icy water. This cracking of the emulsion produces a "craze" pattern, commonly called *reticulation.*

Agitation Agitation is a means of replacing exhausted developer with fresh developer that has not yet been in contact with the emulsion. By guaranteeing that the emulsion is periodically bathed with a fresh supply of developer, agitation ensures that the reaction will continue at a constant rate throughout the development period. The amount of agitation a film receives during development has a marked effect on its density, so agitation must be consistent. Overagitation results in increased grain, especially in high-speed films. Too little agitation yields poor-quality negatives. With careful agitation, all parts of the film will be affected equally by the developer. The size of the film tank you use and the type of film you are processing will determine which type of agitation is best. For roll film processed in a small tank, you might simply invert the tank.

Many of the factors that influence the outcome of a negative are interrelated. As you become familiar with the development process, you will learn to adjust the development procedures to fit certain needs. There is a limit, of course, to how much you can change the rules—the idea is to change them only when and only as much as necessary to make each negative fit your purpose.

Bringing the developer to temperature and setting the time

Before it comes into contact with the film, the developer must first be brought to the proper temperature. The range that most manufacturers recommend for processing black and white film is 65° to 70°F. For example, Kodak D-76, a commonly used developer, has a recommended processing temperature of 68°F (20°C).

Determine temperature by placing a thermometer in a beaker containing the amount of developer in working dilution needed to fill the tank in which the film is being processed. If the developer is too hot, place the beaker in a cold-water bath; if the developer is too cold, place it in a warm-water bath until it reaches the proper temperature. To save time, you can load the developing tank with film while the developer is coming to temperature. (See Figure 6-6.)

A time–temperature chart for D-76 diluted 1:1 is provided in Table 6-2.

To use the chart, find the type of film you are going to develop and the recommended processing temperature of the developer. The time shown at the intersection of the two lines is the one you should use for the developing period. For example, Tri-X film with developer at 68°F should be developed for 11 minutes. Remember: this chart is only applicable for D-76 diluted 1:1. If you use other developers or dilutions, follow recommended times. (See Figure 6-7.)

Set the timer for the amount of time determined from the time-temperature chart. Start the timer as soon as you begin to pour the developer into the tank. Pour the developer as rapidly as you can, and pour enough of it into the tank to completely cover the film. You can pour more quickly if you tip the tank at a 45-degree angle. As soon as the developer is in the tank, tap the tank firmly several times to dislodge any air bubbles that might be clinging to the film. Another method is to place the properly tempered developer in the tank first, then put the film in the tank and tap the tank. (See Figure 6-8.)

Agitating the tank

For small-tank development, agitate for five seconds out of every thirty seconds—in other words, agitate the tank for five seconds, and then put it on the countertop for twenty-five seconds. Repeat this cycle for the

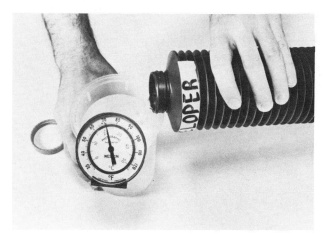

FIGURE 6-6 BRINGING THE DEVELOPER TO TEMPERATURE

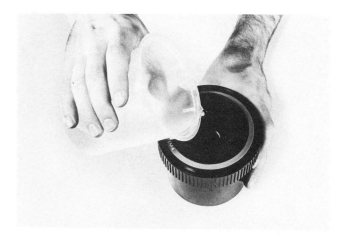

FIGURE 6-8 POURING DEVELOPER INTO TANK

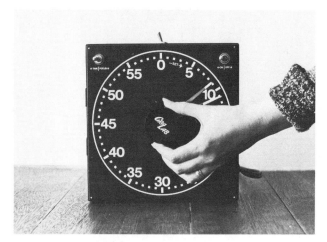

FIGURE 6-7 SETTING THE TIMER

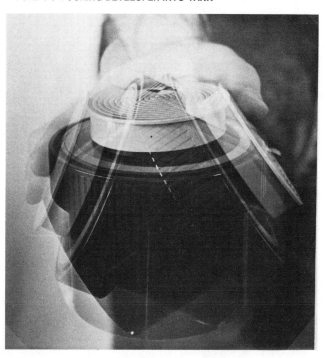

FIGURE 6-9 AGITATING THE DEVELOPING TANK

duration of the development period. Some manufacturers recommend agitation for ten seconds each minute.

Agitation is critical and so should be done with a great deal of care. To ''agitate'' does not mean to shake the tank violently. A tank with a tight-fitting lid can be gently inverted and then placed right side up. A gentle side-to-side circular motion also works well. (See Figure 6-9.) Find a style of agitation that gives good results and make it a part of your developing routine. The main thing is consistency.

Stop bath

As the development period comes to an end, be ready to pour out the

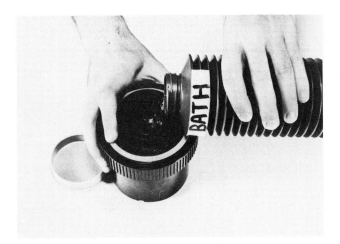

FIGURE 6-10 POURING IN THE STOP BATH

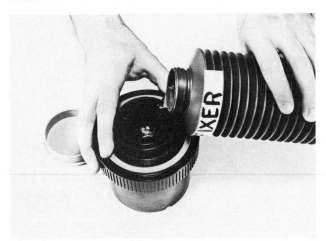

FIGURE 6-11 POURING IN THE FIX

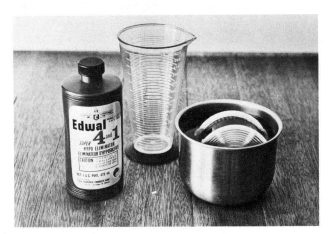

FIGURE 6-12 WASHING AID

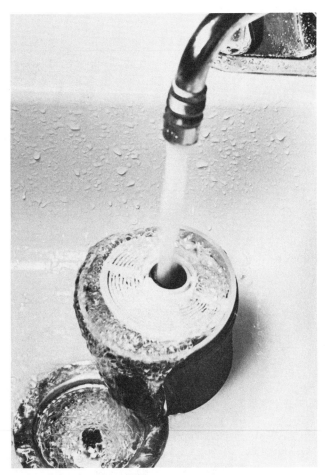

FIGURE 6-13 RUNNING WATER WASH

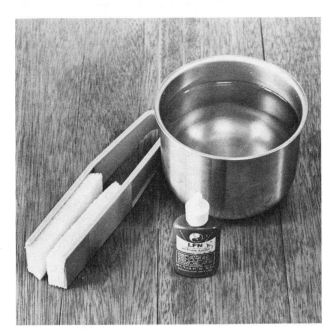

FIGURE 6-14 DRYING AID

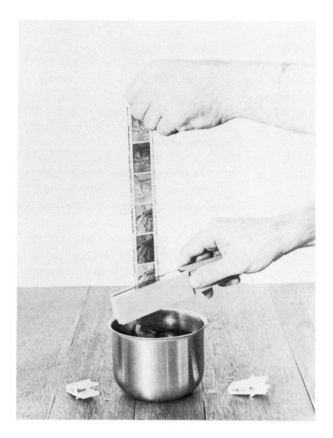

FIGURE 6-15 SQUEEGEEING EXCESS WATER FROM THE FILM

developer as rapidly as possible. Pour in enough stop bath to cover the film. (See Figure 6-10.) Reset the timer for thirty seconds. Swirl the tank a few times and then empty the stop bath at the end of the thirty-second period.

To mix stop bath to working dilution, follow the manufacturer's recommendation or use a 1:20 working dilution of concentrated acetic acid. This will provide a 2 percent solution. Although the temperature of the stop bath is not as critical as that of the developer, it should be between 65° and 72°F.

Fixer

Once you dump out the stop bath, pour the fixer into the developing tank. (See Figure 6-11.) Fix—or "hypo," as it is sometimes called—chemically removes all unexposed and undeveloped silver halide grains, rendering the emulsion insensitive to light. Also,

most commercial fixers contain hardening agents that increase the emulsion's resistance to scratches and abrasions.

The fix should be agitated for five seconds out of every sixty seconds. After the fix period is up (usually from five to ten minutes), pour fix into a bottle marked "used fix." Fix can be used over again many times before it loses potency.

After the fix step, the film is no longer sensitive to light, so take it out of the tank and examine it to make sure it is completely fixed. If the fixer was weak or exhausted, the film emulsion will look milky. Refix the film with freshly mixed fixer for an additional five minutes.

Wash

Fill the tank a couple of times with water and then empty to remove the

fixer so that the washing aid will work more effectively. The temperature of the wash water should be about 65–75°F.

Washing aid The *hypo clear,* or washing aid, is a big time-saver. Hypo clear chemically removes the byproducts of developing, stop bath, and fixing from the emulsion—and it reduces the wash time from thirty to five minutes. The film should stay in the hypo clear for two minutes with occasional agitation. (See Figure 6-12.)

Water wash A running-water wash of at least five minutes' duration (or thirty minutes if no washing aid is used) is an important step because it washes away all traces of the chemicals you have used throughout the development process. You have to use running water to ensure a complete wash. (See Figure 6-13.) If any of the chemicals remain in the emulsion, they will discolor and eventually ruin the negatives.

Drying

Drying aid A drying aid is generally used after the wash has been completed, to prevent water spots from forming and to help the negatives dry uniformly. For best results, mix the chemical with distilled water. (See Figure 6-14.) Put the film in the drying aid solution for about thirty seconds.

Drying Hang up the negatives to dry in a dust-free place. You can use a squeegee to gently remove the excess water from the hanging negatives. (See Figure 6-15.) To keep the negatives from curling while they dry,

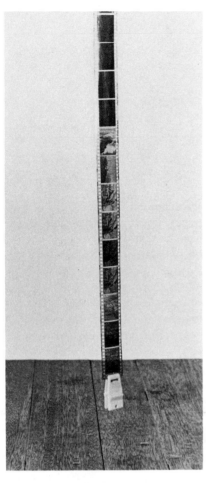

FIGURE 6-16 HANGING THE FILM TO DRY

attach a film clip to the bottom end of the hanging film. (See Figure 6-16.)

Storing the negatives After the negatives are dry, store and catalog them. You will protect them, and you will know exactly what you have. You can store the negatives in plastic sheets, single-paper envelopes, or folded paper envelopes. (See Figure 6-17.) Each method has its advantages and disadvantages.

Table 6-3 summarizes the development process with a list of the major steps and the chemicals vital to each one. A little practice will convince you that the development process is easy to perform. As your experience grows, try to standardize each step so that you can immediately spot what is wrong if you err.

COMMON NEGATIVE PROBLEMS

It is easier to prevent negative problems than to try to correct them later. Some problems can be so bad that it is better to reshoot the pictures than to labor over the damaged negatives. Careful developing is of course crucial for irreplaceable shots, which you will never have the opportunity to recapture on film.

Many things can happen to film. The following are seven of the most common problems.

Too little developer A clear or lighter area along one edge of the negative signals too little developer—the developer in the tank did not completely cover the film. Prevention is easy: make sure you always have enough processing solution in the tank to immerse the film entirely. Most of the time negatives damaged in this way are not salvageable. (See Figure 6-18.)

Fixer exhaustion When the fix has lost its strength, the incompletely fixed negatives will come out looking as if they had been left in a glass of milk. (See Figure 6-19.) To correct the problem, put the unfixed negatives in a bath of fresh fix solution for another five minutes. Most are usable after they have been rewashed and dried.

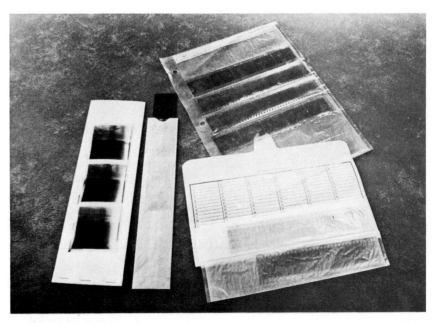

FIGURE 6-17 NEGATIVE STORAGE

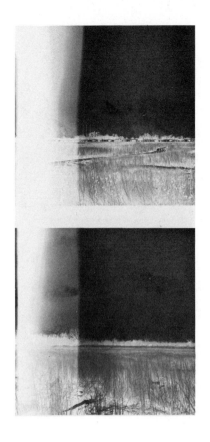

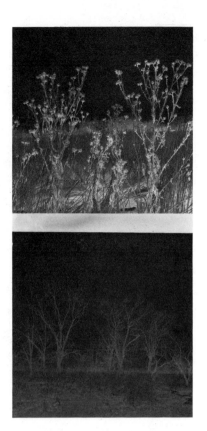

FIGURE 6-18 NEGATIVE PROBLEM: TOO LITTLE DEVELOPER

FIGURE 6-19 NEGATIVE PROBLEM: FIXER EXHAUSTION

TABLE 6-3 □ SUMMARY OF DEVELOPMENT STEPS

STEPS	CARRY OUT IN	TIME	TEMPERATURE		AGITATION	FUNCTION
			°F	°C		
Bring Developer to Temperature	Room light	Varies	68	20	DNA	Developer is ready to use after film is loaded.
Load Film into Tank	Total darkness	DNA	DNA	DNA	DNA	
Determine Development Time	Room light	From table	681	201	DNA	Determine proper development time for film being developed
Pour Developer into Tank	Room light	From table	68	20	Tap tank several times; follow manufacturer's instructions	Develops latent image
Stop Bath	Room light	30 sec.	About 68	About 20	Swirl tank	Stops development
Fix	Room light	4–6 min.	About 68	About 20	5 sec. in each min.	Removes all undeveloped silver halide, making film insensitive to light
Washing Aid	Room light	2 min.	About 68	About 20	DNA	Shortens wash time by chemically removing remains of developer, stop, and fix
Wash	Room light	5–10 min.	About 68	About 20	Water should circulate and be replaced by fresh water	Washes impurities out of emulsion
Drying Aid	Room light	30 sec.	About 68	About 20	DNA	Prevents spots from forming on film during drying
Drying	Room light	30 min.	Room temperature		DNA	Sets the emulsion

FIGURE 6-21A
The film was not exposed in the camera: the film-identification markings and the frame numbers are visible.

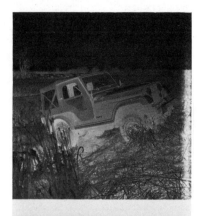

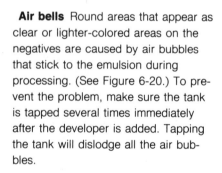

FIGURE 6-20 NEGATIVE PROBLEM: AIR BELLS

FIGURE 6-21B
The developer did not work: there is no image of any kind on the film.

Air bells Round areas that appear as clear or lighter-colored areas on the negatives are caused by air bubbles that stick to the emulsion during processing. (See Figure 6-20.) To prevent the problem, make sure the tank is tapped several times immediately after the developer is added. Tapping the tank will dislodge all the air bubbles.

Clear negatives Two types of error can cause clear frames. First, either the developer was bad or some other chemical was mistakenly used as the developer; or second, the film did not advance through the camera. In order to establish which is the source of the problem, look at the leader and the frame numbers. If the leader is black and the frame numbers are visible, the developer was good but the film was not advanced through the camera. If the entire roll is clear from the leader to the end of the roll, then the developer solution was bad. (See Figure 6-21.) The only cure for this problem is to go back out and reshoot the pictures.

Light leaks Black or dark patches that appear across the roll of negatives are caused by light leaks from a camera back that does not close tightly, a darkroom that is not light-tight, or a lid that was not securely attached to the tank during processing. (See Figure 6-22.) To prevent this problem, make sure that the camera back closes tightly, that the darkroom is light-tight, and that the tank has a tight-fitting lid.

Water spots Light spots with a darker white edge are water spots.

(See Figure 6-23.) You will probably get water spots if you do not use a drying aid or if you forget to squeegee the excess water from the film during drying. Most negatives are usable if you rewash and properly redry the film.

Touch marks An additional hazard to the film is touch marks—marks that occur when the film was loaded onto the reel so badly that the back of one layer pressed against the face of the next. This prevents both the developer and the fixer from working on that part of the film. Unfortunately, there is nothing you can do after the fact. The best prevention technique is to learn how to load the reel correctly and then always be careful when loading. (See Figure 6-24.)

**FIGURE 6-22A&B NEGATIVE PROBLEM:
LIGHT LEAKS**

FIGURE 6-22A
This type of light leak is most common with
roll film; it can be prevented by making
sure that the roll is sealed tightly after it is
removed from the camera.

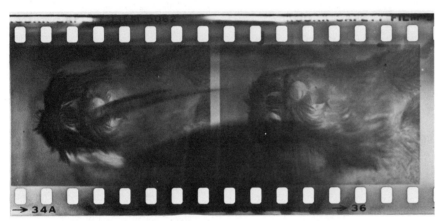

FIGURE 6-22B
Light leaks of this type are caused if the
back of the camera or the developing tank
is not light-tight.

**FIGURE 6-23 NEGATIVE PROBLEM: WATER
SPOTS**

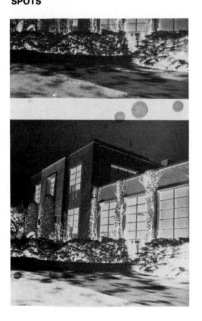

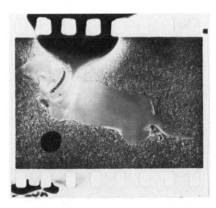

**FIGURE 6-24 NEGATIVE PROBLEM: TOUCH
MARKS FROM IMPROPER FILM LOADING**

SUMMARY

Development, the key to making the latent image visible, is accomplished by a reducing agent that changes activated silver halide grains into grains of metallic silver. The developing solution is complex, and many different effects can be achieved by changing the chemicals in the developing solution.

The secret to producing good negatives is cleanliness and consistency during film processing—a procedure that includes assembling the materials, loading the tank, using the chemistry, washing the film, and drying the film. A good photographer establishes and adheres to a set pattern in order to get the best results in developing film.

Even professionals are sometimes confronted with processing problems. With care and attention to detail, problems can be eliminated before they affect the negatives. If a problem recurs, each development stage should be examined until the mistake is discovered.

Photographers' joy in developing their own pictures comes from the knowledge that they have total control over the end products. Care exercised during development guarantees the most beautiful and dramatic effects, thus richly rewarding photographers for their efforts.

REVIEW QUESTIONS

1 What is the purpose of development?

2 To what class of compounds do film developers belong?

3 What are the two types of developers?

4 What are three common developing agents?

5 How strong a solution of acetic acid should be used as a stop bath?

6 What is the purpose of the fix?

7 Why are washing aids important to film processing?

8 What are the five main steps in processing a roll of film?

9 What are the three variables that affect film processing?

10 What is the most commonly used temperature for developing solutions?

11 List four of the seven most common problems with film or processing.

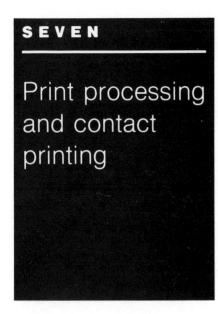

SEVEN

Print processing and contact printing

For many photographers, the printing process is the most rewarding and enjoyable part of the craft—the satisfaction of creating a fine print is the reward for the time and effort expended.

There are two reasons for making a print. One is to transfer the negative image from the film to paper; the second is to change the negative film image into a positive image that represents the original scene more accurately.

The process of printing consists of two phases. *Contact printing* transfers the negative film image onto paper and forms a positive image the same size as the negative. (See Figure 7-1.) Projection or *enlargement printing* projects a negative image much larger than the actual negative. (Enlargement printing will be covered in more detail in Chapter Eight.) The actual processing steps are really the same for both—and once you master the techniques of making a contact print, you can use the same techniques for enlargement printing.

The basic printmaking process is similar to the negative development process. Photographic paper used for printing is special paper that has been coated with a light-sensitive emulsion. A sheet of this paper is exposed to light shining through a negative. The paper is then placed in a developing solution to develop the newly formed latent image. Next the print is placed in solutions of stop bath and fixer. In the final processing steps, it is washed with water and dried. The result is a positive photographic print on paper.

Cameras, lenses, light meters, and developing equipment are all essential for the production of a negative image on film. Producing photographic prints on paper also requires basic equipment—an enlarger, a timer, printing paper, a contact printing frame, an easel, trays, tongs, a magnifier, a safelight and chemicals. (See Figure 7-2.)

THE ENLARGER

An enlarger is a projection device much like a slide projector fastened to a vertical column. (See Figure 7-3.) It is the "camera" of the printing process—the basic piece of equipment in projection printing. It is also frequently used for contact printing, although the enlarger is not essential to this process.

Making an exposure on printing paper with an enlarger is not unlike making an exposure with a camera. The amount of light that is allowed to fall on the printing paper will determine how dark or light the print will be. The lens of the enlarger is equipped with an aperture so that the light intensity can be controlled. A timing device is also attached so that the time of exposure can be limited.

Parts of a typical enlarger

The controls on enlargers are simple and straightforward to use. Figure 7-3B shows the main parts of a typical enlarger: the enlarger head, the support column, and the baseboard.

The enlarger head An enlarger head houses the projection system of the enlarger. It contains a *light source* and a pair of convex lens elements called *condenser lenses*. These lenses focus the light and channel it through the negative. The negative is placed in a holder, or *negative carrier,* that is inserted between the condenser lens and the enlarger lens. A flexible *bellows* that has the enlarger lens at one end moves up and down to focus the image. Just above the focusing lens is an adjustable *diaphragm.* Its function, like that of the camera lens diaphragm, is to regulate the amount of light passing through the lens. The *enlarger lens* bends rays of light passing through the negative to form an enlarged image.

FIGURE 7-1 CONTACT PRINT SHEET

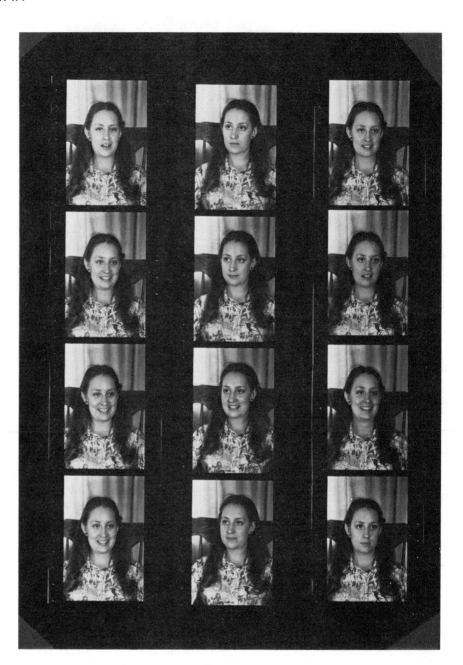

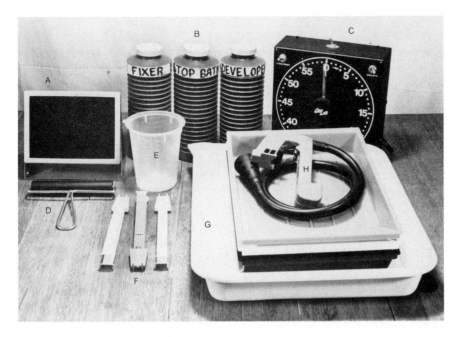

FIGURE 7-2A EQUIPMENT NECESSARY FOR PRINT MAKING

A Safelight
B Chemicals
C Timer
D Squeegee
E Beaker
F Tongs
G Processing Trays
H Wash Siphon

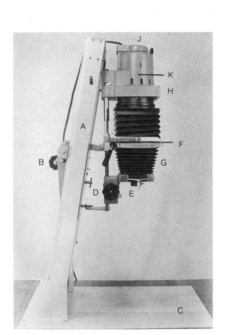

FIGURE 7-2B EQUIPMENT NECESSARY FOR PRINT MAKING

A Enlarger
B Dodging Tool
C Burning Tool
D Negative Envelope
E Contrast Filters
F Timer
G Compressed Air
H Photographic Paper
I Grain Focuser
J Negative Brush
K Printing Easel

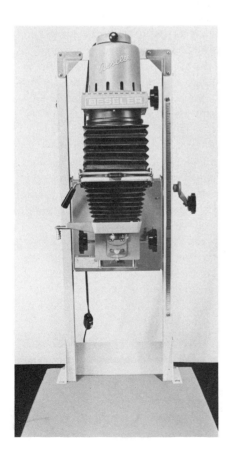

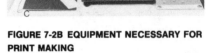

FIGURE 7-3A THE ENLARGER

FIGURE 7-3B ENLARGER, SHOWING THE MAIN PARTS

A Support Column
B Height-Adjustment Knob
C Baseboard
D Focusing Knob
E Lens
F Negative Carrier
G Bellows
H Filter Drawer
I Enlarger Head
J Lamp Housing
K Condenser-Lens Location

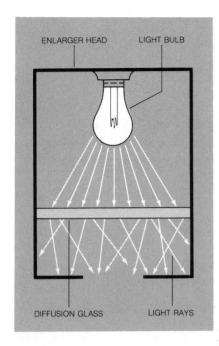

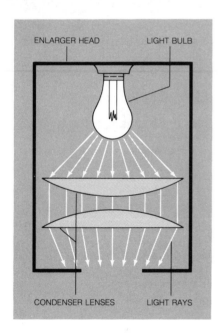

FIGURE 7-4 DIFFUSION-ENLARGER OPTICS

FIGURE 7-5 CONDENSER-ENLARGER OPTICS

The support column The support column holds the enlarger head out over the baseboard and printing paper. It also serves as a rail on which the head can be moved up or down.

The baseboard The baseboard is the foundation that supports the entire unit. It also provides a convenient place for the easel that holds the printing paper.

THE OPTICAL SYSTEM

Although operational details and the location of controls vary on different models, the factor separating enlargers into different classes is the type of optical system they incorporate.

One requirement for any enlarger is that the light falling on the negative must be evenly distributed. The edges of the negative must receive the same intensity of light as the center. This would be impossible if the light source were allowed to shine directly on the negative—the center of the negative would receive more light than the edges, and the print would not be evenly exposed.

Two basic systems are used to spread the light evenly over the negative, and the light source for both of these systems is the same—generally a white or frosted bulb of about 75 watts. The important variation between the two systems is in what happens to the light between the light source and the negative.

Diffusion enlarger A diffusion enlarger employs a ground or frosted glass plate just below the light source to diffuse and scatter the light so that it reaches the negative in a uniform way. A diffusion enlarger has no condenser lens. When light passes through the ground glass plate, it is scattered in many directions; some of this light passes through the negative. This image-bearing light is then magnified by the enlarger lens and focused on the base of the enlarger.

Light from a diffusion-type optical system strikes the negative at numerous angles, softening the projected image slightly and reducing detail. Many photographers like this effect; it is perfect for obtaining the smooth, even skin texture needed for portrait printing. (See Figure 7-4.)

Diffusion enlargers also lower contrast, so they tend to reduce the effects of dust and scratches on the negative. However, lower contrast and a softer image make printing large prints from 35 mm negatives difficult if a sharp, clear image is needed.

Condenser enlarger A condenser enlarger is used to obtain maximum clarity, detail, and contrast from a negative, especially 35 mm and smaller. A condenser enlarger's large convex lenses spread light evenly over the negative. The two saucer-shaped lenses, called *condenser lenses,* are located just below the light source. These two lenses concentrate and direct the light straight through the negative. Condenser optical systems are capable of producing dazzling contrast and of transferring maximum detail and sharpness from the negative to the print. Although condenser systems are very efficient, since most of the light reaches the lens and the printing paper, one distressing feature is that they also magnify any dust or scratches or other negative imperfections that may be on the negative, so that these become glaringly apparent on the the finished print.

Even though the enlarger is a simple machine, it is a vital link in the photographic process. The best camera equipment in the world cannot compensate for a poor enlarger. (See Figure 7-5.)

OTHER PRINTING ESSENTIALS

Although the enlarger is the basic tool, other pieces of equipment and materials are equally necessary.

Equipment and materials

Timer A timer is used to measure exposure and development times for the printing paper. A timer is attached to the enlarger so that the enlarger light may be set for varying exposure times. It is also used to measure the amount of time a print is in each of the processing chemicals.

Printing paper Photographic printing paper is marketed in a wide range of sizes. Various types of paper have different characteristics that make them suitable for particular printing applications. Two basic types of paper that call for different sets of processing steps are *resin-coated papers* (RC) and *fiber-based papers.* Resin-coated papers are plastic-coated, waterproof papers. The main advantage of RC paper is that considerably shorter fixing, washing, and drying times are possible because processing chemistry does not penetrate into the resin-coated paper fibers. Fiber papers must be processed for longer periods, especially during the washing step, to remove the unwanted chemical compounds. (See Figure 7-6.)

Contact printing frame The contact printing frame is like a picture frame in that it has a glass front and a removable back. Contact printing frames are used to press the negative and printing paper together for exposure of the contact print.

Easel A device for holding a sheet of printing paper perfectly flat under the enlarger for exposure, the easel is used for projection or enlargement printing.

Trays Print processing is usually done in trays rather than in a tank. The printing paper is placed flat in each different tray of processing chemicals. Trays vary in size, but must be at least as large as the prints being made. Common tray sizes are 8 × 10 and 11 × 14.

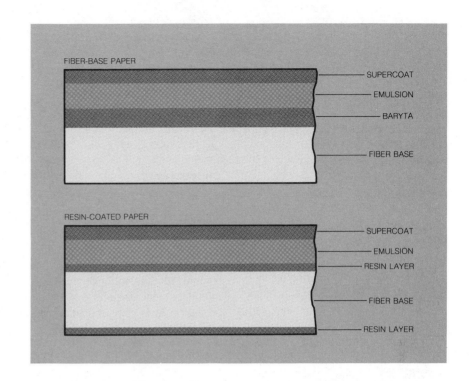

FIBER-BASE PAPER
— SUPERCOAT
— EMULSION
— BARYTA
— FIBER BASE

RESIN-COATED PAPER
— SUPERCOAT
— EMULSION
— RESIN LAYER
— FIBER BASE
— RESIN LAYER

FIGURE 7-6 CROSS-SECTION OF FIBER-BASE AND RESIN-COATED (RC) PRINTING PAPERS

Tongs Printing tongs are used to move the printing paper from one tray of chemicals to another. The important thing to remember about tongs is that they can damage the paper emulsion if they are not used properly. Tongs should *not* be used to submerge paper forcibly in chemicals. Tongs are used to lift prints *by the corners* and hold them to drain. The tongs used to transfer prints from the developer to the stop bath should be rinsed in water before being dipped into the developer again. Since stop bath is used to stop development, stop bath solution on tongs can ruin the developer.

Some workers prefer to process prints by hand rather than with tongs. Photographic chemicals may cause skin reactions, depending on the individual. Rubber gloves or protective hand creams can prevent this problem. If you do use your hands, it is absolutely essential that you make sure your hands are chemical-free and completely dry before you touch a sheet of unprocessed paper or a finished print. Also take care not to contaminate the developer by handling prints in stop bath or fixer and then placing your hands back in the developer without rinsing them.

Print magnifier Sometimes called *a grain focuser,* the print magnifier is used to focus the image precisely from the enlarger onto the printing paper. Grain focusers are often used in enlargement printing to make certain the image is as clear as possible.

Safelights and darkroom Calling the room where printing is done a darkroom is not really accurate—the printing process is not carried out in total darkness. *Safelights* used to illuminate the working area for black and white print processing range in color from yellow-green to amber and cause no harm to the print paper if used properly. Safelights work because most black and white paper emulsions are not panchromatic emulsions and are sensitive only to blue-violet light. (A few black and white and all color papers are panchromatic; these papers must be printed in darkness.) This feature allows you to work with a certain amount of "safe" light in the darkroom.

TABLE 7-1 □ SOME COMMONLY USED BLACK AND WHITE PAPER DEVELOPERS

Cold Tone	Acufine Printofine
	Dupont 53-D
	Edwal Paper Developer
	Ethol LPD
	GAF Vividol
	Ilford Multigrade
	Kodak Dektol
Neutral Tone	Agfa Metinol
	Ethol LPD
Warm Tone	Dupont 55-D
	Ethol LPD
	GAF Ardol
	GAF Miradol
	Kodak Selectol

Ethol LPD varies in tone, depending on dilution and temperature.

Any kind of light-tight place can serve as a darkroom—from a closet or bathroom to a sophisticated professional darkroom. A permanent darkroom is the most convenient place to store and use the equipment necessary for printmaking.

CHEMICALS

The final essential element of the printing process is the photographic chemistry used for printing. Although there are some modifications, the same basic process used for developing the negative is repeated for producing a print. Chemicals used for print processing vary somewhat in composition and dilution from those used for film.

Paper developer Paper developers are available for regular and special applications. Some, called *warm-tone developers,* impart a slightly brownish tone to the print. Other developers have a *neutral or cold tone.* Warm-toned developers are especially useful for portrait work; cold-toned developers are most often used for general-purpose printing. Some developers are formulated to impart higher contrast to the print, while others are low-contrast developers. Table 7-1 provides a list of some common developers and their recommended working dilutions.

Stop bath The same stop bath used for development can be used for printing. The one problem is that since a number of prints may be processed through the same tray of stop bath, the stop bath may become exhausted and lose its effectiveness. By keeping track of the number of prints processed in the tray and by working to the manufacturer's recommended quantities, you can ensure that this problem will not occur. *Indicator stop bath* warns of exhaustion by turning a dark color upon depletion.

Fixer Paper fixer is essentially the same chemical as that used for film, but the solution may be more diluted. Unlike film, prints are usually fixed with two baths. Two-bath fixing is much more efficient and economical than using a single fixing tray. The first tray of fix dissolves most of the silver halide, and the second removes the rest.

Careful fixing is very important for quality prints. Underfixing leaves light-sensitive silver in the emulsion, and overfixing leaves chemical byproducts that are difficult or impossible to wash out. Either can ruin a print, as stains will eventually appear. The best way to avoid underfixing is not to exceed the manufacturer's recommendation for the number of prints to be processed in a given quantity of fix. Another good idea is not to overload the fix tray with prints. As a rule of thumb, no more than twelve 8 × 10 prints can be properly fixed at one time in a half-full 16 × 20 tray. To avoid overfixing simply abide by the recommended times.

Washing aids Washing aids are even more important for prints than for film. Washing removes fixing chemicals and silver compounds. Photographic paper is more porous than film and tends to absorb these chemicals. Washing aids make any remaining fix or other chemicals more soluble in cold water and therefore easier to remove. By chemically eliminating the traces of fixer that would be left by normal print washing, one can shorten the wash time considerably. Wash time also depends on the type of paper being used. Heavy double-weight papers take longer to wash than single-weight papers; resin-coated papers can be washed faster than regular fiber-based papers.

Washing Photographic paper base is somewhat absorbent, so it is difficult to remove the last traces of hypo and silver from prints. Three elements are important for ensuring adequate print washing: the *water circulation* (or rate of flow), the *temperature,* and the *print circulation.*

There are many print washing devices available. To be effective, a device must be designed so that the water completely cycles through at least every three to five minutes and the wash temperature is 65 to 75°F, or 18 to 24°C. Cold water slows the removal of unwanted chemical compounds considerably. However, perfect water temperature and rate of flow are of no value if the prints cannot circulate freely. If prints are stacked on top of one another, the center of the print may not wash completely.

MAKING A CONTACT PRINT

Two of the most important aspects of printing are organization and consistency. A chef follows a specific recipe to make sure that a dish will taste the same each time it is prepared. Following a basic printing "recipe" will help the photographer obtain results that are consistent time after time. Another requirement for darkroom work is that the work areas be clean and organized.

The first step in the printmaking process is contact printing, or making the contact sheet. Contact printing essentially consists of shining light through a negative and exposing this image onto a sheet of printing paper. The exposed sheet is then developed to produce the contact print. From this contact sheet, the photographer will later choose images for enlargement printing.

Preparing the chemistry Mix the paper developer, stop bath, and fixer according to the manufacturer's instructions. The temperature of each should be 65 to 75°F. Fill each of the processing trays full enough to cover the print, but leave enough room for agitation. (See Figure 7-7.)

Assembling the negatives Exercise great care in handling the negatives

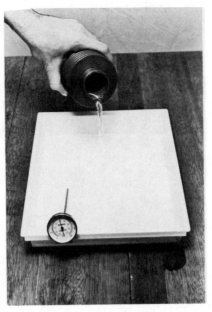

FIGURE 7-7 PREPARING THE CHEMISTRY

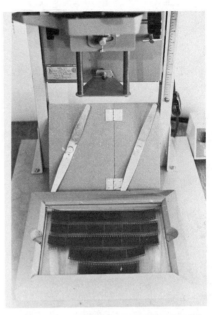

FIGURE 7-9 PLACING THE NEGATIVES INTO THE CONTACT PRINTER

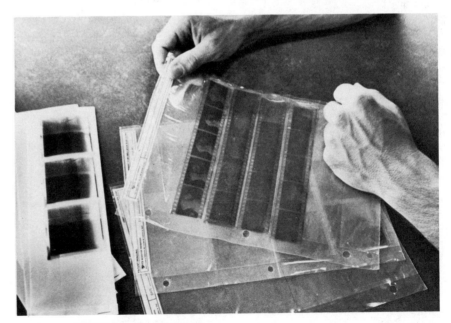

FIGURE 7-8 ASSEMBLING THE NEGATIVES

**FIGURE 7-10 ADJUSTING THE ENLARGER
LIGHT**

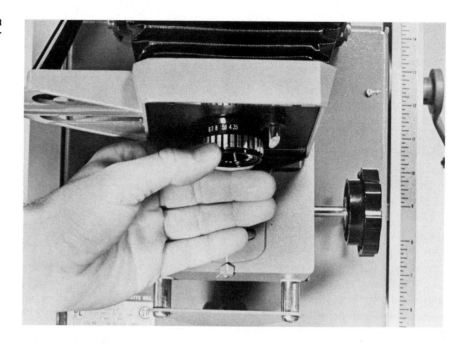

only by the edges. Fingerprints, scratches, and dust left on negatives will show as white spots or marks on a print. If negatives are dusty or dirty, gently clean them with a soft brush. Then identify the emulsion side—film naturally curls toward the emulsion side, which has a dull sheen. If negatives are placed on a flat surface, the emulsion side should be down, so that the curl causes the negatives to rest on their edges. (See Figure 7-8.)

Preparing the equipment Clean the contact printing frame if necessary. Use only water or dilute wetting solution—household glass cleaners often contain ammonia and other harsh chemicals that may harm the negatives.

Placing the negative in the printing frame Place the negatives in the printing frame carefully. A contact sheet is much easier to view if all the negatives are facing in the same direction. Remember that the emulsion side (dull side) of the negative must be facing the paper or the contact print will be backwards. Be careful not to overlap the negatives. (See Figure 7-9.)

Adjusting the enlarger Place the contact printing frame on the enlarger baseboard and turn on the enlarger lamp. Raise the enlarger head until the printing frame is completely covered by the projected light, which should overlap the edges of the printing frame for all sides. Open the lens aperture to allow maximum light through the lens. Be sure the surface of the printing frame is still covered, and turn off the enlarger lamp. Note how far up the column the enlarger head is and mark the spot on the column for future use. (See Figure 7-10.)

Opening the photographic paper With the room light off and the safelight on, remove a single sheet of photographic paper and close the package. (See Figure 7-11.) The emulsion side of the paper may be identified by the way the paper curls—both paper and film tend to curl toward the emulsion side. Place the paper in the contact printer so that the paper emulsion is in contact with the negative emulsion and close the back of the printer. It may require practice to get the paper and negatives together without sliding the negatives out of alignment. Place the loaded printing frame

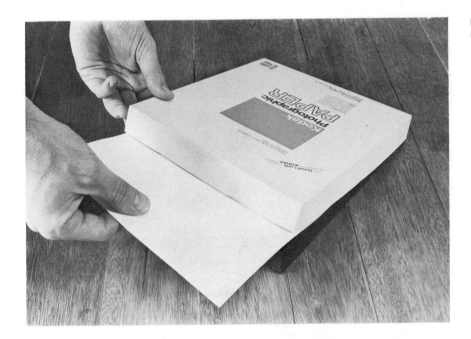

FIGURE 7-11 TAKING OUT A SHEET OF PRINTING PAPER

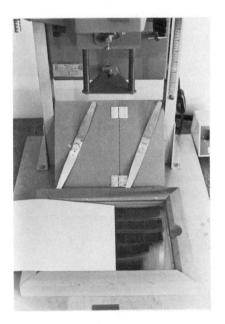
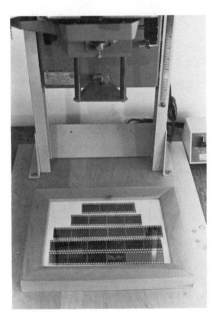

FIGURE 7-12 PLACING THE PRINTING PAPER INTO THE CONTACT PRINTER

FIGURE 7-13 MAKING AN EXPOSURE USING THE CONTACT PRINTING FRAME

under the enlarger so that the light will completely cover the frame. (See Figure 7-12.)

Making an exposure The emulsion side of the paper must face the enlarger lens, or an image will not be made. Set the enlarger timer. You may have to experiment with exposure times. (See Figure 7-13.) When you have found a proper exposure time,

remember it for future use. Start the timer and expose the printing paper.

Developing Remove the paper from the printing frame, but leave the negatives in the frame until after development in case a second exposure is necessary.

Slide the paper into the developer, emulsion side up, covering the entire surface as quickly as possible. (See

Figure 7-14.) Do not attempt to set the paper on the surface of the developer and then force it under with tongs—the sharp edges of the tongs may damage the paper. Fiber-based papers are inclined to curl up out of the developer, so it may take you a while to perfect the technique. Resin-coated papers generally do not curl badly and can more easily be slipped in with the emulsion side up. Agitate the print by

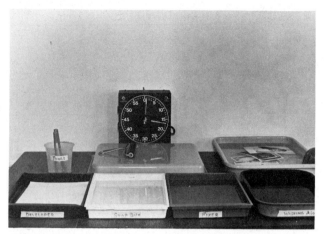

FIGURE 7-14 EXPOSED PRINTING PAPER IN DEVELOPER

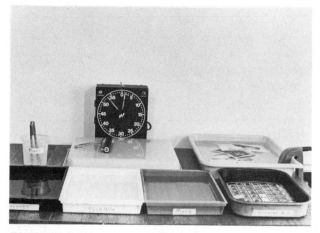

FIGURE 7-17 PAPER IN WASHING AID

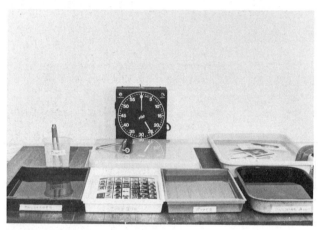

FIGURE 7-15 PRINT IN STOP BATH

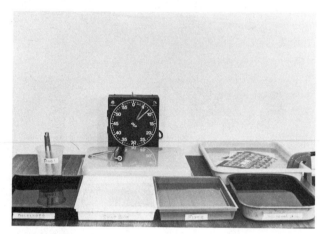

FIGURE 7-18 PAPER IN WATER WASH

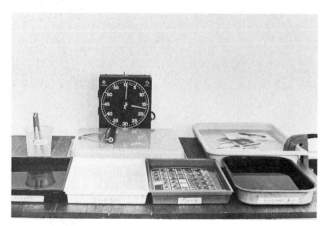

FIGURE 7-16 PAPER IN FIX

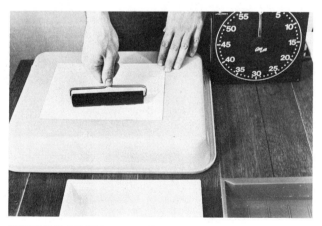

FIGURE 7-19 SQUEEGEEING THE PAPER

raising and lowering one end of the tray slightly every few seconds. Development is usually complete in one to three minutes, depending on the type of paper and the developer you are using.

Stop bath Using tongs, lift the print by one corner out of the developer and let it drain back into the tray for the last ten seconds of developing time. Place the print in the stop bath. Be careful not to put the developer tongs into the stop bath; if you do, rinse them with water before using them again in the developer. Leave the print in the stop bath for fifteen to thirty seconds and agitate. Use tongs to remove and drain the print. (See Figure 7-15.)

Fixer Place the print in the fixer, agitating occasionally. Use two fixer baths. Approximately halfway through the fix step, you may turn on the room lights, after makinge sure all photographic paper is put away first. Use tongs to remove and drain the print. (See Figure 7-16.)

Rinse Place the print in running water to rinse it before placing it in the washing aid solution.

Washing aid Treat the print for the recommended time in a washing aid; use constant agitation. (See Figure 7-17.)

Wash Place the print in a running water wash, 65 to 75°F, for from five minutes to several hours, depending on paper type. (See Figure 7-18.)

Drying You can dry prints in any one of several ways, depending on the kind of paper used. You can air-dry resin-coated papers by hanging them by a corner; both resin-coated and fiber papers may be dried in a blotter book or may be screen-dried. If you have a drying machine, it can be used on fiber papers, but do not use it for resin-coated papers; it can melt the plastic resin and even ruin the machine itself. (See Figures 7-19 and 7-20.) Table 7-2 summarizes the steps in making a contact print.

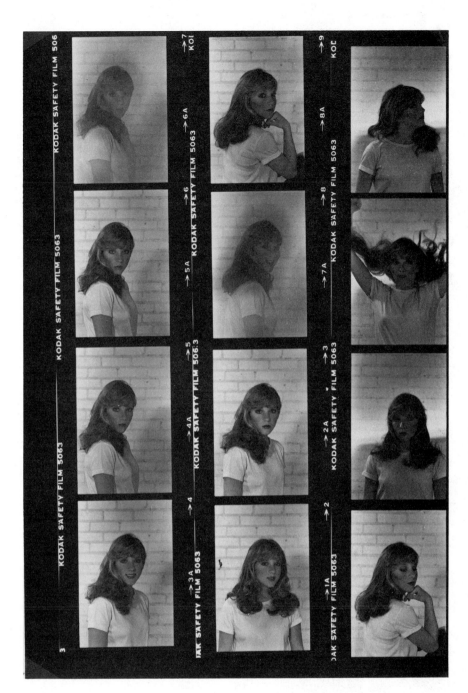

FIGURE 7-20 FINISHED CONTACT SHEET

TABLE 7-2 □ SUMMARY OF CONTACT PRINTING STEPS

| | CONTACT SHEET | |
PROCESSING STEPS	FIBER PAPER	RC PAPER
Developer	1½–3 min.	1–1½ min.
Dilute Acid Stop Bath	30 sec.	10 sec.
Fix	6 min.	4 min.
Washing Aid	2 min.	Not necessary
Wash	15–30 min.	5–10 min.
Print Flat	2 min.	Not necessary
Dryer	5 min. machine dry	5–10 min. air dry

SUMMARY

For many, the best part of photography is the print—the tangible, beautiful evidence of all the time and effort. So invest time and effort well to get the best results. Use the proper chemicals, and take the necessary time to learn the right procedure. The reward for your investment will be the privilege of sharing your message through the magic of your photographs.

REVIEW QUESTIONS

1 What are the two reasons for making print?

2 Why are safelights safe?

3 What are the two most common types of enlargers and what makes them different?

4 What are the two varieties of printing paper?

5 While developing a print, what should you do to the developing tray?

6 Why is it important to remove dust from the negative before printing it?

7 Why is washing prints so important?

8 Why should tongs and hands be rinsed before being placed in further developing solution?

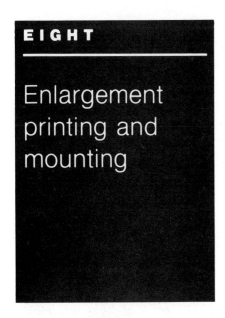

EIGHT

Enlargement printing and mounting

An enlargement is the final reward for your efforts—at last the image is in a form in which it can be viewed and enjoyed. A fine print displays your talent for composition, exposure, and development.

Printing enlargements allows tremendous latitude for creative expression. The difference between a mediocre print and a stunning one depends in part on choices made prior to enlargement, but choosing the right negative and paper can make a real difference in how the finished print turns out.

PRINTING PAPER

The two types of printing paper available were described briefly in Chapter Seven. The following is an in-depth discussion of their characteristics and uses.

You might be confused at first glance by the wide variety of printing papers available, but closer inspection reveals that all fall within two basic groups—resin-coated and fiber-based. *Fiber-based paper* consists of a fiber base, usually of cotton fiber, that is coated with a light-sensitive silver halide emulsion and gelatin. *Resin-coated paper* (sometimes referred to as RC) begins with a fiber base that is sandwiched between two thin layers of a plastic

resin material. The resin surface is coated with the photographic emulsion. (A cross-sectional view of each kind of paper was shown in Figure 7-6.)

Resin-coated paper has a number of advantages. The resin coating helps to prevent the processing chemicals and wash water from getting into the fiber base—a feature that saves time by greatly reducing the fixing, washing, and drying time for the print. Resin-coated paper can also be air-dried, which eliminates the need for costly print dryers. As for disadvantages, resin-coated paper is not available in as many varieties as is fiber-based papers. Also, it does not hold up as well over the long stretch as does fiber-based paper. Table 8-1 lists some typical printing papers.

Paper characteristics

Making black and white prints is like painting with only three colors: black, white, and gray. Many beginning photographers consider black and white prints to be dull and uninteresting, but in the hands of a skilled worker, a black and white print is one of photography's greatest challenges and produces very dramatic results.

Printing papers, especially fiber-based ones, come in such a variety that the shades of gray between black

TABLE 8-1 □ SOME TYPICAL PRINTING PAPERS

Enlarging Papers	Agfa Brovira	neutral-cold	G
	Agfa Record Rapid	warm	G
	Ilford Ilfobrom	neutral-black	G
	Ilford Multigrade	neutral-black	VC
	Kodak Kodabromide	neutral-cold	G
	Kodak Medalist	warm	G
	Kodak Polycontrast and Polylure	warm	VC
	Kodak Panalure	warm	P
Contact Papers	Agfa Contactone	neutral	G
	Kodak Azo	neutral	G
	Kodak Velox	cold	G

G = Graded; VC = Variable Contrast; P = Panchromatic

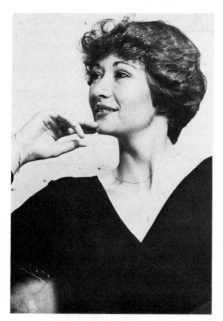

Figure 8-1A On Grade 1 Paper

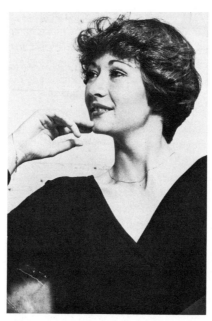

Figure 8-1B On Grade 2 Paper

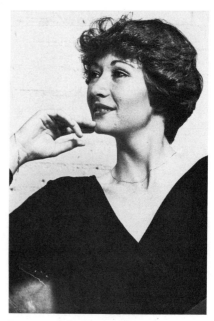

Figure 8-1C On Grade 3 Paper

and white seem infinite. The paper base can be manufactured in many textures, tones, and surface finishes as well. Altering the proportions of the silver halide crystals in the emulsion coating produces warm, cool, or neutral images and controls the amount of contrast in the prints. There are six general characteristics of both fiber-based and resin-coated papers:

Speed The speed of the paper refers to the sensitivity of the paper's emulsion to light; the speed depends on the type of silver halide used. Slow papers (those less reactive to light) are often coated with silver chloride and are primarily used for contact printing. High-speed papers (those most reactive to light) use a silver bromide emulsion and may be as much as ten times faster than silver chloride paper. Regular enlarging paper is frequently treated with a mixture of silver chloride and silver bromide.

Tone The appearance of the metallic silver gives a print its tone. In black and white photography, the tone is always a shade of gray somewhere between pure white and deep, rich black. Black tones may vary between

bluish black and brownish black. A paper that creates bluish blacks is referred to as a *cold* paper; one with brownish blacks is termed a *warm* paper. In the middle is a neutral paper. Cold-toned papers contain either silver chloride or silver bromide in the emulsion; warmer-toned papers are usually a mixture of silver chloride and silver bromide. Tone selection is an important consideration in printing photographs. Cold-toned papers are especially appropriate for such subjects as machinery, winter scenes, or architecture; warmer tones are used for portraits. Choosing the proper paper enhances and adds feeling to the composition.

Tint The color of the paper base is the *tint*. It may be pure white or one of several shades of off-white. Ivory, cream, and buff are the most common off-white shades. Pure white tint is usually associated with cold papers; off-white tints look better with warmer paper. Tones and tints may vary from one manufacturer to another, so you should experiment until you find the tone and the tint best suited to your application. Many photo dealers have sample books available for reference.

Surface texture The look and feel of the printing paper surface determine the surface texture. Paper textures may be *smooth, fine-grained,* or *rough.* Some papers are described by the names of the fabrics that their surface textures simulate—*tweed, silk, tapestry.*

Finish The amount of shine or brilliance the paper will have is determined by its finish—commonly expressed in such terms as *glossy, high-luster, luster,* and *matte.* Both paper finish and texture add to the overall statement of the photograph by helping to create a feeling. Generally the choice is a matter of personal taste, but some applications are limited to specific textures or finishes. For example, a photograph with a smooth texture and a glossy finish is usually required for reproduction in a newspaper. A rough matte paper is a popular choice for large mural photographs.

Contrast The difference between one tone or shade of gray and a slightly darker or lighter one is called *contrast.* The more suddenly and dras-

FIGURE 8-1A–E SERIES OF PRINTS MADE ON GRADED PAPER

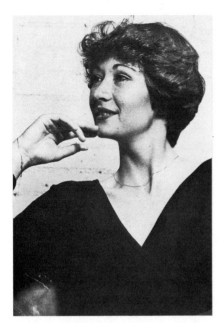

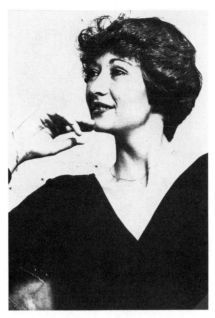

Figure 8-1D On Grade 4 Paper

Figure 8-1E On Grade 5 Paper

tically the tone changes, the higher the contrast; the more gradually and subtly the tone changes, the lower the contrast.

Print contrast is vital to the look of the print. One of the best—although not perfect—ways to study black and white contrast is to experiment with the image on a black and white television set. On the set, locate the tuning knob that is labeled "contrast." As you turn the knob, notice how the image changes from muddy, flat, low contrast to normal and then to harsh, high contrast. This same kind of variation occurs in the contrast of negatives and prints. Negative contrast is largely dependent on development: little development causes low contrast, and a lot of development causes high contrast. Additional factors that contribute to contrast in the negative are the lighting of the original scene and the initial exposure. By selecting a paper emulsion with more or less contrast than the original negative, the printmaker can increase or decrease contrast. Thus careful paper selection can prove to be a powerful tool for enhancing the appearance of the final print.

The contrast of a particular printing paper affects the way various shades of gray will be rendered in the final print. Printing papers treated with contrast-controlling emulsions are divided into two groups: *graded papers* and *variable-contrast papers.*

Contrast grades for graded papers are indicated by numbers from one to five—one signifying "soft" or low contrast, two normal, and five "extremely hard" or high contrast. Figure 8-1 shows a normal negative reproduced on each of these grades of paper.

Variable-contrast paper, capable of producing several different grades of contrast from the same sheet, is made by coating two emulsions on one sheet of paper. A low-contrast emulsion (sensitive to light in the yellow-green part of the spectrum) and a high-contrast emulsion (sensitive to blue-violet light) are combined. The contrast of the paper is varied through the use of colored filters known as *variable-contrast filters.* These filters are numbered from one through four in half-step increments. The filters numbered one and one-and-one-half will lower contrast; the twos are about normal; the threes and fours will

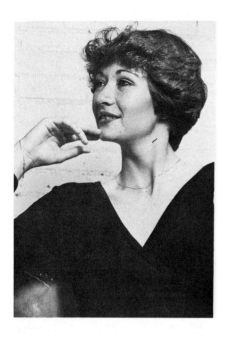

FIGURE 8-2A
With a Number-1 Variable Contrast Filter

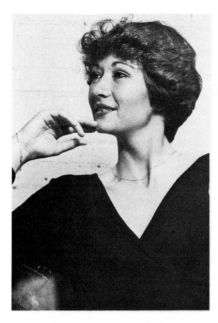

FIGURE 8-2B
With a Number-1½ Variable Contrast Filter

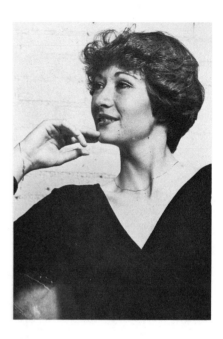

FIGURE 8-2C
With a Number-2 Variable Contrast Filter

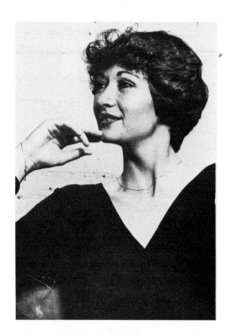

FIGURE 8-2E
With a Number-3 Variable Contrast Filter

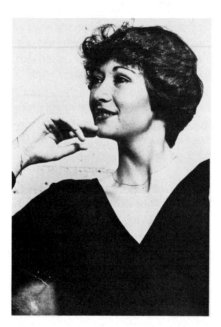

FIGURE 8-2F
With a Number-3½ Variable Contrast Filter

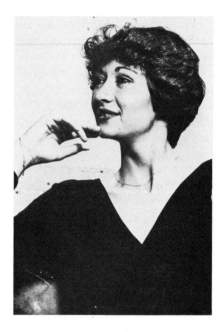

FIGURE 8-2G
With a Number-4 Variable Contrast Filter

**FIGURE 8-2A–G SERIES OF PRINTS MADE
ON VARIABLE-CONTRAST PAPER**

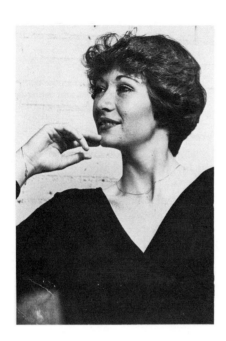

FIGURE 8-2D
With a Number-2½ Variable Contrast Filter

increase the contrast. Each filter changes the color of the light reaching the printing paper and thus varies the contrast by sensitizing one or the other or some of both of the paper emulsions. Since variable-contrast filters are available in half steps, you can attain a finer degree of control over print contrast than is normally possible with graded papers. Figure 8-2 shows how a variable-contrast paper and a set of filters change the contrast of a print.

Changing print contrast To decide whether to use graded or variable-contrast paper, consider the contrast problems of the negative(s) you are going to print. A number three or four graded paper or a number three or four variable-contrast filter with variable-contrast paper will add sparkle to a low-contrast or flat negative. A number one graded paper or a number one through two variable-contrast filter and paper will help soften

the harsh shadows and highlights of a high-contrast negative. It is usually easier to use a graded paper when printing negatives that have about the same contrast; variable-contrast filters and papers work well with negatives that vary in contrast one to the other.

The real advantage of being able to change contrast is that it allows you to improve print quality. The decision as to which type of paper to choose is reached after you consider the contrast problems of the negative. Not every negative that you expose will have perfect contrast, and almost all imperfectly exposed negatives can be improved to some degree.

One of your basic goals in printmaking should be to achieve a long tonal scale—a deep, rich black, a sparkling white, and as many different gray tones as possible in between. Since not all negatives have these qualities, you can compensate by using a different paper contrast. (Figure 8-3 shows the way paper contrast can improve a

FIGURE 8-3A PRINT FROM A FLAT NEGATIVE

FIGURE 8-3B PRINT CORRECTED USING A NUMBER-3 VARIABLE CONTRAST FILTER TO INCREASE CONTRAST

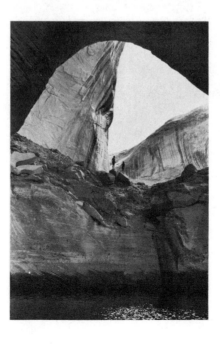

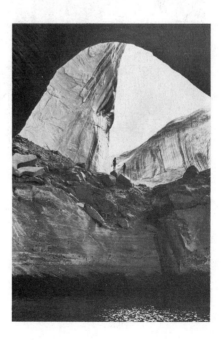

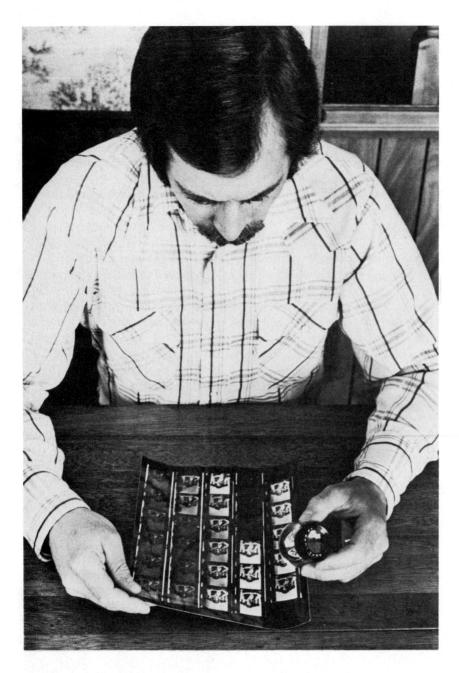

FIGURE 8-4A LOOKING AT THE CONTACT SHEET

negative that suffers from poor contrast.)

MAKING AN ENLARGEMENT

The basic chemical process for enlargement printing is the same as the one used for making contact prints. Instead of exposing the printing paper with the negatives in direct contact, though, you choose one particular negative and enlarge it to the desired dimensions.

Selecting a negative

Analyze your contact sheet to determine which negative will yield the best print. Even from the small positive prints from 35 mm negatives on the contact sheet, it is possible to check lighting, composition, exposure, and overall contrast. Look for technical problems, such as unwanted movement or incorrect camera focus. Slight fuzziness or blurring on the contact sheet print will be magnified when the print is enlarged. Steer away from prints showing scratches, water streaks, or other negative processing problems that can ruin an otherwise good print. If you are selecting 35 mm or smaller format exposures from a contact sheet, use a reading or magnifying glass to help you see the prints more clearly. (See Figure 8-4.)

FIGURE 8-4B CONTACT SHEET WITH THE
SELECTED FRAME CIRCLED

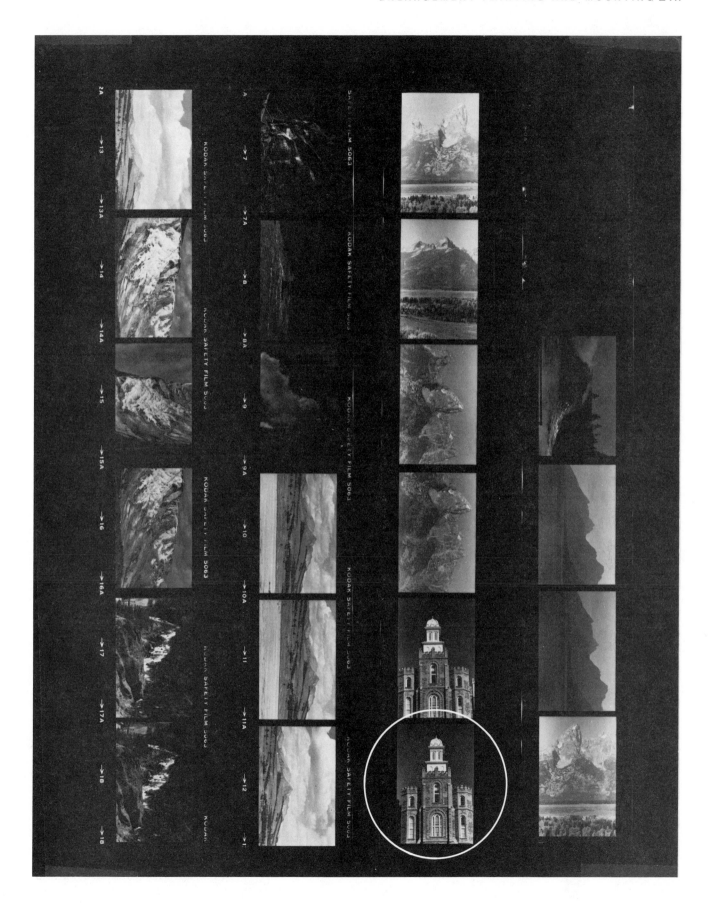

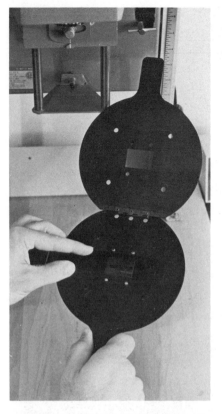

FIGURE 8-5 PLACING THE NEGATIVE IN THE CARRIER

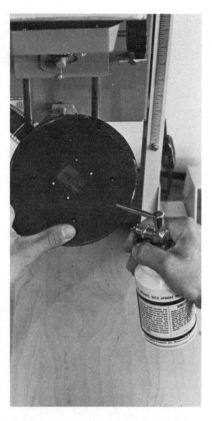

FIGURE 8-6 DUSTING OFF THE NEGATIVE

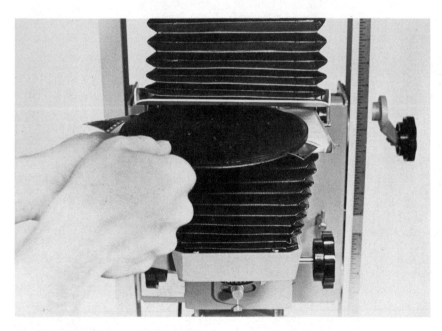

FIGURE 8-7 NEGATIVE IN THE ENLARGER

Placing the negative in the carrier

Once you have chosen the print from the contact sheet, find the negative and place it in the enlarger negative carrier with the emulsion side (dull side) facing down. (See Figure 8-5.) The simple lens system of most enlargers will reverse the negative image from right to left and from front to back. You may need a little practice in order to get the negative to project correctly on the printing easel. Check the position of the negative in the carrier. If it is not centered, do *not* slide the film in the closed carrier to adjust it; you might scratch the negative. Instead, open the carrier, reposition the negative, and close the carrier again.

Dusting the negative

Tiny specks of dust or lint may be attracted to the negative by static electricity. Dust and other particles prevent light from reaching and properly exposing the printing paper in that area. If a small negative is used to make a large print, the dust specks will be enlarged right along with the negative. When the print is developed, the dust spots will appear as small white blotches.

The best way to remove dust from a negative is to use compressed gas designed for photographic use to clean the surface. You can also use a soft brush or a soft, silicone-treated cloth. (See Figure 8-6.)

Focusing

Place the negative in the enlarger. (See Figure 8-7.) Turn on the lamp and focus the image on the printing easel, with the lens aperture wide open to get the brightest image possible. Focus the image carefully, using a grain focuser to make sure the image projected on the easel is sharp and clear. (See Figure 8-8.) Stop down the lens two or three stops, or approxi-

mately halfway, and turn off the
enlarger lamp.

Making a test strip

Two factors, light intensity and time,
determine how much of the image will
be recorded by the paper emulsion. A
test strip will show the effects of various exposures on the print paper you
have chosen. It is critical that you
know exactly how much light must fall
on the paper to produce the best possible print image, and the trial-and-
error technique of a test strip can help
you establish the proper amount of
light.

Place a strip of printing paper, 2
inches wide and 8 inches long for an
8 × 10 print, in the easel. Be careful
not to bump or move the easel. Unless
you are sure that the negative contrast
is either too high or too low for normal
printing, start with a number two paper
or a variable-contrast paper without a
filter. It is much easier to judge the
contrast from the test strip than to try
to outguess the negative. The following steps detail the procedure.

Expose the test strip Work under a
safelight, with the paper emulsion side
up. Position the paper so that it inter-
sects an important part of the image,
such as part of a face. Turn on the
enlarger lamp for two to five seconds
and expose the entire piece of paper.
Next, cover up about a one-inch section of the paper with cardboard and
expose the remaining uncovered
paper for an additional two to five
seconds. Continue moving the cardboard, one section at a time, across
the paper until the entire strip has
been covered. (See Figure 8-9.) Thus
the first section will have been
exposed for the shortest period of
time, the final section for the longest.
Whatever time interval is used for the
step exposures must be consistent for
the entire strip. Test strips are a trial-
and-error process. You may need to
make several before you find the
desired exposure.

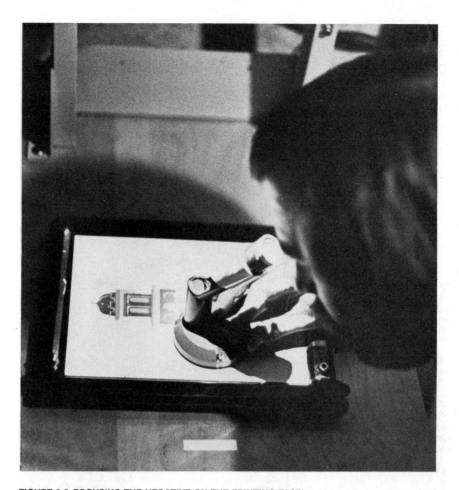

**FIGURE 8-8 FOCUSING THE NEGATIVE ON THE PRINTING EASEL
WITH A FOCUSING AID**

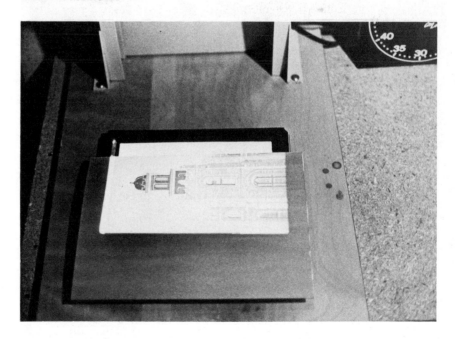

FIGURE 8-9 MAKING A TEST PRINT

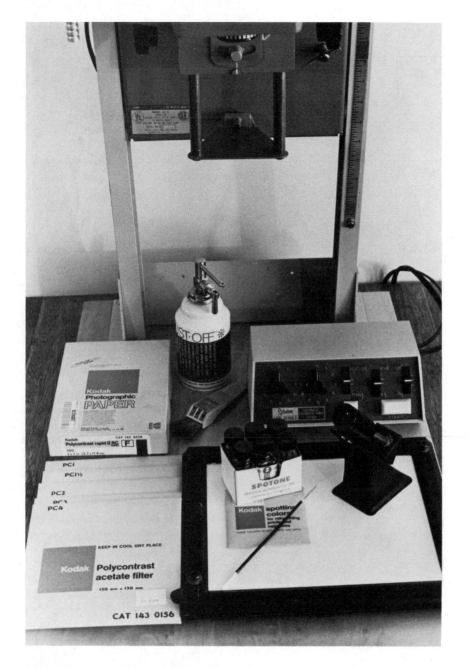

FIGURE 8-10 EQUIPMENT NEEDED TO MAKE THE FINAL ENLARGEMENT

TABLE 8-2 □ BASIC TIMES FOR PROCESSING A TEST PRINT

PROCESSING STEPS	TEST PRINT FIBER PAPER	RC PAPER
Developer	1½–3 min.	1–1½ min.
Stop	10 sec.	10 sec.
Fix	2 min.	2 min.
Wash	1 min.	1 min.

Process the test strip Process the strip, using the same processing steps you followed for the contact sheets. Follow the manufacturer's recommendations for the chemicals you are using. Remember—test strips are temporary and do not require permanent fixing, so fix time can be reduced. A short fix of a minute or so is required so the test strip can be viewed under normal light.

Look at the test strip Examine the strip under a room light. Find the section that most closely approximates the desired exposure and count all the sections up to and including it by the exposure interval, to determine the correct exposure time for the enlarged print. If the exposure interval was five seconds, for example, and the best section was the third from the lightest, then the exposure should be fifteen seconds. The right exposure may be between sections—darker than one and lighter than the next. (See Table 8-2.)

Place a full-sized sheet of printing paper in the enlarger easel and make the exposure using the time found from the test strip. Process the print using the same procedure followed in processing test strips and contact prints, but increase the fix time to the full recommended time. Make sure the washing cycle is completed. For more detailed information, refer to Chapter Seven for print processing procedures. (See Tables 8-3 and 8-4 and Figures 8-10 through 8-12.)

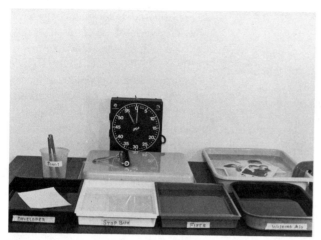

FIGURE 8-11A
Print in the Developer

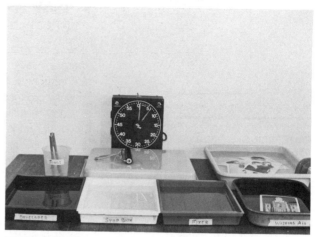

FIGURE 8-11D
Print in the Washing Aid

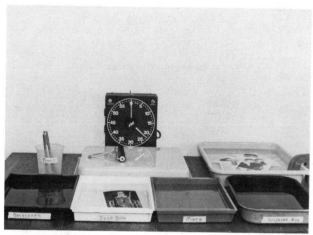

FIGURE 8-11B
Print in the Stop Bath

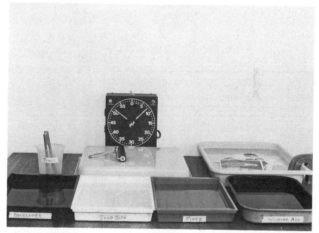

FIGURE 8-11E
Print in the Wash

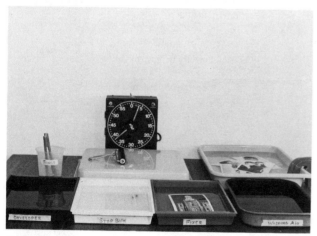

FIGURE 8-11C
Print in the Fixer

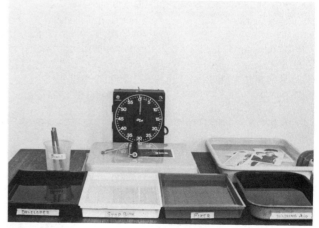

FIGURE 8-11F
Print Ready for Removal of Excess Water Before Air Drying

FIGURE 8-11A–F PROCESSING THE FINAL PRINT

TABLE 8-3 □ BASIC PRINT PROCESSING TIMES

PROCESSING STEPS	FIBER PAPER	PRINT RC PAPER
Developer	1½–3 min.	1–1½ min.
Stop	30 sec.	10 sec.
Fix	6 min.	4 min.
Washing Aid	2 min.	Not necessary
Wash	15–30 min.	5–10 min.
Print Flat	2 min.	Not necessary
Dryer	5 min. machine dry	5–10 min. air dry

These times are general averages. Always check manufacturer's recommended times.

PRINT FINISHING

After a print has been processed, there are several techniques that can further contribute to the quality of the finished product. *Spotting* removes unsightly blemishes from the final print; *cropping* changes the composition by eliminating part of the background; and *mounting* readies the print for display.

Spotting

Spotting is a technique that is very useful for removing small dust and lint spots and small scratches from the finished print. If problems are larger than that, you should reprint. The basic materials are emulsion dyes or paints and a double-zero (00) fine-point artist's brush. (See Figures 8-13 and 8-14.) Emulsion dyes are gener-

ally considered better than paints. They are harder to detect on the print because they are absorbed into the emulsion. Paints remain on the surface of the print, so if the print is held in the right light, paints are easy to see. Mix the colors first on a small square of clear acetate to get the right shade of gray. Apply either type of material with a "dotting" motion—do not stroke or paint it on.

Since spotting can be quite complex, takes a great deal of practice, and is extremely time-consuming, it pays to expend a little extra effort in the darkroom to clean dust off the negative instead of extensively spotting the print. (See Figure 8-15.)

Cropping the print

Cropping is removing from the print part of the image that appears on the

TABLE 8-4 □ BLACK AND WHITE PRINTING PROBLEMS

PROBLEM	CAUSE	CURE
Fuzzy Print	If the grain in the negative is sharp then the enlarger was not focused. If the grain is not sharp then the camera was out of focus.	Make sure that both the enlarger and camera are in focus.
Fogged Paper	Paper has been exposed to light before it was used to print on.	Make sure paper is stored and carried in a light-tight container.
Black Looks Gray	Too little development or exhausted developer solution	Make sure development is carried on for the full length of time, and chemistry is fresh.
Print Discolors on Exposure to White Light	Improper fixation	Make sure fix is not exhausted.
White Dots on the Print	Dust on the negative	Dust the negative before printing from it.
Black or White Lines on Print	Scratches on negative	Handle and store the negatives with care to prevent scratches.
Colored Stains and Blotches on Print	Chemicals on printing paper	Keep printing paper away from chemistry before handling photo paper.
Fingerprints on Print	Handling the paper with wet hands.	Make sure your hands are dry and free of chemistry before handling photo paper.
Pale Image on Print Paper, Reversed Left to Right	Printing paper was placed face down on easel.	Place print paper right side up on easel.
Uneven Print Development	Either there was uneven illumination or print was left partially exposed in the developer solution.	The enlarger should provide even illumination across the negative. Make sure the paper is quickly and fully submerged in the developer.

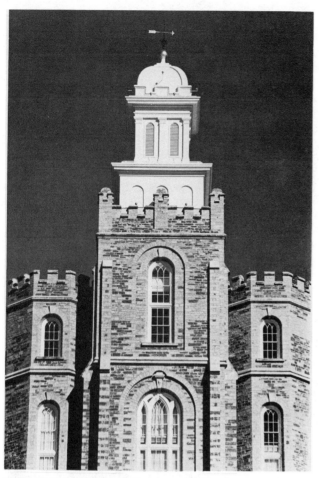

FIGURE 8-12 THE FINAL PRINT

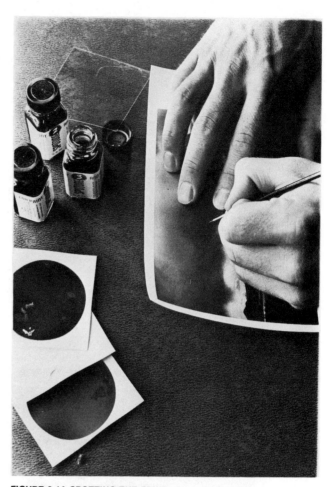

FIGURE 8-14 SPOTTING THE PRINT

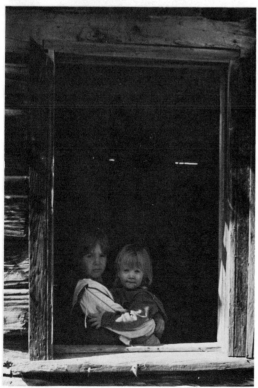

FIGURE 8-13 PRINT THAT NEEDS SPOTTING (Photo: Laird Roberts)

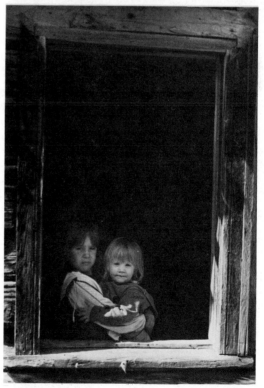

FIGURE 8-15 THE SPOTTED PRINT (Photo: Laird Roberts)

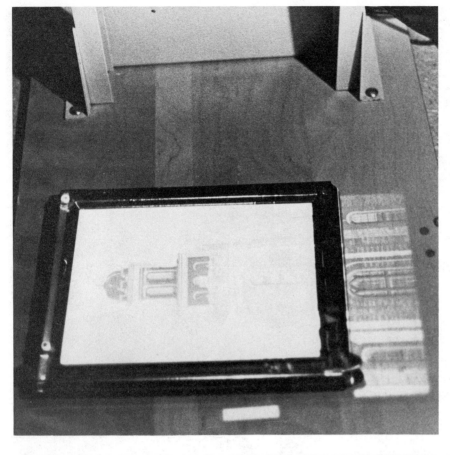

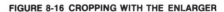

FIGURE 8-16 CROPPING WITH THE ENLARGER

negative. If you decide that the print would be more effective with some of the background deleted, for example, you have two basic choices: either crop or trim the print after it is finished or use the enlarger to crop the image while it is being printed. (See Figure 8-16.)

Cropping Ls are devices that help you decide how to crop a finished print. When you arrange the Ls together in a "frame," the final image is easy to determine. Trim the print to this size, and mount it. (See Figure 8-17.)

During the exposure phase of printmaking, cropping can be done in the enlarger; this technique is explained in Chapter Nine.

Cropping—either on the print or in the enlarger—is not ideal; it should not be a standard printing routine. The best way to "crop" is with the camera viewfinder. If possible, try several different scene compositions in the camera viewfinder, selecting the most pleasing before you take the picture.

Mounting the print

A quality photograph will bring great satisfaction to the photographer and enjoyment to those who view it. Mounting not only makes the print esthetically more beautiful, it protects the print from damage. Good prints should be mounted correctly on good-quality mount board.

How you mount your print is a very personal decisions. You determine the color, dimensions, and print size. Try to visualize the final presentation as you think about how you will mount your print. (For more information on mounting, see Chapter Nine.)

Mount board colors Generally, the three most appropriate colors for mounting black and white prints are black, charcoal gray, and white. The standard is a simple white board, although some prints lend themselves to mounting on a black or charcoal gray. (In certain cases, a black and white print may "demand" some other color.) Remember: you want to draw

the viewer's attention to the print, not the mount.

Mount board sizes There are no hard and fast rules for the size of the mount board, but a few guidelines should be considered. Do not under-size the mount—one that is too big is better—and easier to correct, if necessary—than one that is too small. Standard frame sizes are 8 × 10, 11 × 14, 16 × 20, and 20 × 24. Mount a standard-size print on the next larger size mount board. For example, an 8 × 10 print fits well on an 11 × 14 mount board.

Do not leave the same amount of space at the top and bottom of the mount board; this creates the visual impression that the bottom is "too small." Position the print on the board so there is equal space on the top and sides, with a little extra on the bottom—this gives the print a "base" on which to rest. A vertical 8 × 10 print, for example, would have 1 ½ inches on the top and sides and 2 inches on the bottom border when mounted on an 11 × 14 mount board.

Cutting mount board Before you mount the print, do all cutting and trimming of the mount boards *at a safe distance from the print.* Nothing ruins a print more quickly than a slash mark from a misguided knife. Make careful measurements for print placement before the print is on the board. Use a sharp matte knife and a metal straightedge. Using a paper cutter will ruin both the mount and the cutter.

Dry mounting In dry mounting, the process most commonly used to attach prints to photographic mount board, a heat-sensitive adhesive tissue paper is tacked to the back of the print with a warm tacking iron. Once the dry mount tissue is attached to its back, the print, with tissue, is placed on a mount board of the desired size

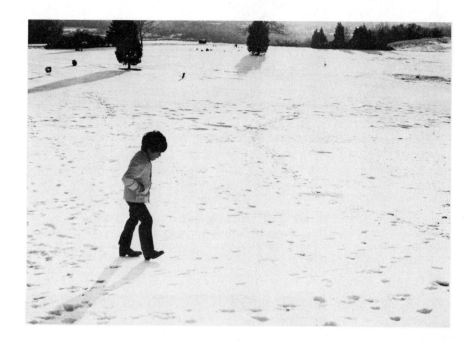

FIGURE 8-17A PRINT WITH DISTRACTING BACKGROUND
(Photo: Brian Bates)

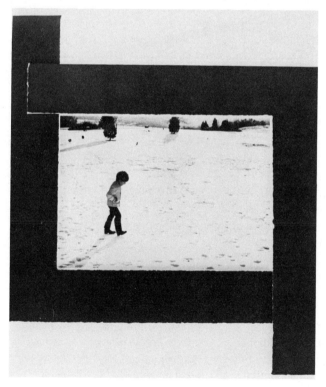

FIGURE 8-17B USING CROPPING LS TO DETERMINE HOW MUCH TO TRIM OFF

FIGURE 8-17C CROPPING LS DRAWN CLOSER TOGETHER TO HELP VISUALIZE COPYING

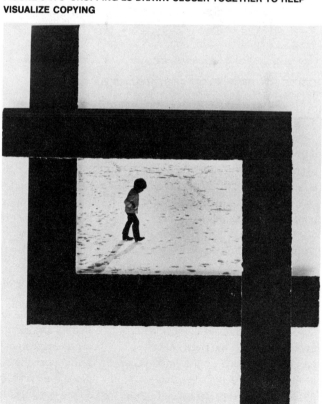

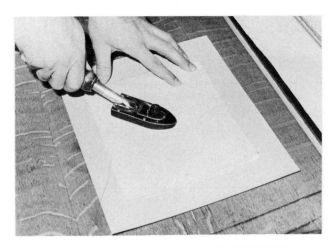

FIGURE 8-18 ATTACHING DRY-MOUNT TISSUE TO PRINT AND BOARD
A hot tacking iron is used to attach the heat-sensitive dry-mount tissue to the back of the print, with care to protect RC paper from excess heat.

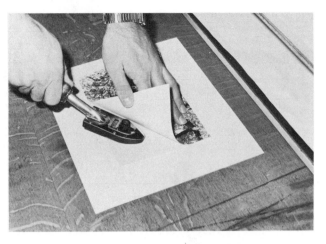

FIGURE 8-20 TACKING DRY-MOUNT TISSUE TO MOUNT
Tissue is tacked to the appropriate size of mount board to prevent the print from shifting from its place on the mount board, as the board and print are placed in the dry-mount press.

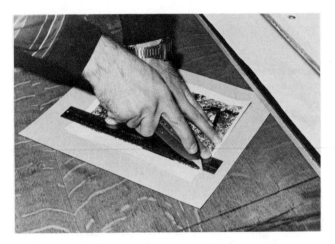

FIGURE 8-19 TRIMMING OFF PRINT AND TISSUE
Trimming tissue and print together gives a smooth, straight edge.

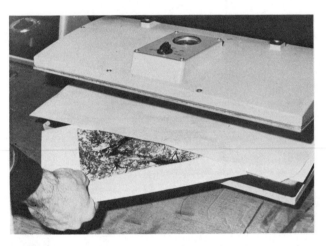

FIGURE 8-21 PLACING PRINT INTO DRY-MOUNT PRESS
The dry-mount press has been warmed to the proper temperature. Always use the lowest posible heat setting for RC paper. Also place a *clean* sheet of white paper over the print to protect it.

and heated in a dry-mount press, which seals the print to the mount board.

When you dry mount, make sure the print and the mount are clean on both sides. Turn the press on, set the temperature at approximately 225°F, or about 105°C. On a table turn the print face down on a clean paper and place a dust-free sheet of dry-mounting tissue on the back of the print. Make sure you have copied any pertinent information onto the back of the mount board. Line up the warm edges of the tissue and the edges of the print. Lightly fasten the tissue to the center of the print with a tacking iron.

(See Figure 8-18.) Turn the print over and trim away any tissue that extends beyond the edges. (See Figure 8-19.) Place the print exactly where you want it on the mount board and then tack the print to the mount board with the tacking iron, by lifting a corner of the print and tacking the corners of the tissue to the mount board. (See Figure 8-20.) Place the resulting sandwich (print, tissue, and board) in a press heated to approximately 250°F, under a protective sheet of board. Center the print under the platen before you close the press. (See Figure 8-21.) Close the press for exactly one minute. Open the press, remove the print,

and place it flat on a table under a weight while it cools. (See Figure 8-22.)

If you mount resin-coated paper, use less heat to avoid melting the resin coating. Follow exactly the manufacturer's directions for using the adhesive sheet you choose. Sheets for mounting fiber papers may not work for RC papers. Generally, temperatures for resin-coated papers are about 200°F, or approximately 90 to 95°C. Once a resin-coated print has been mounted, it must be cooled *immediately* under a weight, or else the print may peel off the mount board.

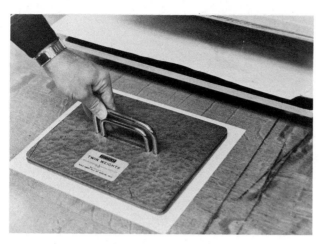

FIGURE 8-22 WEIGHTING THE PRINT
This assures a good bond between the print and mount board.

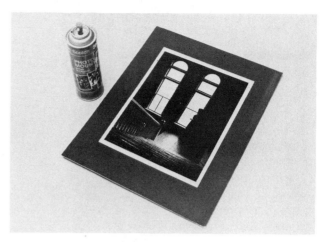

FIGURE 8-24 SPRAY-MOUNTED PRINT
Print is centered on mount board and pressed down to seal.

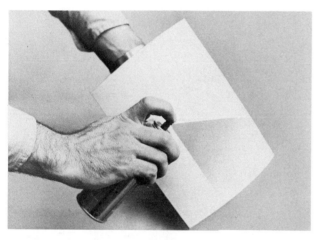

FIGURE 8-23 APPLYING SPRAY ADHESIVE
A light coating is all that is necessary.

Spray mounting Spray mounting is a quick and easy method of mounting prints. It is especially good for resin-coated papers, which can be difficult to dry mount. A number of spray adhesives for mounting prints are on the market. Make sure you choose one that can be used safely for that purpose. A spray adhesive is sprayed onto the back of the print before the print is placed on the mount board.

There are some guidelines you should follow when spray mounting. Make sure the print and the board are clean, or else you will get bumps between the print and the board. Practice spraying the adhesive on a sheet

of clean paper before you try spraying on the print. Use sweeping horizontal strokes to get uniform layers of adhesive. Be sure to swing past the edges of the paper, and keep the can of adhesive six to eight inches away from the print while you spray.

To begin, arrange the print on the board and mark the position of the corners of the print *very lightly* with pencil. Take the print into another room before you spray the adhesive so you do not accidentally get any on the mount board. Place the print face down on a large piece of paper and spray the adhesive evenly over the surface. Wait from thirty seconds to

one minute for the adhesive to dry partially before you try to move the print. When moving the print after applying the spray, be very careful not to get any on the picture side of the print. (See Figure 8-23.) Position the print so that it just fits within the light pencil marks on the mount board. Once the print comes into contact with the board, the bond is permanent, so you must make sure you properly position the print the first time. Place a sheet of paper over the print and work with a rubber roller (or similar tool) from the center of the print out, to smooth the print and make a strong bond. (See Figure 8-24.)

SUMMARY

The process of exposing and developing the film is just the beginning of an exciting procedure. The satisfaction of seeing the print is the photographer's ultimate reward.

The printing process has great possibilities for enhancing the photographic statement. Choice of paper and developer can add to the effect of the print—or detract from it, if care is not used.

The photographer must decide what is desireable and what is not. The difference between an ordinary picture and an effective statement is often a matter of changing contrast or rendering the print in lighter tones. Black and white printing requires disciplined seeing, and the best way to develop this skill is through practice.

REVIEW QUESTIONS

1 What two types of paper are most commonly used in photography?

2 Name three of the six general characteristics of both types of paper.

3 Printing papers come with what two types of contrasts?

4 How many grades are assigned to contrast paper?

5 What filter is used with variable-contrast papers?

6 What kinds of problems may be encountered when one is selecting a negative for enlargement?

7 With what three things can you dust a negative?

8 What is the importance of a test strip?

9 Can spotting be used to retouch large areas of a print? Why?

10 What are two facets of print finishing?

11 What are the two most common mounting techniques?

12 What colors of mount board are appropriate for black and white prints?

NINE

Printing techniques and manipulations

A photographic print is a two-dimensional representation of the three-dimensional world, the end result of what you saw and composed in the camera's viewfinder.

As a printmaker, you have total control over the way this image is portrayed in shades of black, white, and gray. A printed image may closely resemble the light and dark values of the original scene, or it may be very different. Various printing techniques and manipulations provide you with a wide range of means for influencing the appearance of the final image.

Printing techniques are sometimes used creatively to emphasize balance or exaggerate certain photographic elements within the print, improving the impact and statement of the photograph. Printing techniques may also function as "photographic first-aid." A number of problems that often occur during the photographic process—problems involving exposure, contrast, and composition—can be corrected.

Printing techniques, whether creative or corrective, may be used during exposure of the printing paper, during development, or as a part of print finishing.

SELECTIVE EXPOSURE

Modern film is amazing in its ability to capture a very broad range of tones. It can record detail in both dense highlight areas and thin shadow areas of the negative. Unfortunately, printing paper does not share this quality; it shows a much smaller range of printable values. As a result, highlights that are very detailed in the negative will often print pure white; deep, detailed shadows in the negative will print nearly black, showing little or no detail in the print.

Two techniques that can be used to compensate for this problem are burning-in (or burning) and dodging. Burning-in gives more exposure to, and thus darkens, certain areas in the print. In dodging, exposure is held back to lighten the print in certain areas. Burning and dodging are quite personal in their application; skill and judgment are required for pleasing results. The best way to become skillful is to practice.

Burning-in

The basic tools for burning-in are two sheets of cardboard mount board. The first piece of cardboard should be about ten inches square with a hole one-half inch in diameter punched in the center; the second piece should be the same size as the first, but without a hole. These easily obtained tools are all you will need. (See Figure 9-1.)

To determine if there are areas in the print that need burning, make an exposure of the negative onto the printing paper, basing the exposure time on the results of the test strip. Follow the normal printing procedure through the fix step. Remove the print from the fixer and examine it. If the overall exposure seems about right but the highlight areas show little or no detail, burning-in is needed.

To improve the detail, expose another piece of paper, using the same printing time as for the first. After the initial exposure, place the burning tool with the hole in the center between the enlarger lens and the easel. Turn on the enlarger lamp. Hold the burning tool close enough to the lens so that no light can strike the printing paper except through the hole. (Be careful not to bump the enlarger or the easel.) During this second exposure, jog the burning tool back and forth over the highlight areas, allowing additional image-bearing light to reach just those areas that need to be darkened. Burning-in can be applied to other areas besides high-lights: any part of the photograph that would make the composition more pleasing can be burned-

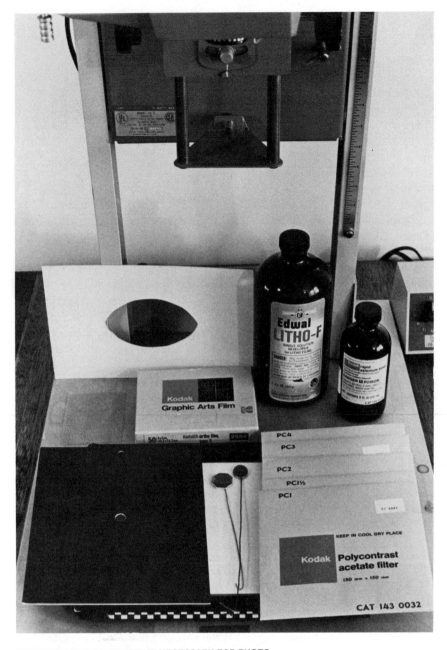

FIGURE 9-1 BASIC EQUIPMENT NECESSARY FOR PHOTO MANIPULATION

A Burning-In Card
B Variable Contrast Filters
C Graphic Arts Film Developer
D Dodging Tools
E Diffusion Screen
F Toner
G Vignette Tool

in. This will give even coverage and extra exposure time to the portions of the print that need it. (See Figure 9-2.)

How much extra time is enough? Accurate estimation of burning time is largely a matter of practice and experience. Small test prints can help, and they also save paper. First, expose the test paper for the time already determined for the rest of the print. Then make additional exposures on the test print in the same manner as for a regular test print. Once you process this test print, it will give you a good idea as to how much additional time is needed for burning-in. With practice, burning-in will become like a sixth sense, and you will not always need to perform tests.

Edge-burning Burning-in may also be used to enhance and emphasize the subject of the photograph. Edge-burning is a burning-in method used to help direct the viewer's eye to the center of the photograph. Edge-burning is done after the initial exposure and any needed spot burning have been finished. Place the plain piece of cardboard under the lens and turn on the enlarger. Burn-in all four sides of the print an inch or so in from the edge. This darkens the edges of the print slightly. As the eye moves toward the center of the print, the tone becomes a little lighter. (See Figure 9-3.) Edge-burning should be done in such a way that it is never obvious to the viewer. The tool must be moved back and forth carefully so there is no line of uneven exposure.

Dodging

Dodging is the opposite of burning-in; it is applied in much the same manner and with the same skills. Dodging entails blocking out some of the light that would form the images in shadow or other areas of the print. The resulting effect is a lightened, more detailed image in these areas. Dodging adds detail to make the composition more effective. (See Figure 9-4.)

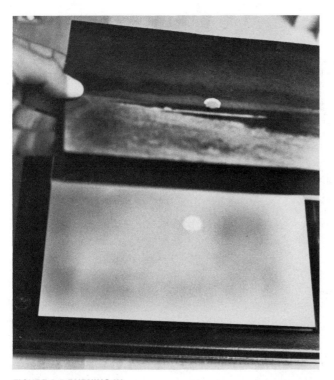

FIGURE 9-2 BURNING-IN

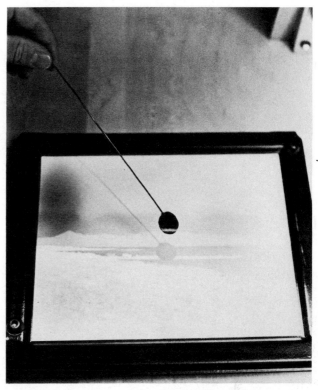

FIGURE 9-4 DODGING

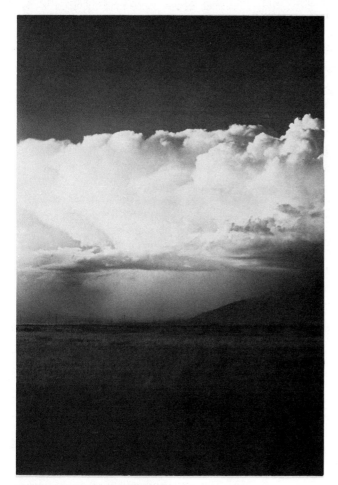

FIGURE 9-3 EDGE-BURNED PRINT

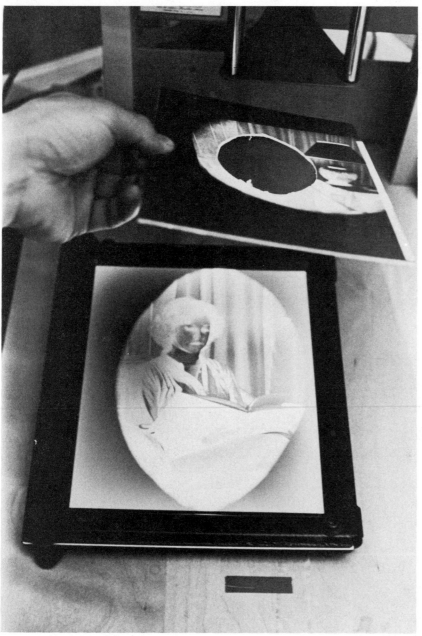

FIGURE 9-5 VIGNETTING

Vignette A specialized type of dodging, vignetting involves removing the background from the print. It is most often used for portraits, but has other creative uses as well. The most common vignetting tool is a piece of cardboard with an oval cut in the center. The size and shape of the oval depend on the print size and the preference of the printmaker. The vignetting tool is kept in constant motion beneath the lens throughout the exposure. This ensures that *only* the desired portion of the negative exposes the paper. (See Figure 9-5.)

Burning and dodging are very effective for balancing the light and dark areas of the print. By using these two printing techniques, one can produce considerably more detail in the print than would otherwise be possible. For best results, these manipulations should be used with exposure times of at least ten seconds. This allows you enough time to work and lessens the effects of errors. A two- or three-second burning or dodging error is not very noticeable when the exposure time is fifteen to twenty seconds. The same error would be much more noticeable with an exposure time of five or six seconds. Remember also that burning and dodging are not cure-all techniques, but rather modifications to the print. They cannot replace accurate exposure; they can only enhance an already good print. Using them to try to save a photograph that has excessively light or dark areas will result only in a muddy effect.

Using burning and dodging

Skill in using selective exposure techniques to their fullest advantage must be developed through practice. The ability to evaluate a test print and determine the exposure that best expresses the feeling of the subject is an important part of that skill.

The best print in Figure 9-6 illustrates a typical printing problem. Each band in the test print represents a three-second exposure, and there is no single exposure that can capture the feeling of the original scene. The foreground of the print should be rendered very darkly; it must show detail, but not so much detail that it distracts from the rest of the print. The nine-second exposure on the test print seems about right for this particular area. The sky must be printed to capture the feeling of a heavy, stormy afternoon; a fifteen-second exposure emphasizes good cloud detail and adds contrast and depth to the image. The water presents a double problem: good detail is rendered by the twelve-second exposure, but the central sunlit area of the lake will require some extra exposure. A good starting point for total print exposure is nine seconds; the sky and foreground can then be burned-in and dodged as needed. A final exposure for the sunlight on the lake will add slight detail. Figure 9-7 shows the print completed according to these specifications.

Cropping with the enlarger

Another technique that may be employed during the exposure phase of the printing process is cropping. This technique allows you to print only a portion of the negative. The best way to deal with some problems, especially those involving composition, is to eliminate them from the print.

In cropping, the head of the enlarger is raised to increase the size of the projected image. Refocus the image and adjust the easel position to frame only the desired parts of the negative. Remember that raising the enlarger head will decrease the amount of light available for that area, so you will need to increase exposure time.

Almost every negative is cropped to some extent, simply because most negatives do not fit standard print and paper formats. No matter how much a 35 mm negative is enlarged, it will never exactly equal or fit on an 8 ×

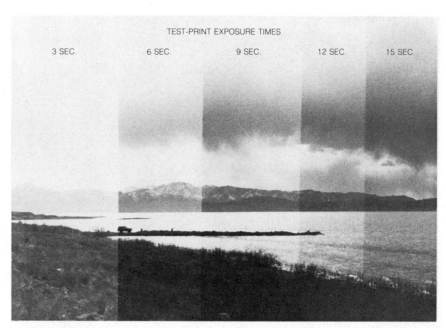

TEST-PRINT EXPOSURE TIMES

3 SEC.   6 SEC.   9 SEC.   12 SEC.   15 SEC.

FIGURE 9-6 TEST PRINT TO CHECK FOR BURNING AND DODGING

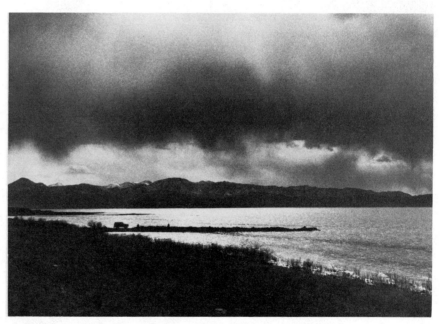

FIGURE 9-7 FINAL BURNED AND DODGED PRINT (Photo: Laird Roberts)

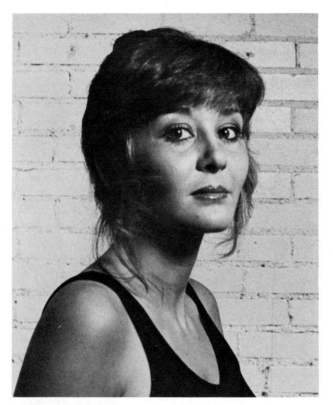

FIGURE 9-8 PRINT WITH NORMAL CONTRAST

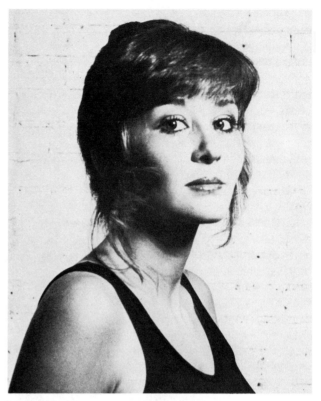

FIGURE 9-9 PRINT WITH INCREASED CONTRAST

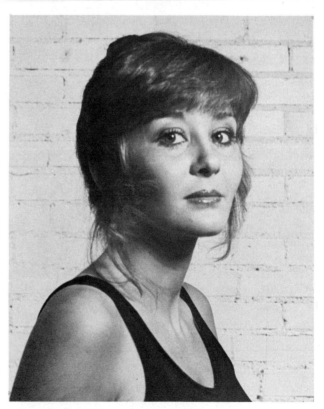

FIGURE 9-10 PRINT WITH DECREASED CONTRAST

10 piece of printing paper. A 35 mm negative is approximately 1 inch wide and 1½ inches long. If the width of the negative is enlarged to 8 inches, the length of the enlarged image will be approximately 12 inches. Therefore, the image will fit widthwise on the paper, but be 2 inches too long. If the length is enlarged to 10 inches, the width will be only 6⅔ inches, which is 1⅓ inches too short.

The same logic may be applied to a 2¼ × 2¼ inch negative. No matter what degree of enlargement is given to the negative, it will always be a square and will not fit a standard paper format. This is not to say that standard paper size should dictate the composition of a photograph. A 35 mm negative can be printed full frame without cropping, to produce a 6½ × 9¾ inch print; the excess of the 8 × 10 inch sheet is then trimmed off.

Cropping is a very valuable printing tool, but it does have some disadvantages. Increasing the size of the projected image increases grain size in the print, magnifying negative defects, dust, and scratches. These are important considerations when one is enlarging small negatives for cropping purposes—unsatisfactory print quality may be the end result. To repeat—try moving in closer for the original shot, cropping with the camera viewfinder.

DEVELOPMENT TECHNIQUES

Techniques other than burning-in or dodging may be required to deal with some printing problems. There are a number of techniques that can be applied during the development portion of the printing process.

Image correction

Many photographs show the approximate relationship of light to dark areas and have good detail in the highlights as well as the shadow areas of the print. Unfortunately, a print may still lack expression, appear lifeless, or be harsh and disconcerting. The problem is contrast.

Controlling contrast is one of the most common problems for beginning photographers. Contrast can be regulated three ways during the printing process: you can use graded paper, you can use variable-contrast paper and variable-contrast filters, or you can increase or decrease the development time. All three are effective methods for either increasing or decreasing contrast.

Graded paper is available in grades of contrast from 1 (soft) to 5 (extremely hard). The effective contrast of graded paper can be adjusted further by altering the development time of the print. A number 3 graded paper may be slightly overexposed in the enlarger and then developed for slightly less than the recommended time to produce a contrast grade of about 2 or 2½. Number 3 paper may also produce contrast similar to that of grade 4 paper if it is underexposed and then overdeveloped by 50 or 100 percent of normal contrast.

Variable-contrast paper can produce a great variety of contrast grades on one paper. By using burning and dodging techniques on variable-contrast paper, you can produce several grades of contrast on the same print. Changing variable-contrast filters during exposure, in combination with selective burning and dodging, will further vary contrast.

Choice of a grade of contrast is a matter of personal preference and depends on the feeling and mood you are trying to express in the print. A print with normal contrast should have some areas of maximum paper black and some areas of pure paper white. A good range of gray tones should be expressed between these two extremes. Generally, increasing the contrast will remove some of the gray values from the middle range. Decreasing the contrast will remove

the black and white accent areas and tend to bring out more gray values. (See Figures 9-8 through 9-10.)

If the print looks muddy and the highlights are not brilliant, you need a higher grade of contrast. If the shadow areas look black and there is a loss of detail in the important highlight areas, use a lower grade of paper or a filter. Printing on a lower grade of paper is easier than dodging all the shadows and burning-in the highlights of a high-contrast negative.

Graded papers and variable-contrast papers were discussed in more detail in Chapter Eight.

PRINTMAKING FOR PERMANENCE

Correct processing and mounting are critical if you are interested in permanence—if you want to create pictures that will endure to become an important photographic record for future generations. Some of the photographs produced by early printmakers have lasted for a century or longer, but many others have begun to deteriorate badly. Unfortunately, it is difficult to determine how long many of today's materials will last and how vivid today's photographs will be years from now. But there are some things you as a printmaker can do to lend stability to your photographs.

Processing for stability

The greatest hazards to permanence are improper processing of film and haphazard printing techniques. It is best to follow the manufacturer's instructions carefully, especially when it comes to fixing and washing.

Development As in all stages of processing, make sure that you adhere closely to the manufacturer's instructions during development. As a rule, you can expect more negative-deterioration problems from images developed for extremely fine grain as opposed to those with normal grain. Greatly overexposed or underexposed images also suffer from this tendency.

Stop bath A very common error is exceeding the recommended strength of the stop bath. The excess acid causes the photographic paper to become brittle as it dries, resulting in blistering and gas bubbles on the surface of the print. After the photographs have been stored for some time, small brown spots appear over the entire surface of the picture. To avoid this problem, make sure the stop bath is fresh and mixed to the right dilution.

Fixing Fixing is critical to stability for two reasons. First, it dissolves the undeveloped silver halides; second, it permits proper washing for removal of unwanted chemicals.

If your fixing bath is fresh, a single sheet of film or paper fixes in a relatively short time. When you are processing a batch of prints or negatives, however, the papers may stick together, preventing the fixing bath from coating the entire surface of each completely. It is critical that you agitate the bath thoroughly, making sure that you separate the photographic materials often during agitation. The result of failure to separate the materials may be a large stain in the center of the photograph. If you do process a batch of negatives at once, the best method is to use film hangers or reels suspended in the tank to keep the negatives separated—the less you handle the negatives during processing, the less chance of damage.

If you process a large batch of prints, make sure the tray you use is large enough to permit easy separation of the prints during processing. Do not ignore the fix bath. Bubbles will tend to form under the floating print, resulting in spots that are only partially fixed and that show up as purplish spots on the finished photograph.

You should never leave paper in the fix bath for longer than recommended; otherwise the chemicals will excessively penetrate the fibers of the paper, making effective rinsing almost impossible. This is especially true of resin-coated paper. If the chemical penetrates between the resin layers, it is almost impossible to wash out. To be safe, carefully follow the manufacturer's instructions for the type of film or paper you are fixing.

If you have enough space, the most effective method for fixing a print is to use two successive fix baths of three to five minutes each.

Hypo clearing agents Hypo clearing agents sharply reduce the washing time required for both prints and negatives. They make it possible for you to wash away chemicals that are almost impossible to remove with water alone. You can also wash the negatives or prints in colder water with better success.

You can transfer prints directly from the fixer to the hypo clearing solution without an intermediate rinse, but an intermediate rinse increases the capacity of the solution and results in better photographs.

Because of the rapid washing characteristics of resin-coated papers, it is not necessary to use hypo-clearing agents with these papers unless water conservation is important.

Washing Washing is essential: it removes the chemicals and silver compounds from the paper or negatives. It is easy to wash negatives, because the chemicals are not absorbed by the film base. Most require only twenty to thirty minutes of washing. This time can be dramatically reduced if you use a hypo clearing agent first. Prints on paper—which *does* absorb chemicals—require about one hour of washing when a hypo clearing agent is not used.

Mounting for stability

No matter what you intend to do with your photographic prints, once you have invested time and effort in the process, from shooting the picture to finishing the print, you want your photographs to last. The following sections explain how to achieve this goal of archival or museum mounting. These steps differ from those given earlier on mounting, in that more care is required in the selection and use of materials and in the actual mounting process itself.

Mount size This is obviously a personal choice, but steer away from prints that are too large—they are more easily damaged and are more difficult to store. Keep a generous margin around the image, and mount the prints on boards of uniform size to simplify storage and lessen the chances of damage.

Mounting Never use rubber cement, animal glue, or starch paste for mounting. Dry mounting is best for all sizes of prints. You should use dry-mounting tissue between the print and the mounting board to protect the print from impurities that may exist on the mount. (Mounting is explained at length in Chapter Eight.)

Mounting board Do not scrimp here. High-quality mounting board is worth every penny you spend on it. Make sure the board is free of ground wood, alum, or alum rosin. It should have a pH of about 6.5 and should be of uniform quality and size.

Borders Wide borders are a guarantee against damage. Survey a group of old photographs—you will find that those with wide borders have held up much better than those with narrow borders. For permanence, mount prints with a 3-inch border on the top and sides and a border of $3\frac{1}{2}$ inches at the bottom. Since damage often occurs during handling, the wide borders allow for some trimming later to get rid of damaged edges.

Frames If you are going to hang a print on the wall, use a sheet of cardboard matte between the print and the glass so that the print is held away from the glass. Otherwise, the print surface may be damaged by condensation. Avoid varnished or oiled frames; aluminum frames are best. If a frame has a plywood backing, discard the plywood—raw wood contains oxidizing agents that will eventually ruin the print—and replace it with a sheet of high-quality mounting board. (See Figure 9-11.)

CREATIVE TECHNIQUES FOR THE DARKROOM

Once you have mastered the basic darkroom techniques, you are ready to experiment with new techniques that can greatly increase your creativity. These creative techniques allow you not only to create better pictures from the negatives you take in the future, but also to create entirely new pictures from negatives you already have.

Texture screens

Dramatic effects can be produced with a texture screen, a device that gives the print a textured appearance. A texture screen can be anything that has translucence and texture—sheer fabric, especially flocked nylon cloth, is often used. The fabric is stretched taut across a frame and placed in contact with the paper in the printing easel. Using a piece of clear glass to hold the texture screen against the paper will prevent a blurred effect.

Another possibility is to use a negative texture screen. Shoot a picture of a textured surface, process the negative, and put that negative with the photograph negative in the enlarger.

You can use dodging and burning with any kind of texture screen. Since texture screens cause a slight loss of contrast, use a higher contrast paper. (See Figure 9-12.)

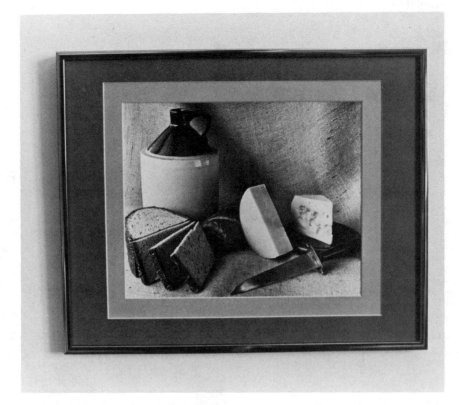

FIGURE 9-11 PRINT READY FOR EXHIBITION

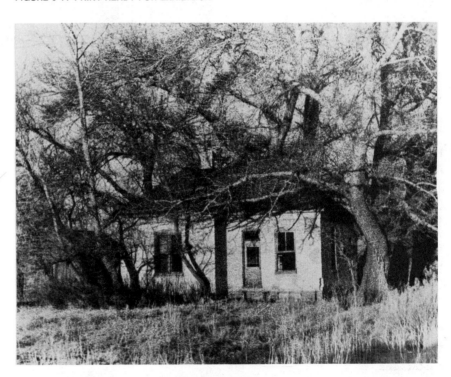

FIGURE 9-12 PRINT MADE USING A TEXTURE SCREEN

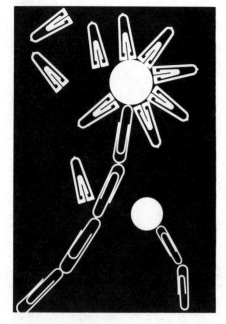

FIGURE 9-13 PHOTOGRAM
This print was made from two kinds of
paper clips, a quarter, and a dime.

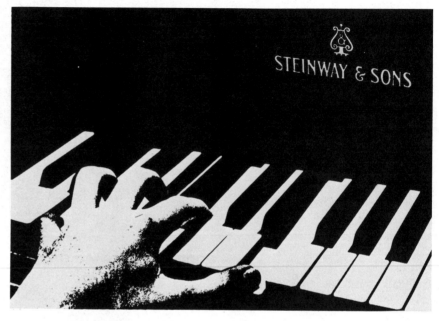

FIGURE 9-14 HIGH-CONTRAST PRINT

Toning

Black and white prints can take on
new interest as a result of toning—
using a chemical to change the color
of the existing images in the picture.
You can re-create the atomsphere and
mood of a scene with toner. Brown
toner, for instance, brings out the
warmth of flesh tones, while blue toner
adds drama to marine and snow
scenes. Use toner according to the
manufacturer's directions during the
processing. Make sure the photograph
will really benefit: toning is a waste of
time unless it will make a real difference in the quality of the photograph.

Photograms

Photograms are photographs made
without a camera. Opaque objects are
placed on a sheet of photographic
paper in the darkroom. The paper is

exposed to light and then processed.
Flat nature objects are popular subjects of photograms. You have probably seen photograms of feathers,
leaves, transparent insect wings,
grasses, or weeds. For a dramatic
effect, you can place objects on a
paper that is being exposed to a negative.

You can make a sophisticated photogram by suspending a sheet of glass
above the paper; this produces a
softer, more blurred effect. If you combine this technique with placing the
objects directly on the paper, you can
get both sharp and blurred objects in
the same photograph. (See Figure
9-13.)

High-contrast prints

A high-contrast print is a black and
white photograph that has no interme-

diate gray tones—the essential shapes
of the photograph are printed in solid
black and white. Cluttered negatives
can be converted into clean, dramatic
photographs by this process. You
need to use high-contrast film and
paper. Most can be used with a safelight. Consult manufacturer's instructions for proper processing times and
techniques. To eliminate small
pinholes that result from dust on the
film, retouch the film using opaque.
You can use either opaque or lithogra-
pher's tape to blot out large areas of
the negative. (See Figure 9-14.)

Combination printing

You can create a stunning photograph
by printing two or more negatives on
the same sheet of photographic paper.
The best candidates for this technique

are negatives with large amounts of blank space where the other images can be imposed. (See Figure 9-15.)

SUMMARY

Once a photographer has mastered the basic printing and darkroom techniques, it is time to venture out—to dare to experiment with new photographic techniques. Prize-winning shots are often those that have been improved by burning-in, dodging, edge-burning, or vignetting or have been altered in the darkroom by any of a number of creative techniques to change the mood and improve the effect. Creative techniques can be used for two purposes: correcting problems and adding impact.

But remember: even the best printing can be a waste of effort if time and care are not taken to use techniques that add stability. Proper processing, printing, mounting, and framing will result in photographs that can provide a vivid history for years to come.

REVIEW QUESTIONS

1 Name the two techniques used in selective exposure.

2 Edge-burning is a specialized type of what technique?

3 Vignetting is a form of what?

4 What is one of the most common problems for beginning photographers?

5 How can you get more contrast from a negative?

6 Which paper produces higher contrast, grade one or grade four?

7 What is the purpose of the hypo clear?

8 What are three creative printing processes?

9 Explain the difference between normal print mounting and mounting for permanence.

10 Why is fixing critical for proper processing for permanence?

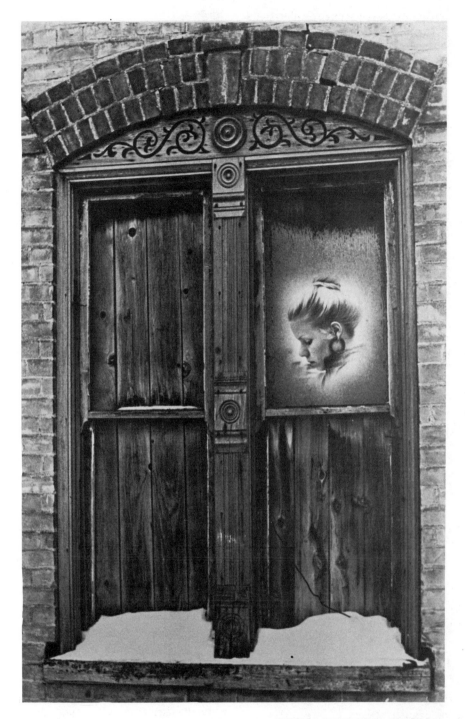

FIGURE 9-15 MULTIPLE-IMAGE PRINT

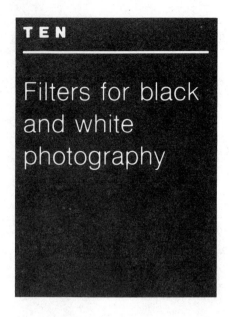

TEN

Filters for black and white photography

When you take a picture, the film records light images reflected from the subject. Both black and white and color pictures are made from reflected rays of colored light. That simple fact creates unique problems for black and white photography. Black and white images are the exceptions in nature—color is the rule. Black and white photography strives to capture and reproduce a vibrant, colorful world only in black, white, and tones of gray.

You can produce more effective black and white photographs by using filters—either glass or gelatin pieces that are attached to the lens of the camera. When filters are properly used, they add a creative touch to ordinary pictures. They can correct for insensitivities of the film, alter the contrast, emphasize certain elements, or create special effects.

LIGHT AND FILTERS

Composition of light

As discussed in Chapter Four, the complete series of electromagnetic waves arranged in order of their wavelengths is termed the *electromagnetic spectrum*. There is no sharp, clear-cut line between one group of waves and another; the electromagnetic spectrum is continuous from the shortest to the longest wavelengths. Photography is mainly concerned with the visible wavelengths. This *visible spectrum* occupies only a small part of the electromagnetic spectrum; it is composed of wavelengths ranging from 400 to 700 nanometers (10.₉ meters). Within these limits the human eye sees a change of wavelength as a change of color. The change from one color to another is not a sharp one, but the visible spectrum can be approximately divided up as shown in Figure 4-2.

We see the colors of the visible spectrum as white light. This white light can actually be considered the sum of the three primary colors of light: red, blue, and green. Any other color of light that we see is a mixture of various amounts of these three. For example, yellow light is made by mixing equal amounts of red and green light.

You can conduct an interesting experiment in color with three projectors. Put a red filter in one, a blue filter in another, and a green filter in the third. Slightly offset the projected images, and see what happens. This is called *additive mixing* of the primary colors. Chapter Fourteen gives more information on the color systems used in photography.

Sensitivity of the human eye to light

It is important to consider *what* the human eye sees and *why*. There are a number of different sensitive regions in the human eye. The eye is most sensitive to green, followed by yellow-green, yellow, and blue-green.

Each of us sees colors in a very personal way. Our perception of one color is influenced by surrounding colors and brightness levels and by the surface texture of the object. Some people suffer from a condition known as color blindness, in which two colors—such as red and green—appear approximately the same. (See Figure 10-1.)

Sensitivity of panchromatic film to light

Unlike the human eye, panchromatic film is most sensitive to blue light. (See Figure 10-2.) Thus, when blue objects are captured on film, they tend to appear brighter than they did in the original scene. Panchromatic film is about equally sensitive to red and green wavelengths, so when red and green objects are photographed they appear as about the same shade of gray in the picture.

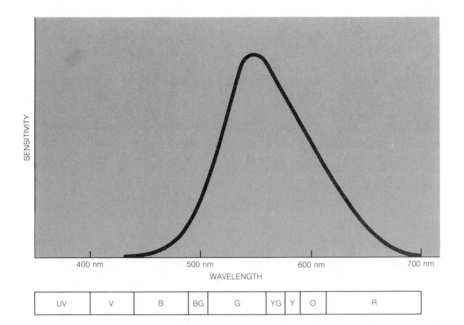

FIGURE 10-1 SENSITIVITY OF THE HUMAN EYE TO LIGHT

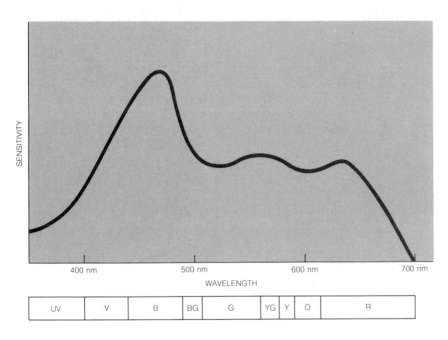

FIGURE 10-2 SENSITIVITY OF PANCHROMATIC FILM TO LIGHT

FIGURE 10-3 ABSORPTION AND REFLECTION
The apple appears red to the eye because its surface absorbs the green and blue wavelengths and reflects the red wavelengths.

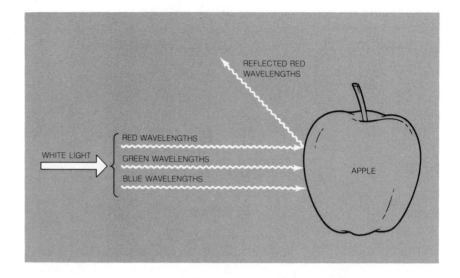

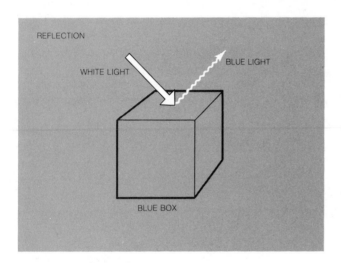

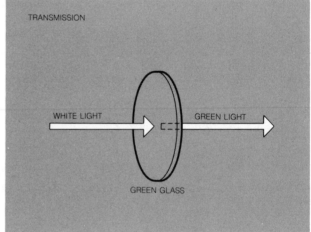

FIGURE 10-4 REFLECTION AND TRANSMISSION
A solid blue box reflects blue light, absorbing red and green.
Green glass transmits green light, absorbing red and blue.

TABLE 10-1 □ ABSORPTION AND TRANSMISSION PROPERTIES OF FILTERS

FILTER	COLORS OF LIGHT ABSORBED	COLORS OF LIGHT TRANSMITTED
Yellow	Blue	Red and Green
Red	Green and Some Blue	Red
Green	Red and Some Blue	Green
Blue	Green and Some Red	Blue

Selective absorption and reflection of light

All matter both absorbs and reflects light. This is why apples are red and leaves are green. Exactly why does an apple look red? White light—composed of red, blue, and green light—strikes the apple. The apple acts as an absorber; it absorbs *most* of the green and blue wavelengths from the white light. It does not completely eliminate any wavelength; very few things are perfect absorbers. The color that is then reflected from the apple, that is, the color the eye sees, is red. The apple selectively absorbs the green and blue wavelengths and reflects the red wavelengths. (See Figure 10-3.)

Colors in nature are usually not pure, because absorption and reflection are rarely complete. Most of the time we see a *mixture* of colors, with one color dominating all the others.

Reflection and transmission

In order to develop an understanding of light and filters, you need to comprehend the difference between reflection and transmission, illustrated in Figure 10-4. Opaque objects, such as desks, chairs, and pencils, *reflect* light; transparent materials, such as colored glass, *transmit* light. In both cases, selective absorption determines the color seen.

COLOR FILTERS FOR BLACK AND WHITE PHOTOGRAPHY

The principle of selective absorption applies to color filters: they always subtract some of the light passing through them. See Table 10-1 for information on the colors of light transmitted and absorbed by different color filters. To get the best results when using colored filters in black and white photography, remember that these filters always subtract something from the image. Get into the habit of thinking of a red filter not as a red filter, but as a filter that absorbs blue and green. This concept—important regardless of the color of filter—defines the way the filter will affect the recording of the image.

When you use a filter, use one designed for photographic use. A handy substitute—a piece of colored glass or film, for example—may have poor optical quality and an uneven or unexpected absorption quality. The result is image distortion. Photographic filters have known absorption characteristics and are manufactured with the necessary optical quality.

You can purchase filters in a number of different forms, the most common being gelatin, acetate, solid glass, and gelatin cemented in glass. Gelatin filters have excellent optical quality. They outperform the best-quality glass filters by producing no image distortion. They are available in a wide range of colors, with various absorption characteristics. Because gelatin filters are easily damaged by handling and heat, it is best to use filters of gelatin cememted between pieces of glass.

The filters used in black and white photography can be classified into three general groups. *Correction filters* change the response of the film to light so that all colors are recorded at approximately the same relative brightness value as the eye sees. *Contrast filters* change the relative brightness values of colors within the scene. *Special-purpose filters* alter the image in ways that neither correction nor contrast filters can.

Correction filters

Panchromatic films respond to all the colors the eye can see, but they do not reproduce them with the same relative brightness as the eye sees. Correction filters correct the image so that it can be reproduced with the same relative brightness as the eye sees. For example, with a filter, green will appear lighter on black and white film than violet does—just as it is viewed by the human eye.

To reproduce the colors in an outdoor scene in the same brightness relationship as your eye sees, use a yellow filter. It will absorb the ultraviolet light and some of the blue light. You can also use a red filter as a correction filter. See Table 10-2 for a list of some correction filters and their uses in black and white photography. Figure 10-5 shows common applications of correction filters in black and white photography.

An object you photograph from a distance may show low contrast because the light that reaches you has been scattered either by the gas molecules that make up the air or by small drops of water in the atmosphere. This scattering does not affect all wavelengths in the same way. It affects ultraviolet wavelengths to the greatest degree,

TABLE 10-2 □ CORRECTION FILTERS FOR BLACK AND WHITE PHOTOGRAPHY

TYPE OF LIGHT SOURCE	BLACK AND WHITE FILM TYPE	UNCORRECTED RENDERING OF COLORS ON PANCHROMATIC FILM		CORRECTION FILTER NEEDED FOR	
		Colors That Appear Too Dark	Colors That Appear Too Light	Partial Correction	Full Correction
Daylight	Panchromatic	Green	Blue	Pale Yellow	Yellow-Green
Tungsten	Panchromatic	Blue	Red	Pale Green-Blue	Blue-Green
Electronic Flash	Panchromatic	—	Blue	—	Pale Yellow

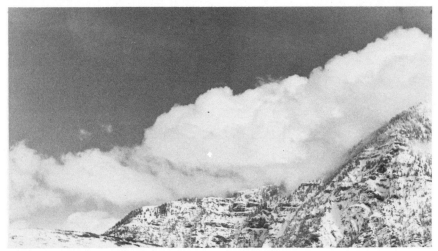

FIGURE 10-5A–C CORRECTION FILTERS
FIGURE 10-5A Taken Without Filtration

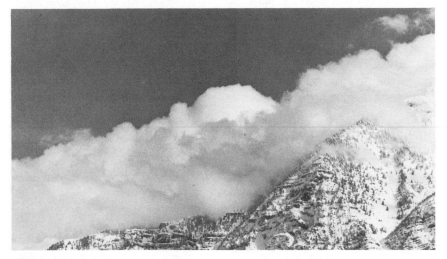

FIGURE 10-5B
Taken with a Yellow Filter

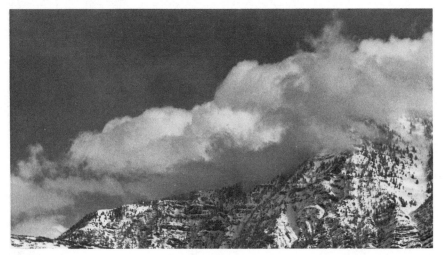

FIGURE 10-5C
Taken with a Red Filter

decreasing steadily in effect through the visible spectrum from violet down to red; it has the least effect on the infrared wavelengths. This means that scattered light has a relatively higher blue content than the original unscattered light. It is also the reason the sky is blue.

All photographic materials have a pronounced sensitivity to the blue and ultraviolet regions of the spectrum, so panchromatic films exposed without a filter give an impression of more haze than the eye sees. To prevent the camera from recording too much haze, you need to use a filter. In order to balance the light properly, the filter must absorb some of the blue wavelengths and transmit most of the red wavelengths. Therefore, a yellow or red filter is best.

Contrast filters

The eye distinguishes between objects by comparing their colors and relative brightness. In a black and white print, these differences are represented by differences in contrast. This can be controlled by contrast filters.

Contrast filters make a color appear lighter or darker than it would normally be recorded by the film; certain contrast filters make one color appear darker and another appear lighter simultaneously. For example, consider a subject that has areas of green, red, yellow, and blue. These areas have considerable color contrast, but the lighting makes the subject appear as though there were little difference in brightness between the colors. An uncorrected rendering would show blue as the brightest color, with little contrast between the shades of gray that record the red, green, and yellow. A contrast filter provides the tone separation necessary to create distinct variations between the shades of gray that represent the different colors. (See Figure 10-6.) Contrast filters allow for the most objective reproduction with black and white film. Table 10-3 lists the most important contrast

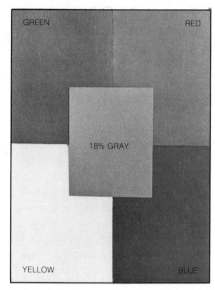

FIGURE 10-6A
Normal Exposure, No Filter

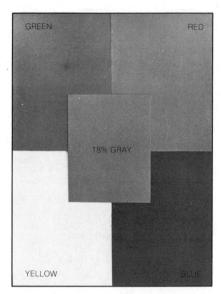

FIGURE 10-6B
Yellow Filter

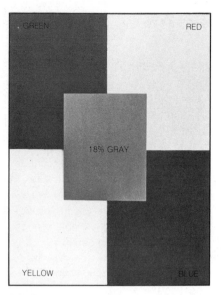

FIGURE 10-6C
Red Filter

FIGURE 10-6A–E RED, YELLOW, GREEN, AND BLUE FILTERS AND THE COLOR BOARD

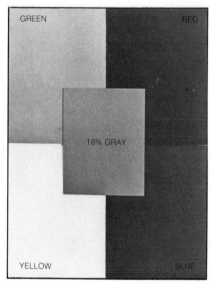

FIGURE 10-6D
Green Filter

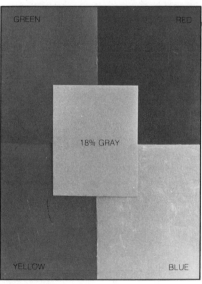

FIGURE 10-6E
Blue Filter

TABLE 10-3 □ CONTRAST FILTERS FOR BLACK AND WHITE PHOTOGRAPHY

SUBJECT COLOR	TO DARKEN TONES	TO LIGHTEN TONES
Yellows	Blue 47	Yellow 8, 15; Yellow-Green 11, 13; Red 25; Green 58
Greens	Blue 47; Magenta 33; Red 25	Yellow 8, 15; Yellow-Green 11, 13; Green 58; Cyan 44
Cyans	Red 25	Green 58; Cyan 44; Blue 47
Blues	Red 25; Green 58; Yellow 8, 15; Yellow-Green 11, 13	Blue 47; Cyan 44; Magenta 33
Magentas	Green 58; Yellow-Green 11, 13	Blue 47; Magenta 33; Red 25
Reds	Green 58; Cyan 44; Blue 42	Red 25; Magenta 33; Yellow 8, 15
Oranges	Green 58; Cyan 44; Blue 47	Red 25; Magenta 33; Yellow 8, 15

Numbers are those of Kodak filters.

filters used in black and white photography.

When you are selecting contrast filters to use in black and white photography, it is important to make a critical distinction: *monochromatic filters* are used to change the contrast between objects of different colors when one is shooting pictures; variable-contrast filters are used to change the contrast grade of variable-contrast photographic printing papers. You cannot use a variable-contrast filter to add or subtract contrast while you are shooting the picture, nor can you use a monochromatic filter to boost contrast while you are printing. Make sure you use the right kind of contrast filter for the job.

Two basic guidelines will help you in your selection of correction or contrast filters:

1 To lighten a color in the final print, use a filter that transmits that particular wavelength.

2 To darken a color in the final print, use a filter that transmits that particular wavelength poorly or not at all.

See Table 10-4 for a summary of color filters for black and white photography.

Filters for special purposes

Ultraviolet-absorbing filters The human eye is insensitive to ultraviolet (UV) radiation, but, as previously mentioned, all photographic materials possess considerable sensitivity to it. Since UV radiation is strongly scattered by haze, black and white photographs taken in hazy conditions lose contrast and color photographs show a strong blue cast.

Usually, the farther you are from the subject, the more haze or blueness will be recorded on film. To reduce such an effect, use an ultraviolet filter (sometimes called a skylight filter). Besides eliminating the hazy or blue cast, an ultraviolet filter reduces the effect of excessive scattered ultraviolet light in blue sky. This type of filter works equally well with color and with black and white film.

Most ultraviolet filters are colorless or very pale pink or yellow. Many photographers use them as optical lens caps to protect the front element of the camera lens from damage—it is less expensive to replace even a high-quality filter than it is to replace or repair a lens. (See Figure 10-7.)

Polarizing filters Light rays travel in straight lines, vibrating in all directions

TABLE 10-4 □ SUMMARY OF FILTERS FOR BLACK AND WHITE PHOTOGRAPHY

IF YOU ARE SHOOTING THIS:	USE THIS FILTER:	TO GET THIS EFFECT:
Blue Sky	Yellow 8	Natural
	Deep Yellow 15	Darkened
	Red 25	Spectacular
	Deep Red 29	Very Dark
	Red 25 with Polarizing Screen	Night
Marine Scene with Blue Sky	Yellow 8	Natural
	Deep Yellow 15	Dark Water
Sunset	None; Yellow 8	Natural
	Deep Yellow 15; Red 25	Increased Brilliance
Distant Landscape	Blue 47	Increased Haze
	None	Slightly Increased Haze
	Yellow 8	Natural
	Deep Yellow 15	Decreased Haze
	Red 25; Deep Red 29	Greatly Decreased Haze
Stone, Wood, Brick, Sand, Snow, Cloth, etc. in Bright Sunlight	Yellow 8	Natural
	Deep Yellow 15; Red 25	Increased Texture
Nearby Foliage	Yellow 8; Yellow-Green 11	Natural
	Green 58	Light
Flowers and Leaves	Yellow 8; Yellow-Green 11	Natural
Outdoor Portraits	Yellow-Green 11; Yellow 8; Polarizing Screen	Natural

Numbers are those of Kodak Filters.

FIGURE 10-7A
Without Filter

FIGURE 10-7C
With a Medium Yellow Filter (Kodak Number 8)

FIGURE 10-7B
With a UV Filter

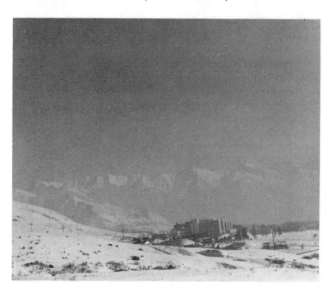

FIGURE 10-7D
With a Red Filter (Kodak Number 25)

FIGURE 10-7A–D HAZE PENETRATION

FIGURE 10-8 POLARIZED AND UNPOLARIZED LIGHT
Unpolarized light can vibrate at any angle. Polarized light vibrates in only one plane. Long arrows show the direction of the light's motion—i.e., radiation, reflection, or refraction. Short arrows show the direction of the light's vibration.

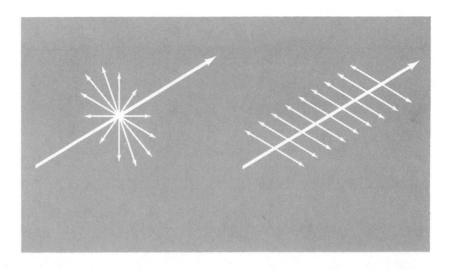

FIGURE 10-9 HOW A POLARIZER WORKS
When the polarizing filter is oriented in the direction of vibration, polarized light can pass through. When the polarizer is oriented against the direction of vibration, polarized light cannot pass through.

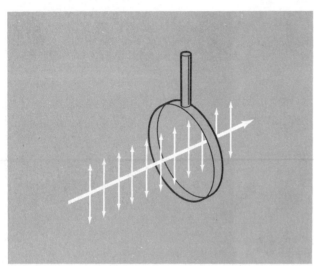
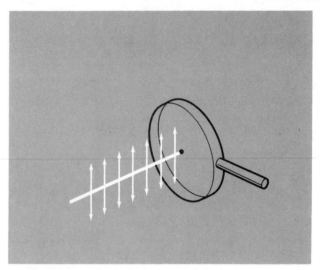

FIGURE 10-10 HAND INDICATOR FOR SKY SHOTS

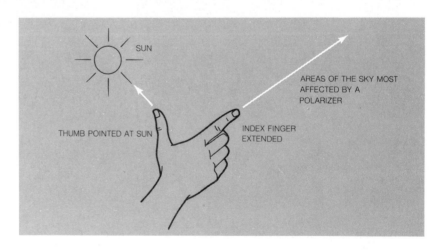

perpendicular to their direction of travel. When light rays hit a nonmetallic surface, only the vibrations in a single plane are reflected. The others are reduced or sometimes eliminated completely. The light reflected in a single plane is called *polarized light.* An interesting example of polarized light is sunlight that has passed through the atmosphere: as each ray of light is reflected from a nonmetallic molecule or particle in the atmosphere, that ray becomes polarized. (See Figure 10-8 and 10-9 .)

There are two major applications of polarizing filters:

1 *To control the rendering of the sky.* In a clear blue sky, the light that comes from opposite the sun is partially polarized. You can quickly locate the partially polarized area in the sky by forming an L shape with your thumb and index finger. When your thumb is pointing at the sun, your index finger will be pointing at the partially polarized area of the sky. (See Figure 10-10.) Placing a polarized filter over the camera lens will make the sky in this region darker than normal. (See Figure 10-11.) The advantage of a polarizing filter over a normal filter is that it does not distort the color rendering—a fact that makes it extremely useful in black and white photography as well as in color photography.

2 *To reduce unwanted reflections.* Light that is reflected from a shiny nonmetallic surface can be considered to be polarized, so polarizing filters can control reflections from most such surfaces. The filters are commonly used to reduce reflection from glass, wood, paint, paper, and any wet surface. You can use a polarizing filter to reduce the glare from swimming pools or other bodies of water and from windows and other glass-fronted objects. (See Figure 10-12.)

You can find out what effect the polarizing filter will have by looking through the filter at the subject. If the filter is on a single lens reflex camera, you can easily see the effect through the viewfinder. Rotate the filter slowly until you obtain the best effect. Then

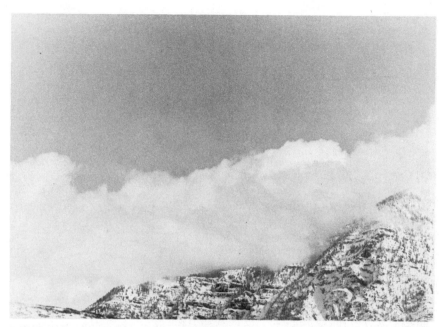

FIGURE 10-11A WITHOUT A POLARIZING FILTER

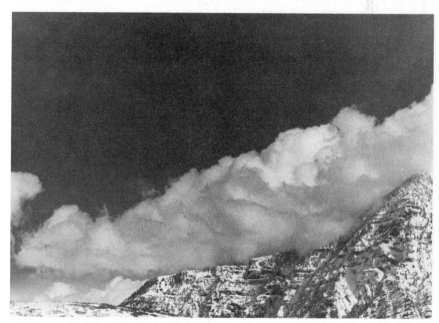

FIGURE 10-11B WITH A POLARIZING FILTER

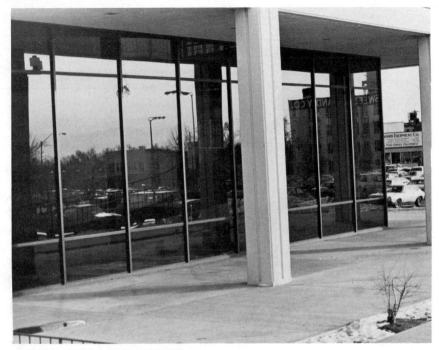

FIGURE 10-12A WITHOUT A POLARIZER
Note the reflections on the glass wall.

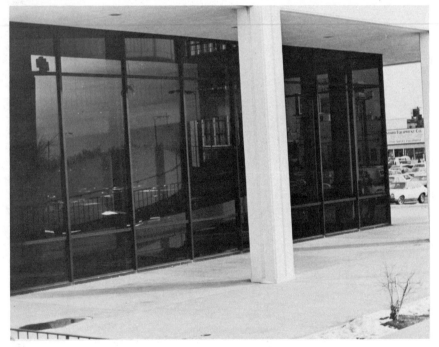

FIGURE 10-12B WITH A POLARIZER The polarizer eliminates most of the reflection.

note the position of the marks on the edge of the filter. When you take the photograph, make sure these marks are in the position noted.

Polarizing filters only work with polarized light, such as sunlight or artificial illumination that has been passed through polarizers, and can be rotated for different effects. When held parallel to the plane of vibration, the polarizing filter will transmit the polarized light and thus will not affect the reflections. If you rotate the filter 90 degrees, the filter will eliminate the polarized light, removing the reflection or darkening the sky.

Soft-focus attachments Soft-focus attachments are popular in certain types of photography, such as portraiture, because they give a soft misty effect by spreading the highlights of a subject into adjacent areas. The softening of the image is caused by the filter's scattering, refraction, and diffraction of the light. Some soft-focus filters have a clear center area and soft edges. Others render the entire image in soft focus. (See Figure 10-13.)

An inexpensive way to experiment with soft focus is to use an ultraviolet or skylight filter with a very thin layer of petroleum jelly on it. To achieve a more delicate effect, spray an ultraviolet or skylight filter with aerosol hair spray; the thickness of the coating will determine the softening effect. Make sure you apply either the petroleum jelly or the hair spray on the filter surface closer to the subject and *before* you put the filter on the camera.

Cross-screen or star-burst filters Closely spaced lines engraved on glass will cause diffraction of the image. The diffraction produced by a cross-screen filter elongates small, intense highlights, giving a star effect. This procedure does not seriously affect overall image definition, and can create a dazzling effect at night or after a rainstorm. (See Figure 10-14.)

Neutral-density filters Neutral-density filters absorb all wavelengths of light equally and thus appear gray in color. They reduce the amount of light that passes through the lens, but they do not change the rendition of the colors in the scene. They are available in varying densities; you may need to combine two of them to achieve the density you need for photographing a certain scene. (See Table 10-5.)

Two common applications of neutral density filters are

1 When you photograph a subject in brilliant sunlight, the filter protects the picture from being overexposed by the bright light.

2 When you photograph fast-action shots, the filter allows you to pan and follow the action for a sharply focused subject and an out-of-focus background.

DETERMINING CORRECT EXPOSURE USING FILTER FACTORS

In order to achieve properly exposed results when you are using any kind of filter, it is necessary to increase the exposure, because a filter always absorbs some of the light that passes through it. To increase the exposure, you either increase the exposure time or use a larger aperture.

To help you determine exposure when you use a filter, all filters are assigned a number based on the ratio of filtered exposure to unfiltered exposure. This number is called the *filter factor*. For example, a yellow filter has a filter factor of 2, and a dark red filter has a factor of 16. The equation is simple:

$$\text{Filter Factor} = \frac{\text{Exposure with Filter}}{\text{Exposure without Filter}}$$

The filter factor tells you the number of stops you need to open up to compensate for use of the filter. In other words, it tells you how much extra exposure is necessary to make up for the light that is absorbed by the filter.

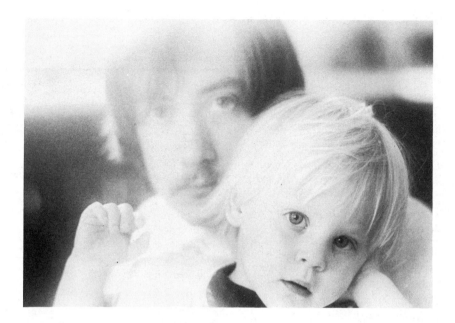

FIGURE 10-13 SOFT FOCUS
(Terry Ashe)

FIGURE 10-14 CROSS-SCREEN FILTER
(Joseph C. Lawless)

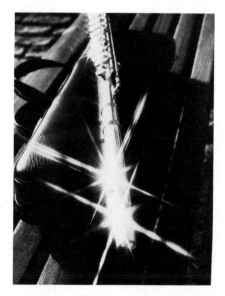

TABLE 10-5 □ NEUTRAL-DENSITY FILTERS

FILTER	PERCENTAGE OF INCIDENT LIGHT TRANSMITTED	FILTER FACTOR	INCREASE IN EXPOSURE (STOPS)
0.1	80	$1\frac{1}{4}$	$\frac{1}{3}$
0.2	63	$1\frac{1}{2}$	$\frac{2}{3}$
0.3	50	2	1
0.4	40	$2\frac{1}{2}$	$1\frac{1}{3}$
0.5	32	3	$1\frac{2}{3}$
0.6	25	4	2
0.7	20	5	$2\frac{1}{3}$
0.8	16	6	$2\frac{2}{3}$
0.9	13	8	3
1.0	10	10	$3\frac{1}{3}$
2.0	1	100	$6\frac{2}{3}$
3.0	0.1	1000	10
4.0	0.01	10000	$13\frac{1}{3}$

Some common filters with their factor numbers and appropriate exposure compensations are listed in Table 10-6. To determine how many additional stops to open up your exposure when using a filter, follow these steps:

1 Determine how many times two would have to be multiplied by itself to equal the filter factor number.

2 Increase the exposure by that many stops.

If a filter has a filter factor of two, then a one-stop increase in exposure is needed to yield an exposure equivalent to that of the unfiltered scene (2 = 2). A filter factor of four requires a two-stop increase in exposure (2 × 2 = 4). If the factor number is eight, then you would have to open the aperture by three stops (2 × 2 × 2 = 8). See Table 10-7 for a summary of this relationship. If the exposure compensation is calculated to be a fraction, the closest whole number should be used.

You should note that a filter has a different factor number for daylight than for tungsten light. *Daylight* is considered to be any type of lighting that originates with the sun; *tungsten* is any kind of artificial illumination. The factor numbers are not the same, because the different kinds of light contain differing amounts of the primary colors, red, blue, and green.

EXPOSURE METERS

A single lens reflex camera with a built-in light meter has an advantage when you are working with filters. When the filter is placed in front of the lens, the meter automatically makes the necessary exposure adjustment. In other words, you do not have to worry about figuring out the exposure using filter factors.

Cameras incorporating through-the-lens exposure metering should give the correct compensation for neutral density and correction filters, but you

TABLE 10-6 □ FILTER FACTORS

FILTER	DAYLIGHT FILTER FACTOR	DAYLIGHT INCREASE EXPOSURE (F/STOPS)	TUNGSTEN LIGHT FILTER FACTOR	TUNGSTEN LIGHT INCREASE EXPOSURE (F/STOPS)
Light Yellow 3	1.5	$\frac{2}{3}$	None	None
Yellow 4	1.5	$\frac{2}{3}$	1.5	$\frac{2}{3}$
Light Yellow 6	1.5	$\frac{2}{3}$	1.5	$\frac{2}{3}$
Yellow 8	2	1	1.5	$\frac{2}{3}$
Deep Yellow 9	2	1	1.5	$\frac{2}{3}$
Yellow-Green 11	4	2	4	2
Deep Yellow 12	2	1	1.5	$\frac{2}{3}$
Dark Yellow-Green 13	5	$2\frac{1}{3}$	4	2
Deep Yellow 15	2.5	$1\frac{1}{3}$	1.5	$\frac{2}{3}$
Light Red 23A	6	$2\frac{2}{3}$	3	$1\frac{2}{3}$
Red 25	8	3	5	$2\frac{1}{3}$
Deep Red 29	16	4	8	3
Blue 47	6	$2\frac{2}{3}$	12	$3\frac{2}{3}$
Deep Blue 47B	8	3	16	4
Deep Blue 50	20	$4\frac{1}{3}$	40	$5\frac{1}{3}$
Green 58	6	$2\frac{2}{3}$	6	$2\frac{2}{3}$
Deep Green 61	12	$3\frac{2}{3}$	12	$3\frac{2}{3}$
Gray Polarizing Screen	2.5	$1\frac{1}{3}$	2.5	$1\frac{1}{3}$

Numbers are those of Kodak filters.

TABLE 10-7 □ FILTER-FACTOR CALCULATIONS

FILTER-FACTOR CALCULATION	NUMBER OF STOPS TO OPEN UP	SAMPLE EXPOSURE COMPENSATION F/NUMBER	SAMPLE EXPOSURE COMPENSATION SHUTTER SPEED
$1 = 2^0 = 1$	0	f/5.6	60
$2 = 2^1 = 2$	1	f/5.6	30
$4 = 2^2 = 2 \times 2$	2	f/4.0	30
$6 \approx 2^{2.5} \approx 2 \times 2 \times 1.5$	$2\frac{1}{2}$	f/3.5	30
$8 = 2^3 = 2 \times 2 \times 2$	3	f/2.8	30
$16 = 2^4 = 2 \times 2 \times 2 \times 2$	4	f/2.8	15

should quickly check them against the filter factor numbers because the sensitivity of certain measuring photocells varies.

SUMMARY

Trying to photograph a vibrant, colorful world with black and white film presents some unique challenges for the photographer. A keen understanding of the properties of light and the primary colors will enable the photographer to use filters and other equipment that will render black and white photographs brilliant in message and contrast.

Many professionals use filters extensively for black and white photography, either for such obvious purposes as lightening leaves and darkening apples on a tree with a green filter or for more subtle purposes that require a trained eye to recognize. Filters provide creative possibilities for enhancing the rendition of a scene. These important parts of the photographer's tool kit help make the final print more like the visualized scene.

REVIEW QUESTIONS

1 What are the three primary colors of light?

2 Which wavelengths of light is the human eye most sensitive to?

3 Which wavelengths is panchromatic film most sensitive to?

4 On what principle do color filters work in black and white photography?

5 What two rules should you use when selecting a color filter to use in black and white photography?

6 What do correction filters do?

7 What do contrast filters do?

8 Name three special-purpose filters.

9 What is assigned to each filter to help a photographer determine the correct exposure compensation?

10 If a filter had a filter factor number of eight, how many stops would you have to open up to compensate for use of the filter?

11 Give an example of a correction filter and a contrast filter.

12 What type of filters helps prevent the effects of haze in photos?

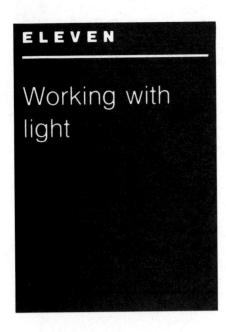

ELEVEN

Working with light

Light, that amazing form of energy that makes vision possible and colors our world so vividly, is the very essense of photography. A photographer must study light carefully, giving it as much attention as is given the people, buildings, and other objects captured on film. An actor's face exists without makeup—but makeup emphasizes certain characteristics, covers up others, and gives form, volume, and definition to the face. The same is true of photography and light. While your scene exists on its own, you must use light to stress its striking points, deemphasize the ordinary, and give form, beauty, and volume to the whole.

Creative photographers see more than subjects when they shoot; they see the light that creates and enhances the subjects' appeal. Simply stated, photography is painting with light. It is critical that you know how to use light to your advantage and how to create photographs with the light that is available.

Eyes are designed to see nothing but light. But sometimes it is difficult to determine exactly what the light is doing. Our eyes jump lazily from place to place, never focusing on any one thing long enough to really capture and understand what the light is doing. One of the most important things you as a photographer can do is learn to slow down and really study light. What kind of contrast exists? How solid is the object? Is there a way to capture a feeling of separation and depth? You will find this to be exhausting at first, but persevere—the rewards are great.

Technically, to *see* is simply to take in light rays through the eye and to interpret what the light rays mean. During fleeting moments when it is necessary for day-to-day survival or when we see something unusually interesting, most of us become aware of the visual elements around us. The rest of the time, seeing is rather a per-functory act. We see, but we rarely think about it. As a photographer, you must learn to become visually aware of all the light around you. You must learn to recognize color, texture, tone, line, and contrast, and you must learn how they relate to one another in what you see. Most important, you must develop a profound awareness of how you feel when you see the world around you. You need to realize what emotions the visible world creates in you. Photography is a way to share with others what you see and what you feel.

SOURCES OF LIGHT

Basically, there are two sources of light: primary sources emit light, and secondary sources reflect light. Anything that is not totally black is either a primary or a secondary source of light. (Most of the references in photography to "source light" refer to primary sources of light, such as the sun or a spotlight, but everything you see that is not black emits or reflects some kind of light.) Primary sources of light can be divided into two broad categories: natural and artificial.

Natural light sources

The ultimate source of all natural light is sunlight; all photographic light, whether natural or artificial, either uses or imitates the light of the sun. But natural light includes more than just direct sunlight.

Daylight consists of two elements: sunlight and skylight. On a clear day, daylight is approximately 80 to 90 percent sunlight, that is, light coming directly from the sun, and 10 to 20 percent skylight, or sunlight that has been scattered in the atmosphere. On a cloudy or hazy day, the percentages change to mostly skylight and very little sunlight. The intensity of the shadows and the luminance range of a scene are determined by the ratio of sunlight to skylight.

Artificial light sources

Often, natural light is the only choice you have. It would be impractical, for example, to shoot a distant mountain peak with anything but natural light. Other subjects, however, lend themselves better to the use of artificial light—any light source that is contrived, controlled, and manipulated by the photographer. The most common artificial light sources include electronic flash units, flashbulbs, floodlights, spotlights, studio strobes, tungsten lightbulbs, and fluorescent tubes.

EXISTING LIGHT

Existing light is the light that falls on a scene or subject. It can be provided by either natural or artificial sources. Whatever the intensity, quality, or type of illumination, existing light—also called available light—is what you have to work with at the scene.

Working with light

One of the challenges of photography is visualizing what the film will see before the picture is exposed. As you try to create the desired rendition of the subject in the viewfinder, you must consider the direction and quality of the existing light.

Light direction is determined by the relationship among the subject, the light source, and the camera, that is, by their relative positions. It influences how the texture, modeling, and illusion of depth and dimension appear in the photograph. *Light quality,* or the evenness of illumination, plays an equally important role. Direct sunlight is quite different illumination from the light in the shade of a building, for instance.

Frontlighting

Frontlighting a subject means placing the light source either at the camera position or directly behind and above the camera. (See Figures 11-1 and 11-2.) The closer the light source is to

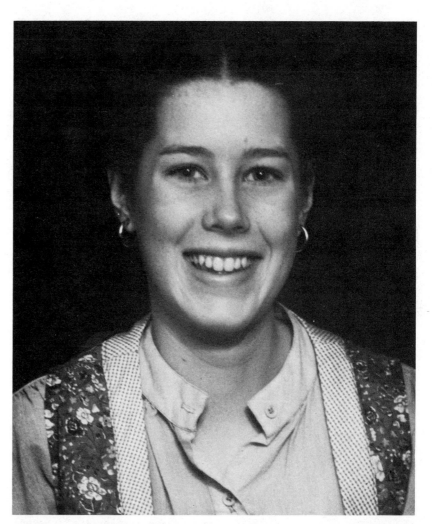

FIGURE 11-1 FRONTLIGHTING (Photo: Laird Roberts)

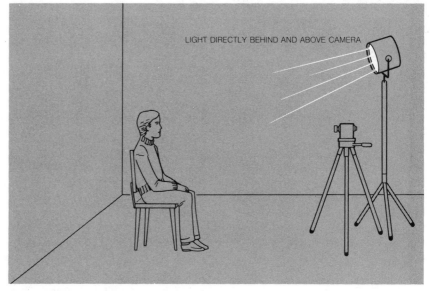

LIGHT DIRECTLY BEHIND AND ABOVE CAMERA

FIGURE 11-2 FRONTLIGHTING DIAGRAM

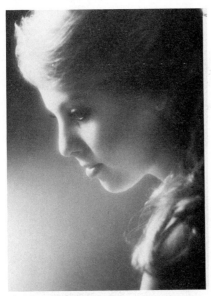

FIGURE 11-3 THREE-QUARTER LIGHTING

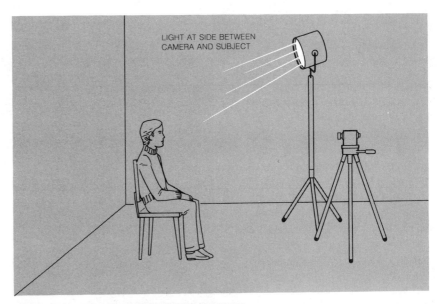

LIGHT AT SIDE BETWEEN CAMERA AND SUBJECT

FIGURE 11-4 THREE-QUARTER LIGHTING DIAGRAM

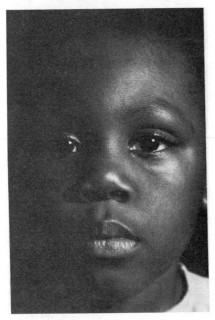

FIGURE 11-5 SIDELIGHTING
(Kenneth C. Jennings Jr.)

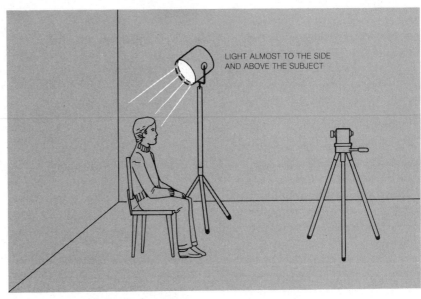

LIGHT ALMOST TO THE SIDE AND ABOVE THE SUBJECT

FIGURE 11-6 SIDELIGHTING DIAGRAM

the camera position, the more severe the frontlighting. With frontlighting, the light strikes the subject head-on.

A classic example of natural frontlighting is positioning a subject facing a morning or afternoon sun.

Frontlighting tends to reduce texture, roundness, and volume in subjects. Many necessary shadows are eliminated, and the subject does not seem to occupy space. The three-dimensional feeling in the photograph is lost.

Three-quarter lighting

The famous "Rembrandt" lighting—a small triangular patch of light on one cheek just below the eye—is especially effective in portrait photography. To create the effect, place your light source above and to one side of the camera. For best results, the light source should be about 45 degrees away from and above the camera position, as measured from the subject. (See Figures 11-3 and 11-4.)

Sidelighting

In sidelighting, the light source can come from either the right or the left side of the camera position. The light

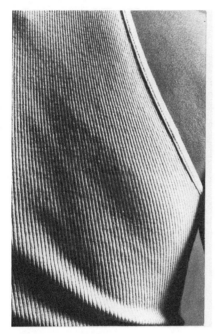

FIGURE 11-7 CROSSLIGHTING
(Debra M. Jacob)

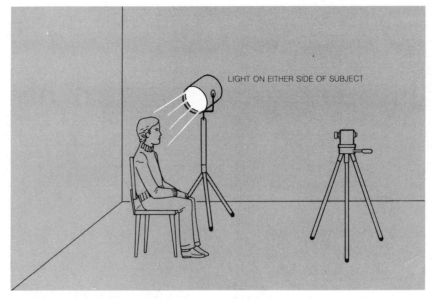

FIGURE 11-8 CROSSLIGHTING DIAGRAM

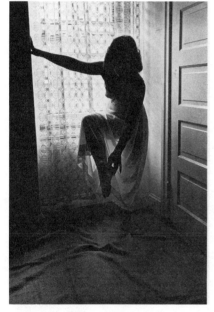
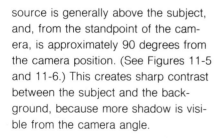

FIGURE 11-9 BACKLIGHTING
(Diane Biondi)

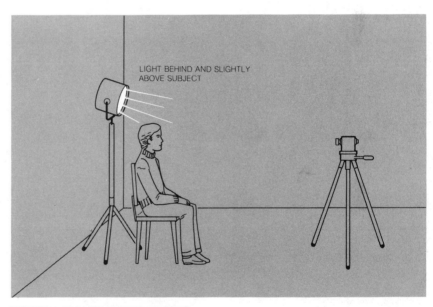

FIGURE 11-10 BACKLIGHTING DIAGRAM

source is generally above the subject, and, from the standpoint of the camera, is approximately 90 degrees from the camera position. (See Figures 11-5 and 11-6.) This creates sharp contrast between the subject and the background, because more shadow is visible from the camera angle.

Crosslighting Extreme sidelighting, in which the light source is about 90 degrees from the camera position and level with the subject, is called *crosslighting*. Crosslight virtually skims the surface of the subject, producing maximum texture and illuminating even the smallest detail on one side, while casting a long, dark shadow on the other side. (See Figure 11-7 and 11-8.)

Backlighting
As the name implies, backlighting means that the light comes into the camera from behind and above the subject. (See Figures 11-9 and 11-10.) Backlighting offers numerous creative possibilities.

Because backlight shines into the camera and surrounds the subject with light, it casts a shadow toward

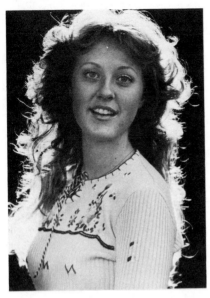

FIGURE 11-11 BACKLIGHTING WITH A FILL
(Photo: Laird Roberts)

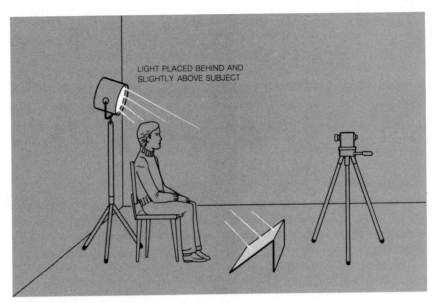

FIGURE 11-12 BACKLIGHTING WITH A FILL DIAGRAM

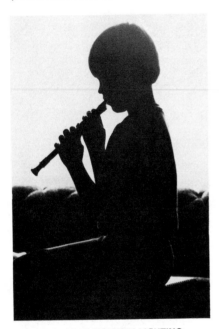

FIGURE 11-13 SILHOUETTE LIGHTING
(Photo: Laird Roberts)

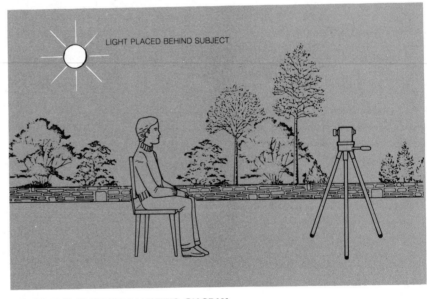

FIGURE 11-14 SILHOUETTE LIGHTING DIAGRAM

the camera. When the subject is seen in its own shadow, exposure meter reading can be difficult. Make sure the exposure meter is in approximately the same light as the subject. Backlight shining into the meter will cause it to make incorrect recommendations. (Backlighting with direct sunlight is also extremely difficult, since there is marked contrast between the highlight and shadow areas.)

Backlighting with fill-in The contrast in backlighted subjects can be reduced by brightening or lightening the shadow areas with a flash, reflectors, or both. Reflectors may be a sheet of white mount board, cardboard covered with gold or aluminum foil, the wall of a building, sand, or snow. Whatever kind of reflector you use, its purpose is to reflect some of the light back into the shadow areas of the subject, reducing the contrast. (See Figures 11-11 and 11-12.)

Photographing people in backlight with fill-in can yield especially effec-

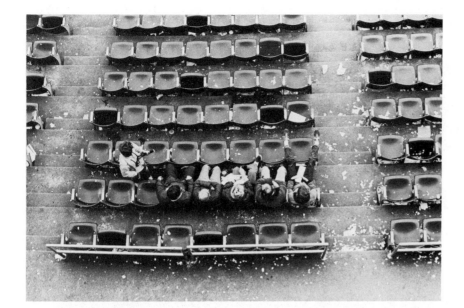

FIGURE 11-15 DIFFUSE LIGHT
(Linda P. Montague)

FIGURE 11-16 DIFFUSE LIGHTING DIAGRAM

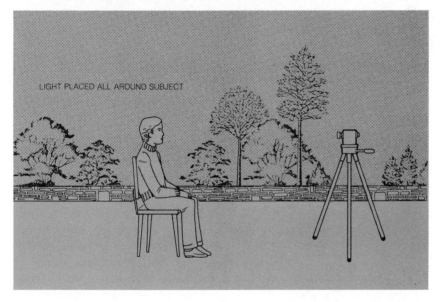

LIGHT PLACED ALL AROUND SUBJECT

tive, interesting photographs. The background has the same backlighting as the foreground: leaves on trees, especially in autumn, become a brilliant color backdrop; grasses and flowers in a field take on a soft glow; and sunlight reflected on water is transformed into diffused circles.

Silhouette lighting Silhouette lighting is a special application of backlighting. Silhouette meter readings are taken from the sky or the backlight source, so the subject is purposely underexposed. This makes possible dramatic sky exposures, with the subject appearing as a black silhouette against a sunset or skyline. (See Figure 11-13 and 11-14.)

Diffuse lighting

Diffuse light is light that comes from many directions. A good example of natural diffuse light is skylight on an overcast day. Depending on the density of the clouds, sunlight is diffused to various degrees through the clouds, shadows are softened, and the contrast between highlight and shadows decreases. Diffuse light produces soft natural shadows and textural highlights. (See Figures 11-15 and 11-16.) Light diffused by mist or fog is excel-

lent for capturing a soft, somber mood.

Once you learn to use light to your advantage, you will become aware not only of the changes in light quality but also of subtle changes produced by using various lighting arrangements.

FLASH PHOTOGRAPHY

Although many of today's films and cameras make it easy to take pictures in any kind of light, you will probably find that using a flash provides you with extra options you don't have with

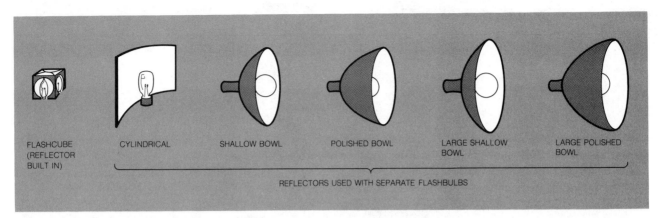

FIGURE 11-17 SOME COMMON TYPES OF REFLECTORS

FLASHCUBE (REFLECTOR BUILT IN)

CYLINDRICAL

SHALLOW BOWL

POLISHED BOWL

LARGE SHALLOW BOWL

LARGE POLISHED BOWL

REFLECTORS USED WITH SEPARATE FLASHBULBS

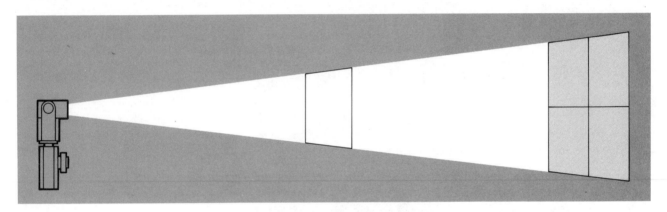

FIGURE 11-18 INVERSE-SQUARE CHART
At double the distance, there is one-fourth the illumination ($\frac{1}{2}^2 = \frac{1}{4}$); at triple the distance, there is one-ninth the illumination ($\frac{1}{3}^2 = \frac{1}{9}$); at four times the distance, there is one-sixteenth the illumination ($\frac{1}{4}^2 = \frac{1}{16}$); etc.

FIGURE 11-19 LIMITATIONS OF FLASHES
Flashcubes can illuminate a subject 8–10 feet from the camera; large flashes can go out to about 75–100 feet.

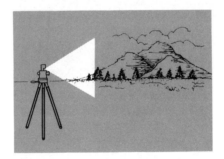

According to the inverse-square law, the following shows how much light is left at the indicated distance. Note that these amounts are relative to the amount at a distance of one foot, which has been given the value of one.

DISTANCE FROM FLASH TO SUBJECT	AMOUNT OF LIGHT ON SUBJECT
1'	1
5'	$\frac{1}{25}$
10'	$\frac{1}{100}$
20'	$\frac{1}{400}$
40'	$\frac{1}{1600}$
80'	$\frac{1}{6400}$

natural lighting. A flash allows you to take pictures in near or total darkness, to stop action, and to create greater depth of field. With a flash, you can use auxiliary lenses with smaller maximum apertures and you can use slower speed, fine-grained film. Although flashbulbs are still available and can be used on many cameras, electronic flash units are generally easier and less expensive to use. (See Figure 11-17.)

Inverse square law and guide numbers

An understanding of the inverse square law will let you more accurately calculate your flash needs as you take pictures. The amount of light falling on the subject is inversely proportionate to the square of the distance. In other words, the farther the light gets from the source, the more it spreads out. The light will cover four times as much area at twelve feet as it will at six feet, so exposure for a subject that is twelve feet from the flash must be four times (two f/stops) what it would be if the subject were only six feet from the flash. With each doubling of the distance, we lose two f/stops. If the subject is twenty-four feet from the flash, there will be sixteen times as much area to cover (four f/stops) as there would be at six feet. (See Figure 11-18.)

If all this seems a little complicated to you, you should be relieved to find out that film and flash manufacturers provide guide numbers. These guide numbers are calculated by a formula that considers the speed of the film, the reflector factor (determined by the shape and surface of the globe or flash), and the lamp's effective light output at a particular shutter speed. The guide numbers are printed on a chart that comes with the flash equipment, flashbulbs, or film. If you know your film speed and the shutter speed you will be using, you can consult the chart and find the guide number. To determine the correct f/number, divide the guide number by the distance in feet from the flash lamp to the subject.

Remember, guide numbers are just that: guides based on averages. They give you instructions based on an indoor shot taken in an average-sized room with light-color walls and ceiling. If you take a picture in a small, dimly lit room or in one with many bright, reflecting surfaces, you will have to make adjustments—open up one stop for large rooms, dimly lit rooms, or pictures taken outside at night; close down one stop for a small room or for one with many bright reflective surfaces. (See Figure 11-19.)

Electronic flash

The flash from electronic flash units is so fast—usually less than $\frac{1}{1500}$ second— that it is quicker than even the fastest shutter speed. The basic electronic flash unit is a flash tube, powered by a battery-fed capacitor. Energy is stored in the capacitor and is released to produce the flash.

Most inexpensive cameras have flash units powered by conventional batteries, so you have to replace them when their energy is drained. If you forget, you will not have a flash when you need it. More expensive units are powered by nicad (nickel-cadmium) batteries. Even though they can be recharged many times, they drain relatively quickly and do not recycle through the capacitor as fast as conventional batteries do. As a result, with many nicad-powered flashes, you cannot shoot pictures in rapid-fire succession. You have to wait a few seconds between pictures while the capacitor charge builds up.

Despite the disadvantage of slow recycle time, nicad batteries are preferred by most professional photographers. Many nicad units are available with tilting heads that allow the light to be bounced off objects easily, with attachments such as cords and diffusers, and with zoom heads that change the lighted area to match different lenses.

Synchronizing the flash

Because the flash of an electronic unit is extremely rapid, it is very important that the flash and the shutter be synchronized so the shutter opens at the precise instant of the flash. In many of the new cameras, when you plug in the flash cord or insert the flash unit into the hot shoe, the synchronization is automatically set. If your camera does not automatically adjust for synchronization, consult your instruction manual. Many older cameras have a hot shoe that can be adjusted for electronic flash; some have a pair of flash-cord sockets. A socket marked M or FP is intended for a flashbulb; a socket marked with an X is usually intended for an electronic flash unit. Your instruction manual will give you details about setting synchronization for your particular camera.

The flash and exposure time

When you use electronic flash equipment, it is the length of the flash that determines exposure—not the camera's shutter speed. If you are shooting with a flash, then, your shutter speed will remain constant, and you will need to adjust only the aperture. With a simple, manually operated camera, you can use guide numbers to determine the aperture opening. Use the formula explained under "Inverse Square Law": divide the guide number by the distance from the subject to the flash unit to obtain the correct f/number. Since guide numbers are based on averages, run a test of your own electronic flash unit to determine its power, then make any necessary adjustments. Table 11-1 gives typical guide numbers for an electronic flash.

Automatic electronic flash

You will not have to bother with guide numbers if you have an automatic electronic

TABLE 11-1 □ GUIDELINES FOR ELECTRONIC FLASH WITH ASA 125 FILM

BCPS	GUIDE NUMBER
350	45
500	55
700	65
1000	80
1400	95
2000	110
2800	130
4000	160
5600	190
8000	220

BCPS = Beam Candle Power Seconds, the measure of the light output of the flash unit.
For example, if your flash unit has a rate output value of 1000 then, with ASA 125 film, your corresponding guide number would be 80. Dividing the guide number by the distance in feet from the flash unit to the subject gives the correct f/number to use. In this example, the distance is 10 feet:

$$\frac{\text{Guide Number}}{\text{Flash-to-Subject Distance}} = \text{f/number}$$

$$\frac{80}{10} = 8, \text{ i.e., f/8.0}$$

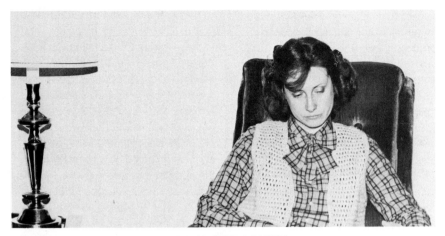

FIGURE 11-20A FRONTLIGHTING A SUBJECT WITH A CAMERA-MOUNTED FLASH
This produces a flat, two-dimensional picture.

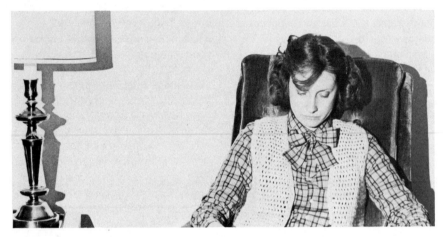

FIGURE 11-20B OFF-CAMERA FLASH
This gives a somewhat more three-dimensional picture.

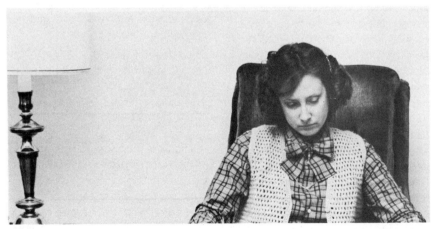

FIGURE 11-20C FLASH BOUNCED OFF THE CEILING
This creates a softer, more natural picture.

flash unit. Light-sensitive cells on the front of the unit instantaneously measure the amount of light flashed onto and reflected back from the subject and adjust the duration of the flash for proper exposure. A close or bright subject will produce a short flash; a dark or distant subject will elicit a longer flash. Besides the fact that it will do the brainwork for you, there are other advantages to automatic elecronic flash units: the choice of several f/stops increases your options; the faster recycling time allows you to take shots in more rapid succession; and since the flash does not always have to use its full capacity, the batteries last longer.

Attaching the flash The most common place to attach the electronic flash unit is on the camera's hot shoe. This is the easiest and most convenient place, since you don't have to use a cord. But there are disadvantages—when the flash is aimed directly at the subject, the subject appears flat and even, so the photograph lacks a three-dimensional feeling. If you are using color film, the tiny red spots in the subject's eyes are reflections of the flash. (See Figure 11-20.)

You can overcome these disadvantages by moving the flash above and to the side of the camera with a bracket that attaches to the camera. Brackets come in various sizes to hold the flash at various heights above the camera.

Following are several other alternatives for the placement of the flash:

1 Hold the flash unit in your hand. This gives you the option of holding the flash unit close to the camera or high above your head. However, you may find it difficult to hold the flash with one hand and control the camera with the other.

2 Place the flash unit on a stand near the camera. This allows you the double advantage of having an indirect flash and having both hands free to handle the camera.

3 Diffuse the light from the flash. Many electronic flash units are equipped with diffusers. If yours does not have this accessory, you can diffuse the light from the flash by taping one or more layers of matte acetate or white tissue over the head of the flash. Since this reduces the amount of light that the flash gives off, you will need to increase your exposure, usually by half an f/stop number per layer of material. You should run a test to make sure of the exposure time.

4 Bounce the flash off a neutral-colored (preferably white) surface. You can hold the flash in your hand, buy an angling bracket that tilts, or use the tilting head of your flash unit. Again, you will have to increase exposure—usually by two f/stops. Again, too, it is a good idea to experiment by bracketing, especially if there are bright, reflecting surfaces in the area.

5 Use a photographic umbrella or other commercial reflector with the flash unit. (See Figure 11-21.)

Multiple flash You can achieve the greatest balance of light and the best dimension in your photographs if you use two or more electronic flash units at a time, directing the light from different angles. One common ratio is 2:1—the main flash should provide two units of light for every one unit of light provided by fill-in flash equipment. This means that the illumination of the fill flash is 50 percent, or one f/stop, less than that of the main flash.

If the fill and main flashes are of equal power, the 2:1 ratio can be achieved using the inverse square law. Place the fill flash 1.4 times as far from the subject as the main flash is from the subject, because the square root of 2 is about 1.4. For example, if the main flash is 4 feet from the subject, then a fill flash of equal power should be placed 1.4 × 4 = 5.6 feet from the subject.

You can connect the flash units with Y-shaped terminals, but this is messy and inconvenient. The best method is to connect the units with "slave" photocells, using a photocell for each flash unit not directly attached to the

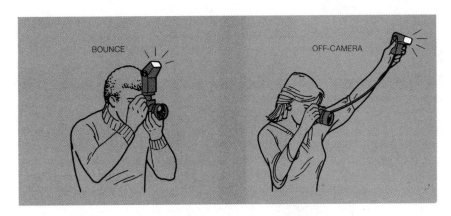

FIGURE 11-21 POSITIONS FOR BOUNCE AND OFF-CAMERA FLASH
The tilting-head unit on a hot shoe bounces the flash off the ceiling. This suffuses the room with soft light.
A direct off-camera flash gives a more three-dimensional appearance than the on-camera flash. There still may be harsh shadows, however.

camera. When the main flash is fired, the slave photocells detect the flash and fire the fill unit(s).

Using the flash unit outdoors It might seem odd, but the best place to use an electronic flash is outdoors in direct sunlight. It helps capture detail in shadow areas. Set the aperture as recommended by the flash's guide number, and then use the light meter to set the correct shutter speed for the sunlight. If you have a single lens reflex camera, set the shutter speed for direct sunlight and set the aperture as indicated on the camera's meter.

Then move back and forth until you find a subject-to-flash distance that uses the settings you have chosen and that guarantees that the flash will be weaker than the sunlight. Instead of moving, you can use several layers of white tissue to diffuse the light. Estimate a half-stop change in f/number for every layer of tissue.

If you use the flash outdoors at night, increase the exposure by one or two f/stops to compensate for the lack of reflective surfaces. If the weather is cold (regardless of whether it is day or night), keep the flash unit warm under your coat—cold temperatures drastically reduce the power of flash batteries.

PICTURING PEOPLE

Photographing a person is a tremendous challenge. A major part of a person is his or her personality: attributes, character, soul, what he or she means to us. Still another major part of a person is the way that person moves and talks. When you capture the image of a person on film, you get a static shot of his or her physical appearance only. The photograph must somehow convey all that makes up that person who is now on film. Sound impossible? Not necessarily, because you have at your disposal props, backgrounds, and settings to help communicate your message.

Most of the time, you should shoot a portrait at eye level. Shooting too high or too low distorts the facial features. If you are shooting a full-length picture, however, you might want to angle the camera slightly to provide drama or to make the subject appear taller. Shoot at close range to eliminate distracting backgrounds, and use a simple, appropriate background—the sky, a plain wall, or seamless photographic paper works well. Use casual conversation to help the subject relax. Decide on a pose that will best cap-

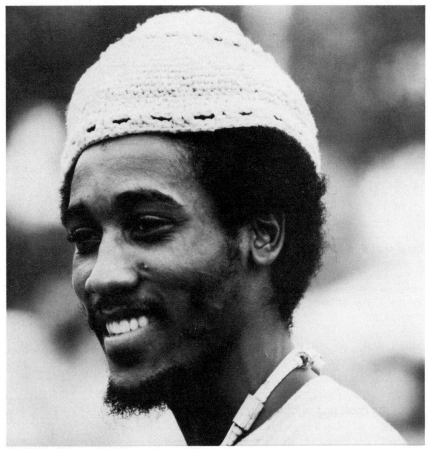

FIGURE 11-22 OUTDOOR PORTRAIT (Photo: Laird Roberts)

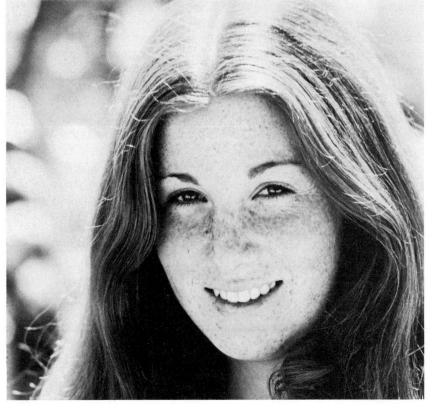

FIGURE 11-23 OUTDOOR PORTRAIT (Photo: Laird Roberts)

ture the essence of the person's personality: profiles are dramatic, pictures taken straight-on are stiff and formal, turning the person slightly to the side results in a more relaxed view.

Lighting is critical when you are photographing people. As the most important element, it can determine the mood of the photograph. You can use light to emphasize certain features. Sidelighting enables you to bring out the texture of the person's skin, hair, and clothing and allows for subtle shadowing that gives a three-dimensional, rounded appearance to the subject. On the other hand, you can use lighting to soften harsh features or to completely obscure others; light aimed directly at the subject tends to wash out details and flatten the subject. If the light is too bright, it will cause shadowing on one side of the subject's face. Eliminate the problem with a less powerful, diffused light or with extra reflection—by using a reflector, by moving the subject close to a light-colored wall, or by having a third person hold up a sheet of white paper that reflects light into facial shadows. Try to avoid strong, intense, direct light; soft, indirect lighting works better and is more flattering for a portrait.

Necessary tools for portrait work

You need some tools that you might not normally need for ordinary still life or scenery photography.

Telephoto lens A medium telephoto lens will enable you to soften a distracting background and to shoot effective photographs in dim indoor light. Choose a lens with a focal length between 75 and 135 mm and an aperture of f/2.8 or larger. A medium telephoto lens (80 to 105 mm) is sometimes called a portrait lens; with it you can maintain a comfortable distance from the subject and yet achieve a detailed, flattering likeness. You will probably need a normal or a wide-angle lens if you want to photograph a group or if you decide to capture a subject in his or her surroundings.

Film A slow- or medium-speed film (ASA 25 to 125) is best because the image such a film produces is less grainy, sharper, and more detailed. However, there will be times when you will need a faster film—especially when you are working with restless subjects, such as animals or children, or when you are forced to shoot in dim light.

Reflector Outdoors, you can use an electronic flash as your reflector. Indoors, you can use it to bounce light off walls, ceilings, or photographic umbrellas. You can easily construct your own reflector: paste crinkled-up aluminum foil on cardboard for a bright reflector; mount a large white card on a simple stand for a more subtle reflector.

Other equipment While other equipment is not essential, a few additional items are extremely useful and will increase the quality of your portrait work. An *automatic winder* advances the film automatically so you can capture rapidly changing facial expressions. This is especially useful for candid and informal portraits of children. A *tripod* guarantees that the camera is stationary during slow exposure times. If you shoot a portrait outdoors in open shade, a *skylight filter* will reduce the bluish hue. You can soften the image and minimize blemishes, freckles, and wrinkles with a soft-focus or *diffusion filter*.

Taking portraits outdoors

Outside, the background can be anything from a mountain peak to a flower garden, from a distant harbor to a sandy beach. The most difficult tasks are choosing a background that will complement—not compete with—the subject and determining the best lighting for the circumstances.

The best light for photographing people—whether indoors or outdoors—is diffused light. It enables you to use a wider aperture, resulting in a softly blurred background and a sharply focused subject. There are several kinds of natural diffused light of which you can take advantage: the shade of a tree, mist, fog, and cloudy skies all diffuse light for a soft, flattering effect.

If you decide to shoot a portrait outdoors and you cannot use diffused light, you can do some things to soften the effect of bright, direct sunlight. Pose the subject so that the sun is coming from slightly above and to the side of the camera. Never face the subject into the sunlight. To soften harsh shadows created by bright sunlight, use a reflector—water, foliage, and walls all help soften harsh shadows. As mentioned previously, an electronic flash softens the effects of sunlight and acts as a reflector; with the proper meter readings, you can achieve sharp focus of the face without washing out the background. (See Figures 11-22 and 11-23.)

Taking portraits indoors

Taking a portrait indoors eliminates the problem of harsh sunlight, but it presents its own set of problems. As always, lighting is critical. The best light for a portrait, regardless of setting, is diffused light; the best light for an indoor portrait is diffused sunlight that filters through a porch or window with a northern exposure. Make sure you take your light reading from the subject's face, not from the window—the bright light coming from the window can cause incorrect readings and faulty exposure. At night indoors, you can use whatever kind of artificial light best flatters the subject.

Shooting portraits inside with color film presents an additional set of challenges. Make sure your fill-in light is color compatible to the portrait, and make sure you use the right kind of film for the predominant light source. (See Figures 11-24 and 11-25.)

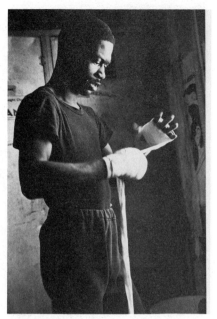

FIGURE 11-24 INDOOR PORTRAIT
(Mike Fasone)

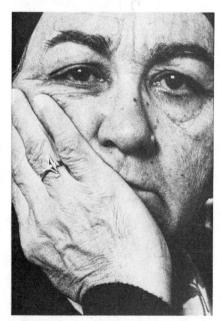

FIGURE 11-25 INDOOR PORTRAIT
(Janet Fornia)

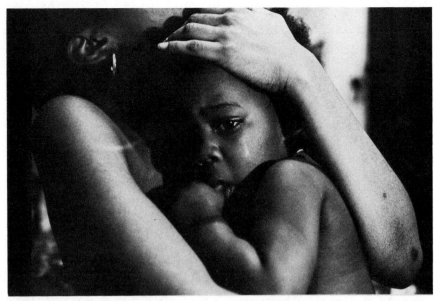

FIGURE 11-26 CHILD PORTRAIT (Monica Rohn-Turner)

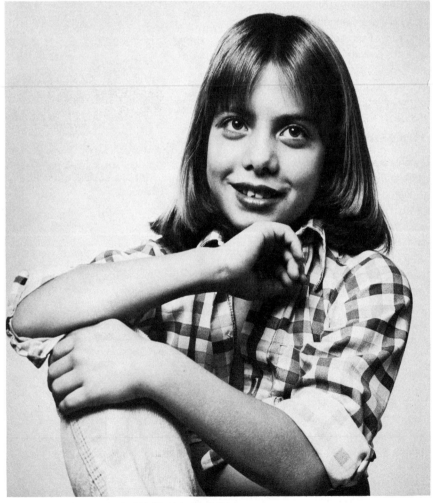

FIGURE 11-27 CHILD PORTRAIT (Patricia M. Artis)

Photographing children

Some children are delightful in front of a camera, but many are bored, self-conscious, or stubborn when posing for a photographer. Some basic rules will help you capture the spirits and personalities of children on film.

First, try to photograph a child when he or she is occupied—playing with something or involved with other children. If this is not possible, talk to the child as you photograph him or her, or ask someone else to talk while you concentrate on taking the picture. For shy children, ask questions that require more than a yes or no answer. Get up close enough to capture the detail of the child's face. If you cannot get close enough without threatening the child, use a telephoto lens. Kneel or squat so you are on the child's level.

A child's attention span is short and mood shifts are sudden, so you will not be able to spend much time determining the perfect background, camera angle, and lighting. Use an electronic flash, but bounce or diffuse the flash to give a soft effect. (See Figures 11-26 and 11-27.)

Photographing the elderly

Photographing old people provides you with the opportunity to capture in a single facial expression the joys and sorrows decades of living.

As in other portrait work, lighting presents the most important and most difficult challenge. To capture the lifetime that is represented in age spots, wrinkles, and facial lines that give so much character to the elderly, use a harsh, direct sidelight. If you want to stress the skin texture without overemphasizing it, use soft light from the side as the main source of light and fill in with diffused light. You may need to supplement diffused light with a flash bounced off the ceiling.

You can create a soft, flattering effect with a diffusing attachment. If the person's skin is pale, use a skylight filter to eliminate the bluish tinge that can

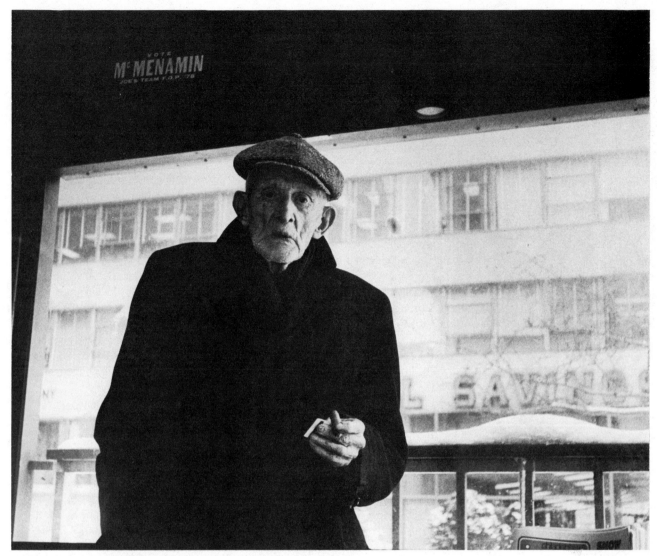

FIGURE 11-28 ELDERLY PERSON PORTRAIT (Richard Osborn Jr.)

result when a portrait is shot in the shade. Three-quarter and profile views are usually the most effective for portraits of the elderly. (See Figure 11-28.)

SUMMARY

Light, the essence of all photography, can either inhibit you as a photographer or become your creative medium. Learning to work with light will allow you to capture the work-worn hands of an elderly farmer, the delicate veins of a bumblebee's wing, or the fiery brilliance of an autumn meadow.

First, learn to see the scene as your camera will see it and as it will be recorded on film. Dare to experiment with different combinations of shutter speeds and aperture openings until you find the one that best emphasizes the subject.

Illuminate your subject with existing light, or capture facial expressions and movement with an electronic flash unit—modern technology's solution to the once difficult problem of achieving lighting balance. Just as the proper light can communicate the softness of a bride's anticipation or the delight in a child's eyes, it can enable you to produce memorable photographs that will communicate with a language all their own.

REVIEW QUESTIONS

1 What is the very essence of photography?

2 What is natural light?

3 What is artificial light?

4 In frontlighting with natural light, where is the light source located?

5 What does sidelighting increase?

6 Name one special application of backlighting.

7 List three common artificial light sources.

8 What is flash synchronization?

9 What is the inverse square law?

10 What is the most important element in portraiture?

11 What are two ways of filling facial shadows in portraiture?

12 What is a 2:1 lighting ratio?

TWELVE

Basic photographic tone control

When Niépce and Daguerre began making photographic innovations, they did not devote much attention to achieving maximum print quality—the unrefined technical and physical aspects of the art made attainment of such a goal extremely difficult. It was the magic of the process and the production of a printed image that appealed to the imaginations of early photographers. But as technology developed, maximum print quality became a primary goal of photographers.

Today recognition in the field of photography is dependent upon technical excellence of both the print and the negative. Negative density range and the corresponding print tones are a determining factor in the impact and quality of the printed image. Printed highlights must be bright and clear, but not featureless; shadowed areas must be rich, yet detailed. Middle gray tones must be well separated and defined.

All too often, the ideal negative density range that produces good tonal quality in the printed image is not achieved. The key to good tonal quali-

ty is controlling the tonal values of the subject throughout the process, from initial exposure to the final print.

There are several schools of thought on gaining quality control. The best-known method of photographic tone control is the *Zone System*, developed largely by Ansel Adams during the late 1920s and early 1930s. Adams manipulated the exposure and development processes in order to control negative density and print tone. Since then, many refinements and changes have been made in the system, and new approaches offer alternatives to the Zone System. (See Figure 12-1.) A number of texts have been written on the subject of tone control and the variables of the photographic process. All the research is aimed at one goal: excellence within the boundaries of the photographic medium.

A basic overview of tone control theory and some ideas about its development will help you to see photographically as you try to previsualize your photographs. Explaining tone control fully would take an entire text—not just a single chapter. This chapter describes simple basics. Some tone control elements are skipped

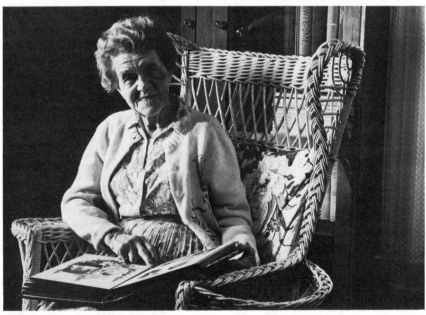

FIGURE 12-1 ZONE-SYSTEM SHOT (P.W. Hayes)

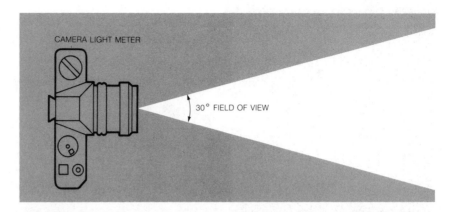

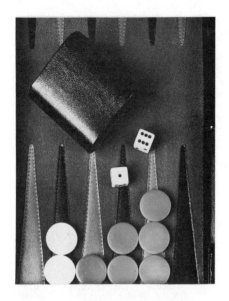

FIGURE 12-2 GOOD LUMINANCE RANGE
(John W. Clifton)

FIGURE 12-3 LIGHT-METER ANGLE-OF-SENSITIVITY COMPARISON

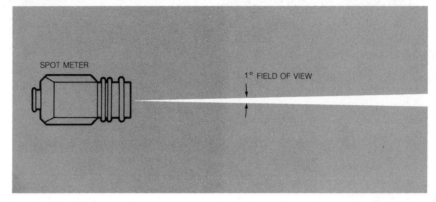

entirely, and a few others are only mentioned briefly. One of the most important concepts you can gain from this material is that you can—and sometimes should—deviate from manufacturers' instructions in order to develop a personal photographic style. To be able to know almost exactly how a photograph will look before the shutter ever clicks, to be able to create freely, and to be able to control the photographic medium are goals of all serious photographers. Tone control provides this freedom and, at the same time, permits this control.

Any tone control system depends on the photographer's ability to manipulate the relationships among three important photographic elements: *luminance range* (subject contrast change), the differences in the brightness of the light reflected from various parts of the scene or subject; *negative density range*, the difference between the blackest and the least blackened areas of the negative; and *printing paper response range*, the maximum

negative density range to which the printing paper is responsive. (Response range is a given characteristic of any printing paper, and it cannot be altered by darkroom techniques. For best results, you need to match negative density range to printing paper response range.)

Each time an image progresses through the photographic process, from exposure to finished print, these three factors are related in some way. You can control the relationships by using various photographic tools and techniques.

LUMINANCE RANGE

Scene luminance, also called subject contrast or subject brightness, indicates the range or difference in brightness among various elements of reflected light in the scene or subject. An exposure or light meter measures luminance range.

A conventional exposure meter measures light reflected from various parts

of the scene; the meter readings register as numbers on the face of the exposure meter dial. These numbers are valuable for determining luminance range—for example, if the meter needle records 12 when aimed at a highlighted portion of a scene and 9 when aimed at a shadow, the luminance range would be 3. (See Figure 12-2.) If the meter is built into a camera, it may convert these readings into recommended f/stops or shutter speed settings. In the above example, there are three f/stops of difference between the highlight and shadow areas.

What light meters do

Scene luminance range becomes more meaningful once you understand how light meters function. Built-in, reflective-type camera meters "read" the light within an angle of about 30 degrees. Specialized spot meters read a much smaller angle—usually 1 degree. (See Figure 12-3.) The meters

FIGURE 12-4 WHITE, 18 PERCENT GRAY, AND BLACK CARDS

interpret the light within the angle to determine what the exposure values should be.

Light meters cannot think for themselves. Within its field of view, a meter performs one simple function: it receives light impulses and converts these impulses into average exposure data in terms of f/stop, shutter speed, or both. Even the most sophisticated meter does not know what it is reading—it cannot tell whether it is reading highlights, shadows, or midtones. The meter merely reacts to the light reaching its metering cell, and for this reason all meters are designed to recommend exposure based on one average tone of gray.

Eighteen Percent Gray. Every scene has some highlights, some midtones, and some shadows. Light meters recommend exposures based on the midtones. Light meters assume that, if exposure is based on an average or middle luminance, the highlights and shadows will fall correctly into place in the final print.

If you follow the recommended exposure, you will get an average gray value in the midtones of the final print. This average gray reflects 18 percent of the light that falls on it. The 18 per-

cent gray value is the basis for exposure meter recommendations and is the key to the entire system of tone control. (See Figure 5-8.)

For many applications, this light-averaging system works very well; for others, it does not. If a light meter reads only *one* luminance level, that value—whether it is highlight, shadow, or midtone—will be exposed to print as 18 percent gray. The following illustration will clarify this concept. Three evenly illuminated cards (white, 18 percent gray, and black) are placed together and are read individually by a camera's exposure meter. (See Figure 12-4.) The recommended exposure is f/16 at $\frac{1}{60}$ for the white card, f/5.6 at $\frac{1}{60}$ for the 18 percent gray card, and f/2 at $\frac{1}{60}$ for the black card.

The recommended exposure was followed in each case, and prints were made. The results can be seen in Figure 12-5. It is no surprise that the shot with the meter reading the 18 percent gray card printed the white as white, the 18 percent gray as 18 percent gray, and the black as black. But the shot with the meter reading the white card printed the white card at about 18 percent gray, with corresponding distortions of the tones of the other two cards. Also, the shot made with the meter reading the black card shows the black card as approximately 18 percent gray, with the other cards lighter. The light meter read the luminance from each card and recommended an exposure that would print that area at 18 percent, whether the card was white, black, or gray.

Previsualization

Imagine you are shooting a picture of a dark brown vase full of flowers against a white wall in bright sun. Within its field of view, the light meter will measure light from the wall and from the vase. The meter will recommend an exposure based on the average luminance of the scene. In this case, since the wall reflects much more light than the vase, most of the light the meter reads will come from the wall. Thus the white background will be rendered as 18 percent (or middle) gray, not white, and the vase will be very dark and the scene underexposed.

It is the light meter's function to recommend an exposure that is an average for the mid-range luminance of the subject; it is your job as photographer to decide which elements of the scene will be recorded as this tone value.

The photographer needs to *previsualize:* to see in the mind's eye how a colored subject will appear when it is rendered in shades of gray. You need to identify which shadow areas are important to the scene, where the midtones fall, and how the highlights should be recorded for greatest impact.

Gray scale

The gray scale was developed by Albert Munsell (1858–1918). This color reference system is based on ten equal steps of gray tone. Step 5 is approximately 18 percent gray. (See

FIGURE 12-5A–C CARD-EXPOSURE SHOTS
FIGURE 12-5A
The exposure was made by taking a meter reading from the 18 percent gray card.

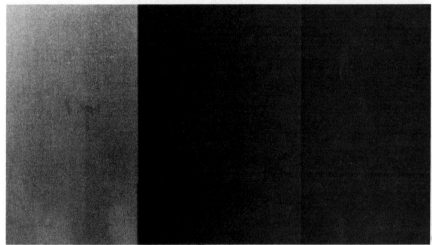

FIGURE 12-5B   The exposure was made by taking a meter reading from the white card.

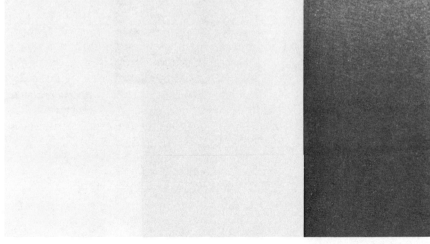

FIGURE 12-5C   The exposure was made by taking a meter reading from the black card.

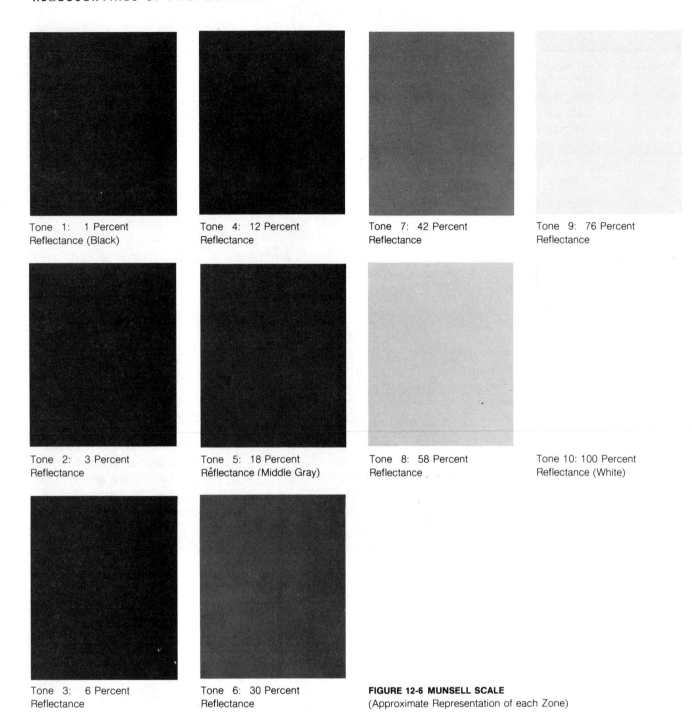

Tone 1: 1 Percent Reflectance (Black)

Tone 4: 12 Percent Reflectance

Tone 7: 42 Percent Reflectance

Tone 9: 76 Percent Reflectance

Tone 2: 3 Percent Reflectance

Tone 5: 18 Percent Reflectance (Middle Gray)

Tone 8: 58 Percent Reflectance

Tone 10: 100 Percent Reflectance (White)

Tone 3: 6 Percent Reflectance

Tone 6: 30 Percent Reflectance

FIGURE 12-6 MUNSELL SCALE
(Approximate Representation of each Zone)

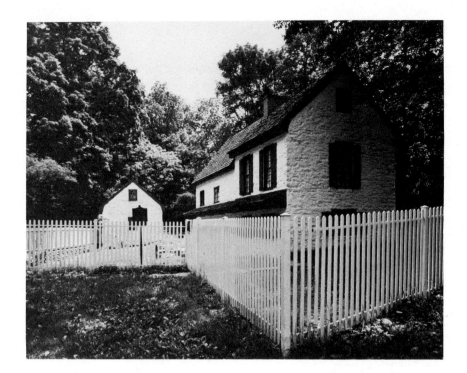

FIGURE 12-7 PREVISUALIZATION SHOT
(Randi Lyn Schor)

Figure 12-6.) Each step is the equivalent of a change of one f/stop of exposure, or an increment of shutter speed.

Previsualization practice

Figure 12-7 represents a subject of about average luminance. Comparison with the gray scale helps illustrate the various tone values in this photograph.

Determining exposure for a subject requires previsualizing the tones in which the subject will be rendered. This is called *placing* the subject. For example, if the subject or an area within the subject is to be rendered in the print as 18 percent gray, or tone 5, then simply meter that subject or area and follow the exposure recommendation. If the subject is light and therefore should be represented as lighter than 18 percent gray, tone 7, for instance, meter the subject and then open the aperture or change the shutter speed to increase exposure by two f/stops.

NEGATIVE DENSITY RANGE

The most important tool controlling negative density range is the film development procedure.

If you refer to the discussion of development in Chapter Six, you can see that increasing development time increases negative density range and decreasing development time decreases negative density range.

Scene luminance range does not always fit into the previsualized gray scale of ten tones or stops—extremely bright subjects may have a much greater luminance range (12–15 stops, perhaps), and low-contrast scenes may display short luminance ranges of only two or three stops. To achieve full zone range without sacrificing something else, you need to adjust development time.

Personal development time

As you acquire proficiency, film development becomes a very personal technique. Due to individual methods (styles of film agitation, for example) and other variables in the development process, it is not realistic to expect all photographers to adhere to uniform standards of development. Each individual photographer must develop a personal standard development time

for each film he or she uses; this personal time may or may not agree with the time recommended by the manufacturer. Personalized development time makes it possible to adjust the negative density range based on exposure conditions. It also allows much greater freedom and variation in shooting and light conditions.

Compaction / expansion

With a broad luminance range, placing the main subject in Zone 5 could cause the print values to exceed the paper's ability to record them; thus, important shadow areas might print as nearly black or highlights might be rendered as featureless white. To avoid this problem, simply decrease your development time from the personalized standard. This will *compact* the tone range to more correctly convey the previsualized scene. Conversely, tone range may be *expanded* beyond the normal by increasing development time. Expansions are necessary when subjects have a low luminance range—otherwise the print will be gray, flat, and uninteresting.

Concise testing procedures are avail-

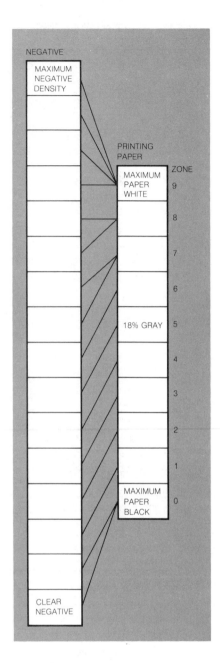

NEGATIVE

MAXIMUM
NEGATIVE
DENSITY

PRINTING
PAPER

ZONE

MAXIMUM
PAPER
WHITE

9

8

7

6

18% GRAY   5

4

3

2

1

MAXIMUM
PAPER
BLACK   0

CLEAR
NEGATIVE

**FIGURE 12-8 COMPARISON OF MAXIMUM
NEGATIVE-DENSITY RANGE AND MAXIMUM
PAPER-RESPONSE RANGE**

A black-and-white negative can have as
many as 16 or 17 tones.

able for determining personalized
development time. Similar testing procedures also determine how many
zones or steps are needed to increase
or decrease development in order to
compact or expand tone range by a
certain number of zones or stops.

PRINTING PAPER RESPONSE RANGE

Negative density range may vary with
development time, but paper response
range is a built-in characteristic of
each particular printing paper.
Although printing paper can have
either a fixed or a variable contrast,
the range of print tones for each kind
of paper cannot be noticeably
changed (that is, expanded or con-
tracted) by darkroom technique.

Printing paper is the limiting factor in
the tone control process. Modern film
is capable of recording a much
greater luminance range than is printing paper. Therefore, it is important to
match exposure and negative density
to the maximum paper range. If paper
response range is not considered,
important highlight areas of the original scene may print without detail.
Shadow areas of the print are not
affected as much, but they also may
suffer from a lack of detail. See Figure
12-8 for an illustration of the relationship between negative density range
and paper response range.

SUMMARY

Tone control systems allow photographers to get an extra amount of satisfaction and pleasure from the
photographic medium. Any tone control system must be a very personal
one; no two photographers apply a
system in the same way.

In simple and basic terms, tone control involves three measurable factors
of the photograpic process: scene
luminance range, negative density

range, and printing paper response
range. These factors must be skillfully
blended to control tone. The exposure
meter, the film development process,
and the inherent characteristics of various printing papers are the tools used
to control tone.

Two distinct steps are followed in
tone control. First, the subject must be
previsualized—seen in the mind's eye
so that a decision can be made on
how to render it in tones of gray. Second, the available tools must be used
to expose, develop, and print the subject as it was previsualized.

Tone control cannot be learned
merely by reading. The testing, the
trial and error, and the successes and
frustrations that come from truly per-
sonalizing photographic technique
must be experienced firsthand. After
all, the technique is the photographer's—not a textbook author's or a
film manufacturer's—and one of the
photographer's joys is learning to
make that technique his or her own.

It is not always bad to deviate from
recommended development times, if
you know what to expect and are
planning on the results you will get.

REVIEW QUESTIONS

1 What is tone control?

2 List three elements that must be
successfully related for a technically
correct print.

3 What is 18 percent gray?

4 What is a gray scale?

5 Define scene luminance range.

6 What is the limiting factor of a tone
control system?

7 What controls negative density
range?

8 What does it mean to *previsualize* a
subject?

9 To what standard or value does a
light meter recommend exposure?

10 Why must negative density range
be matched to paper response range?

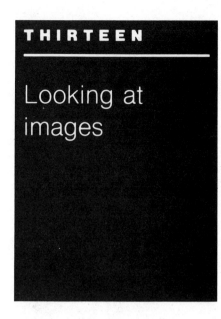

THIRTEEN

Looking at images

Have you ever wondered why all the frames on a roll of film do not turn out successfully? The answer is not a simple one—there are usually a number of reasons. One of the prime reasons is inaccurate exposure or development, which leads to loss of detail. Another possibility is poor composition; or your picture may not have good depth of field. You may even get a bad picture simply because your purpose in taking it was not clear.

THE EXPOSURE–DEVELOPMENT MATRIX

The exposure–development matrix (chart) helps to define the relationship between exposure and development. Nine possible combinations of exposure and development have been assembled on one chart. With this matrix you can describe what happens to three important, interrelated functions: negative density, negative detail, and negative contrast. (See Table 13-1.)

As exposure and development are carried to extremes, the number of possible degrees for each combination is limitless. However, the exposure–development matrix is an effective way of bringing together basic information. The matrix can help you to analyze your negatives and prints and consequently become more efficient as a photographer.

When you compare the information in the exposure–development matrix (E–D matrix) with your negatives and prints, you can easily see the effects of the nine combinations of exposure and development. (See Figures 13-1 and 13-2.)

Underexposed negatives lack *density* and look "thin"; detail is lost from the shadow areas. Normally exposed negatives have normal density that shows detail in all tones. Overexposed negatives have increased density and lack detail in highlight areas.

Development controls the amount of *contrast* in a negative. Underdeveloped negatives are "soft" or "flat"; normally developed negatives display

TABLE 13-1 □ THE EXPOSURE–DEVELOPMENT MATRIX

| DEVELOPMENT | **EXPOSURE** | | | |
	UNDER	NORMAL	OVER	
OVER	Thin	About Normal	Dense	Negative Density
	Loss in Shadows	Good Shadow and Highlight	Loss in High-light	Negative Detail
	Contrasty or Hard	Contrasty or Hard	Contrasty or Hard	Negative Contrast
NORMAL	Thin	Neither Too Thin or Dense	Dense	Negative Density
	Loss in Shadows	Excellent Shadow and Highlight	Loss in High-light	Negative Detail
	Slightly Less Than Normal	Neither Too Soft or Too Hard	Slightly More Than Normal	Negative Contrast
UNDER	Thin	About Normal	Dense	Negative Density
	Loss in Shadows	Good Shadow and Highlight	Loss in High-light	Negative Detail
	Soft or Flat	Soft or Flat	Soft or Flat	Negative Contrast

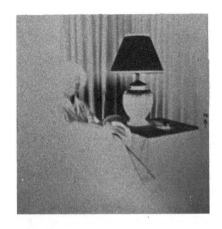
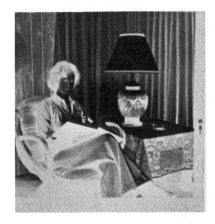
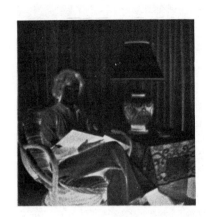
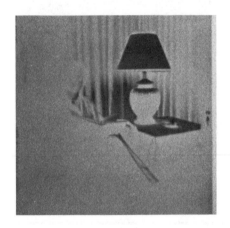
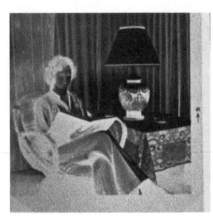
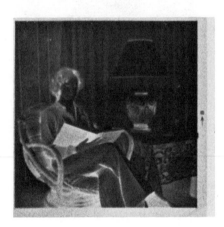
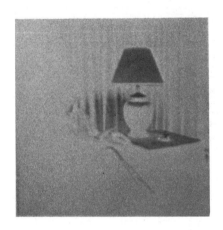
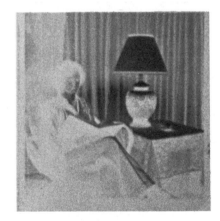
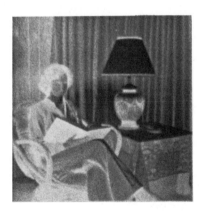

FIGURE 13-1 NEGATIVES FROM THE E–D MATRIX

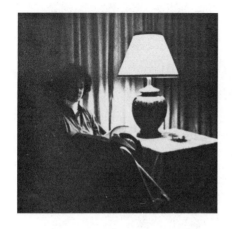
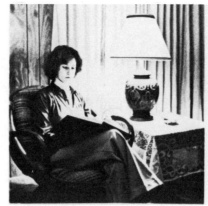
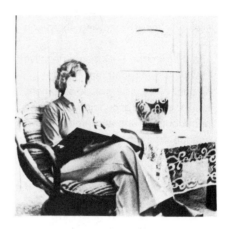
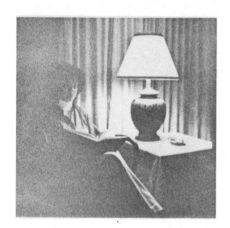
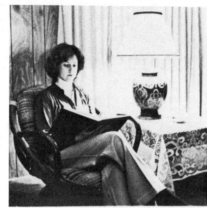
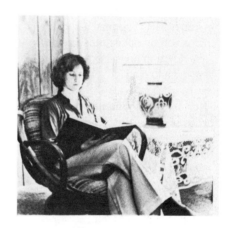
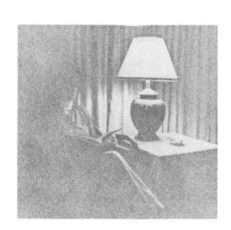
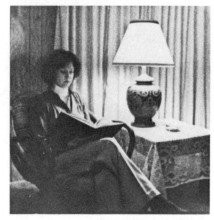
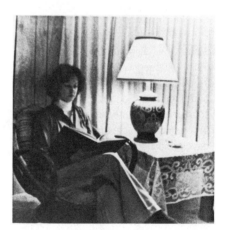

**FIGURE 13-2 PRINTS FROM THE E–D
MATRIX**

good contrast. Overdeveloped negatives are "hard," showing sharp contrast.

Prints from the E–D matrix negatives clearly show that increasing the amount of exposure or development results in a corresponding increase in print contrast—the abruptness of tonal change from areas of print contrast. The more gradual the change, the lower the contrast; the more extreme and abrupt the change, the higher the contrast.

Definitions

Normal exposure For the purposes of Table 13-1, "normal" exposure is that which produces a negative with a wide range of densities and good shadow and highlight detail.

Normal development For the purposes of Table 13-1, "normal" development uses the developing time recommended by the manufacturer.

Prints. Prints are made on number 2 paper and undergo normal exposure and development without any kind of manipulation.

Using the matrix

The matrix serves two purposes. First, it shows what will happen to a normally exposed and developed negative if you decide to try one of the other combinations. Second, it can suggest solutions if you are having problems producing consistently exposed and developed negatives.

Certain procedures can be used to compensate for some of the problems created by various combinations of the E–D matrix. For example, in the case of push processing, the film is intentionally underexposed and then given greater than normal development. To produce a negative that is more printable than one developed by regular push processing, you might process the film in a developer such as Diafine or Acufine, which helps reduce the

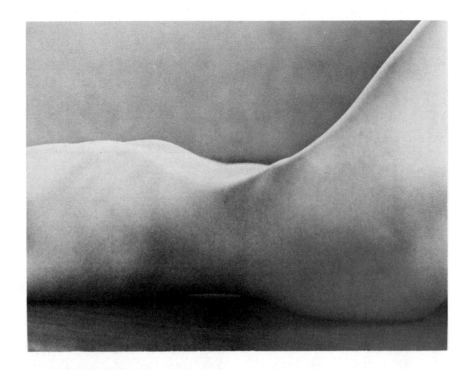

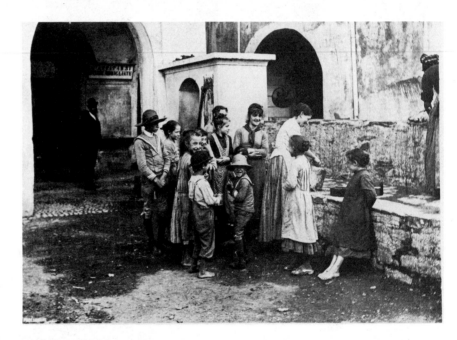

FIGURE 13-3 WESTON: NUDE
(International Museum of Photography at George Eastman House)

FIGURE 13-4 STIEGLITZ: A GOOD JOKE, 1887
(International Museum of Photography at George Eastman House)

contrast and bring out more shadow detail. Note that, even with special processing, a push-processed print will not be a substitute for a normally exposed and developed one.

A normal print of good quality is made by printing a normal-contrast negative on a normal-contrast paper. A normal-looking print can also be made from a moderately high-contrast negative if you use a low-contrast printing paper or from a low-contrast negative with a high-contrast paper. You can also use variable-contrast filters and printing papers to achieve the same results.

Another way to manipulate the matrix is to alter the development time so that, when overexposure occurs, the highlight densities still come out in the normal range. This does not completely correct the overexposure problem, but it does make the highlights more printable.

For each combination in the matrix, appropriate values are given for negative density, detail, and contrast. When you analyze the matrix prints and negatives, watch for changes in density, detail, and contrast. With careful study of the matrix, even beginning photographers can easily learn to tell the difference between over-, under-, and normally exposed or developed negatives and prints. The matrix can help you avoid some common mistakes—such as thinking that greater than normal development will compensate for underexposure. Both exposure and development are critical, and one cannot compensate completely for error in the other.

EIGHTEEN KEY QUESTIONS

The previous section of this chapter reviewed how exposure and development combine to produce a good photograph. The following questions serve as a summary of other topics covered throughout the text; they will help you analyze your own and other people's

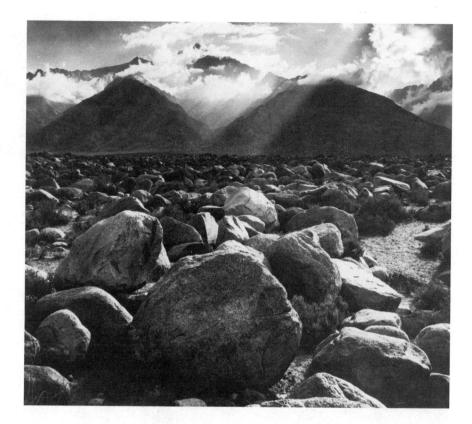

FIGURE 13-5 ADAMS: MT. WILLIAMSON—CLEARING STORM, 1944
(International Museum of Photography at George Eastman House)

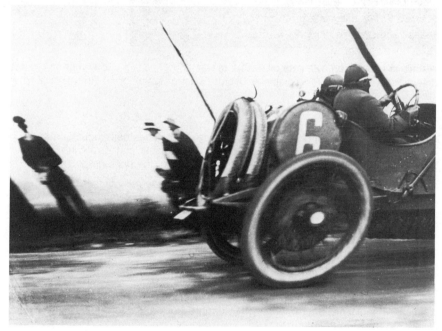

FIGURE 13-6 LARTIGUE: GRAND PRIX OF THE AUTO CLUB OF FRANCE, 1912
(International Museum of Photography at George Eastman House)

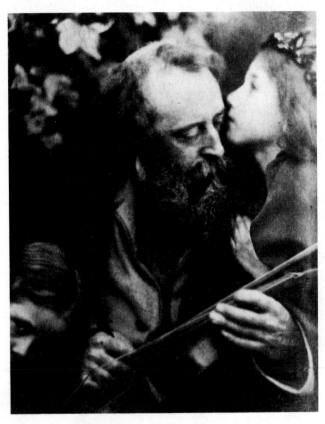

FIGURE 13-7 CAMERON: THE KISS OF PEACE, C. 1867
(International Museum of Photography at George Eastman House)

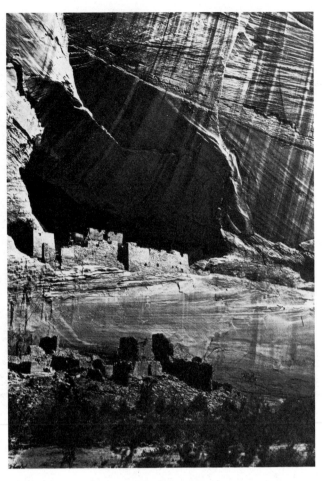

FIGURE 13-8 O'SULLIVAN: CANYON DE CHELLY, ARIZONA, 1873
(International Museum of Photography at George Eastman House)

photographs. Judge the photographs shown in this chapter on the basis of these eighteen key questions to see how well the photographers did. You should also ask yourself these questions every time you take a shot or analyze a print.

1 *What was the photographer's purpose in taking the picture?* Was the photographer trying to report an event, tell a story, create a mood, or make a political or social statement? What was he or she trying to do—and why?

2 *Is the picture effective because of the subject matter, the treatment, or both?* Sometimes brilliant execution makes a picture striking even though the subject is ordinary and really quite uninteresting. In other cases, crude technique results in a stunning photograph because the subject is fascinat-

ing. Sometimes both technique and subject matter play a role in the effectiveness of the photograph.

3 *Can you tell whether the picture was contrived or spontaneous?* Try to determine what approach the photographer used and why. Was the picture carefully planned ahead of time, or did the photographer catch a sudden burst of life that was completely spontaneous?

4 *What role did luck play?* Sometimes luck is the key—especially in candid or action shots. But *a good photographer creates luck from knowledge and experience.*

5 *Is the composition effective?* Does the composition help relay the picture's message, or does the composition work against what the picture is trying to say? What was the photographer's purpose in using that specific

angle and those lines?

6 *Does the lighting contribute to or detract from the photograph?* Try to determine the source, direction, and quality of the lighting. If it contributes to the photograph, decide why; if it detracts, decide how it could have been improved.

7 *Did the photographer use exposure to control the contrast of the picture?* Was the exposure based on the middle tones, on shadow, or on highlight? Why?

8 *Was depth of field used to create a special effect?* Where did the photographer focus—and why? Is the subject isolated or emphasized by this technique?

9 *If the picture is an action shot, did the photographer use a fast shutter speed to control blurring?* Sometimes

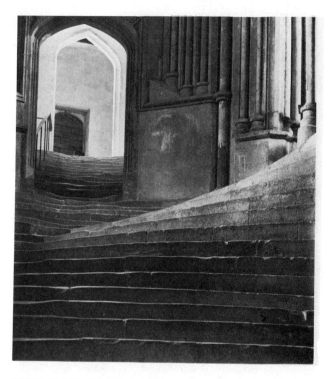

FIGURE 13-9 EVANS: SEA OF STEPS, WELLS CATHEDRAL, ENGLAND, 1903
(International Museum of Photography at George Eastman House)

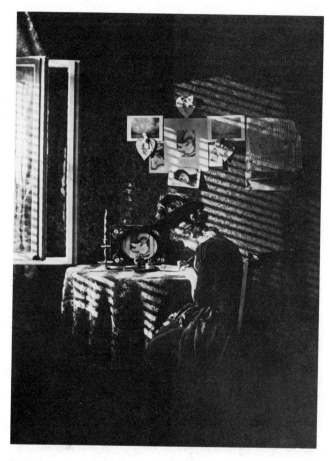

FIGURE 13-10 STIEGLITZ: PAULA, 1889
(International Museum of Photography at George Eastman House)

blurring of an action shot is effective, because it communicates action. Other times action shots are most effective if motion is frozen. How did this photographer handle action? What could his or her reasoning have been?

10 *Did the photographer use a telephoto or wide-angle lens? Why?* Could the subject have been shot better with another type lens, or did the lens used contribute to the photograph's overall effectiveness?

11 *Did the photographer use a filter? What kind? Why?*

12 *Was the photographer's timing precise?* Did the photographer trip the shutter at precisely the right instant, or was the timing off? Was the moment captured, or was it lost by a fraction of a second? Would the picture have been better if the photographer had acted a second earlier or later?

13 *Did the photographer control contrast during printing?* Are there rich blacks, clean whites, and a sharp image? Or did the photographer fall down during printing?

14 *Did the photographer use any special techniques?* Can you tell if petroleum jelly was smeared on the lens? If so, why did the photographer do it? Did he or she use any other special gimmicks? Why?

15 *Did the photographer overcome any technical difficulties?* Maybe the picture had to be shot in poor light, or perhaps an exceptionally fast shutter speed had to be used. Realize the extra skill used to overcome these difficulties.

16 *Is the picture like others you have seen of similar subjects?* A photographer whose work is patterned after the work of others may lack creativity and imagination. Look for photographs with a fresh approach or a dramatic effect; look for a photographer who has succeeded in developing a unique style.

17 *Is the picture worth a second look? Why?*

18 *How well was the photographer's purpose accomplished?* This is the most important question of all—and the answer depends on the answers you got to the first eighteen questions.

LOOKING AT IMAGES

Look at the images in Figures 13-3 through 13-13. Analyze them, using both the exposure–development matrix and the eighteen key questions.

FIGURE 13-12 STRAND: PORTRAIT, NEW YORK, 1915
(International Museum of Photography at George Eastman House)

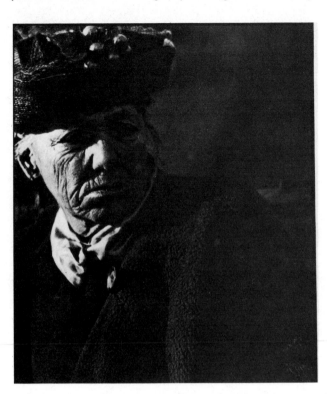

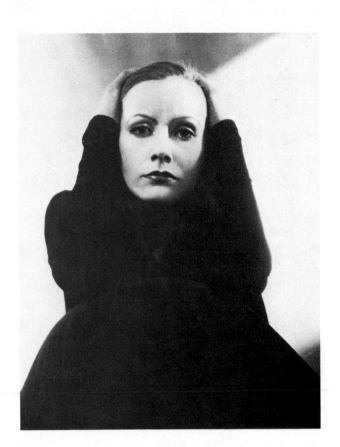

FIGURE 13-11 STEICHEN: GRETA GARBO, 1928
(International Museum of Photography at George Eastman House)

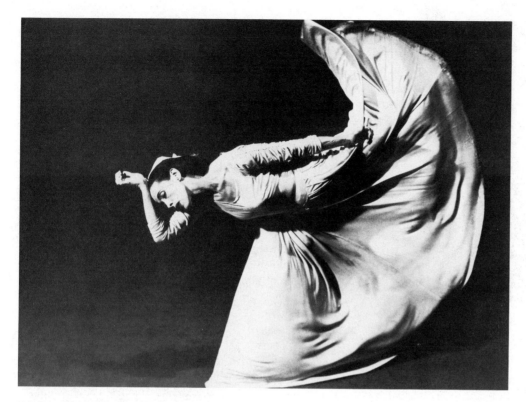

FIGURE 13-13 MORGAN: MARTHA GRAHAM, 1944
(International Museum of Photography at George Eastman House)

SUMMARY

As your skill in photography increases, you will notice a subtle change in yourself: no longer will you be a casual, uninformed observer of photographs. You will find yourself looking at photographs with a new interest, a new awareness. You will search for meaning, for communication; you will analyze technique. You will try to second-guess the photographer; you may even have ideas about how you could have treated the same subject in a more effective way.

Most of all, you will learn from every photograph you see. Keep looking at photographs—drink in all you can. Analyzing and appreciating photographs—those taken by others, and those you take yourself—is the most valuable learning process of all.

REVIEW QUESTIONS

1 A normally exposed negative has good detail in both the _____ and the _____ .

2 A print made from an underexposed, normally developed negative will show a loss of detail in the _____ . The print will also show overall _____ contrast.

3 A print made from an overexposed, normally developed negative will show a loss of detail in the _____ . The print will also show _____ contrast.

4 A print made from a normally exposed, underdeveloped negative will show _____ ; print contrast will be _____ .

5 A print made from a normally exposed, overdeveloped negative will show _____ ; print contrast will be _____ .

6 The negative of an underexposed, underdeveloped scene will have a _____ density. A print made from such a negative will lose detail in the _____ and be _____ in contrast.

7 The negative of an overexposed, overdeveloped scene will be _____ . A print made from such a negative will lose detail in the _____ and have _____ contrast.

8 The negative of an underexposed, overdeveloped scene will be _____ . A print from such a negative will show a loss of _____ and a _____ in contrast.

9 The negative of an overexposed, underdeveloped scene will exhibit _____ . A print from such a negative will show a loss of _____ and have _____ contrast.

10 Can overexposure completely compensate for underexposure?

11 What is necessary for a print to have a full range of tones and detail?

12 On what personal, somewhat random value does normal exposure depend?

FOURTEEN

Fundamentals of color photography

In 1935, after more than seventy-five years of experimentation, a practical process for color photography was introduced for mass use. Before then, the practice of color photography had been limited to a handful of professionals and a few dedicated amateurs. In the years since, color film has soared in popularity, outselling black and white film by a wide margin.

One reason for the phenomenal growth in color film use is that color adds an exciting dimension to almost every kind of subject. Another reason is that it has become increasingly easy to shoot and process color film. Perhaps the most important reason of all, though, is that color photography is not just a black and white picture to which color has been added—instead, it is a challenging medium of expression in its own right.

Of all the processes available to the photographer, color may well offer the ultimate challenge. A color photograph can come closer to the illusion of reality than a black and white shot. However, there are some drawbacks: shooting color film increases exposure problems and requires exacting processing procedures. Color composition and the psychology of color also combine to challenge the photographer's skills and abilities.

If you wish to add the dimension of color to your photographs successfully, you must understand two ideas. First, you must understand how the eye sees and the brain interprets color; second, you must comprehend how light and color film react.

COLOR FUNDAMENTALS

Color vocabulary

To understand the color process, you need to be familiar with the terminology of both black and white and color photography. The basic terms *hue, brightness,* and *saturation* are useful in explaining the color process.

Hue Hue is the name of the color—red, blue, green, cyan, magenta, or yellow, for example. Hue is the attribute of color that is also the essential quality that distinguishes one color from another—green from orange, brown from pink.

Each hue varies over a continuous range of purity. Crimson, for example, is a highly saturated color; when white light is mixed with crimson, it becomes pink—a *tint* of the original hue.

Saturation Another attribute of color, saturation refers to the brilliance of the color or the amount of dye in the color. Saturation varies with the intensity of the hue. A high-saturation red, for example, would be crimson or "fire-engine" red; a low-saturation red would be a pale pink. Saturation is sometimes referred to as *chroma*.

Brightness The third important quality of any color is brightness: the lightness or darkness of any color, which is a result of the amount of light reflected by a surface of that color. Brightness is also sometimes referred to as "tone" or "value." A light red, for example, has a higher value than does a dark red.

In 1915 Albert Munsell published a system that arranged colors in three dimensions, corresponding to hue, brightness, and saturation. Each color is arranged cyclically around a central spine. The colors on the spine are the achromatic shades of gray, in ascending order from black to white. As each hue moves out from the spine, it becomes more vivid as it is mixed with less gray. Since Munsell, others have devised various methods of representing the possible combinations of hue, saturation, and brightness. (See Figure 14-1.)

Color vision

In Chapter Four we saw that light is electromagnetic radiation of various wavelengths. Blues and greens are

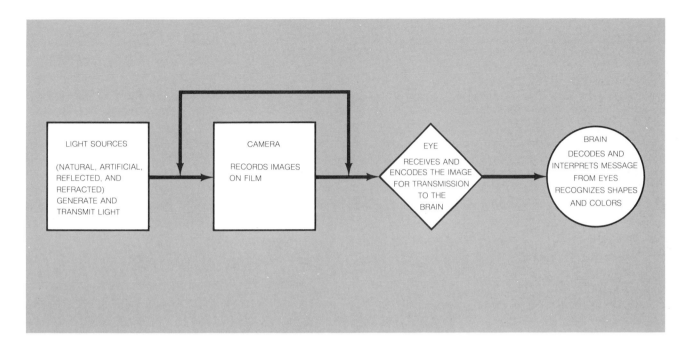

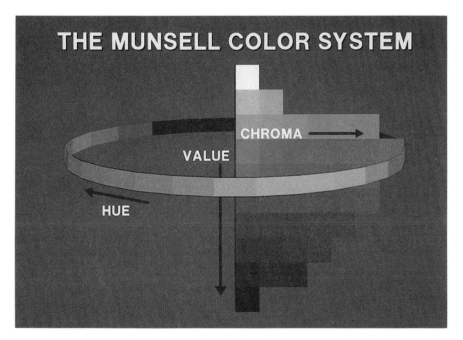

FIGURE 14-1 PSYCHOPHYSICS OF COLOR VISION
The process of vision can be divided into four general steps. The first two, light sources and cameras, depend on physical properties to function. The eye's physiological make-up gives it the ability to perform its job of receiving and encoding the images. The brain decodes and interprets the messages from the eyes, based on principles of psychology. Therefore, the whole process is referred to as the *psychophysics* of color vision.

FIGURE 14-2 COLOR SOLID
(AV Computer Graphics Inc.)

shorter wavelengths than reds and yellows, and the entire spectrum of visible light is composed of the wavelengths between 400 and 700 nm.

Color photography is not as concerned with the physical description of color as with the psychophysics of color vision: how light reaches the eye, how colors are seen by the eye, and how colors are interpreted by the brain. (See Figure 14-2.)

How the eye works The human eye works much as a radio does. The eye receives various wavelengths (colors) of light; this light energy is transformed by the retina of the eye into electrical impulses that move along the optic nerve to the brain. The brain translates these impulses into the col-

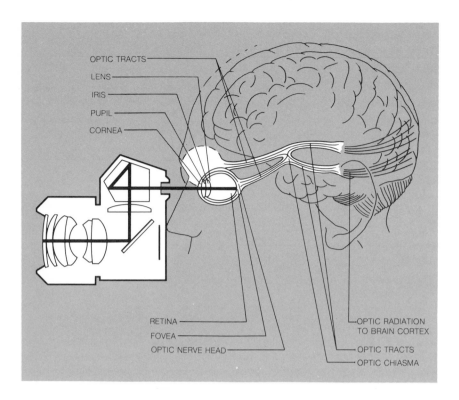

FIGURE 14-3 ANATOMY OF VISION

ors we see. (See Figure 14-3.) Unlike a radio, which can receive only one station at a time, the eye can see all wavelengths in the visible spectrum simultaneously. For example, imagine a yellow balloon. The balloon is not "really" yellow; it does not have any intrinsic color at all. (Nor does any other object, for that matter.) The yellow pigment in the rubber of the balloon absorbs blue wavelengths of light and reflects green and red wavelengths. This reflected red and green light reaches the retina of the eye, where it is transformed into electrical impulses that travel to the brain, which interprets the impulses as "yellow." The balloon is not yellow, but it does reflect light energy that causes you to see yellow.

Science does not completely understand *how* the eye and the brain perform the magic of color vision. We do know that the retina of the eye contains light-sensitive cells in two shapes, the *rods* and the *cones*.

These cells send the electrical impulses, which the brain interprets as sight, along the optic nerve. Rods act as a type of light meter, only indicating more or less light. The rods are color blind; you could see well with just the rods, but the images would be in black and white. Human vision in dim light depends on rods, but normal daylight vision and the ability to see color differences depend on the cones.

Cones are the "radio receivers" of the eye. Cones are color-sensitive and apparently form three separate systems for color reception, with each cone system being sensitive to approximately one-third of the visible spectrum. Some cones are sensitive to the red end of the spectrum, some to green frequencies, and some to blue frequencies.

Adaptations of the eye

Part of the difficulty in color photography is that the film system and the brain system do not always see things the same way. The brain has the ability to adjust both color and brightness, so that what we see is quite different from reality.

Brightness adaptation The eye and the brain work to maintain maximum vision in any situation. For example, consider the light of a flashlight at night—the eye and brain adapt to this level of illumination so that it seems rather bright, and you are able to see quite well. Now consider the flashlight outside on a bright, sunny day. Compare the light from the flashlight with the sunlight—the sunlight, of course, is hundreds of times brighter, yet we can see rather well in each situation.

Brightness adaptation is controlled by the eye. The iris of the eye dilates and contracts to admit more or less light, much as a camera aperture does. The rods and cones of the retina also automatically change to become more or less sensitive. For example, by the light of a flashlight at night, the iris is open wide and the retina is very sensitive; bright sunlight causes the iris to "stop down" and the retina to become far less sensitive. The ability to have approximately equal vision in situations of widely varying light intensities is called *brightness adaptation*.

The eye may take several minutes to adjust for brightness levels in extreme situations. When you go from a brightly lit room, for example, into a darkroom illuminated only by safelights, your eyes require a minute or two to adjust. Brightness adaptation happens much more quickly in less extreme situations, such as those that occur as the eye moves from one scene to another. In such cases, you can see detail both in highlight and shadow areas of the different scenes.

Unfortunately, color film cannot make this adjustment; you must consider the brightness adaptation of your eyes when you are exposing color film.

Color adaptation Most light sources you encounter contain all or nearly all of the wavelengths of the visible spectrum in varying degrees. Many light sources are stronger in certain wavelengths than in others. Daylight is white light that contains approximately equal amounts of red, blue, and green wavelengths. Ordinary room light from a tungsten light bulb is high in yellow wavelengths; light from fluorescent tubes has a greenish tint because it contains a predominance of yellow-green wavelengths.

Color adaptation means that, although light sources may differ, you still see objects as you know they "should" appear under white light. A white shirt is actually yellow under incandescent light, but your brain tells you the shirt is still white—so that is what you see. By training your eye to see what is really there, you can overcome color adaptation. Try walking from bright sunlight into a room that is illuminated with incandescent light bulbs; before your eyes have the chance to adapt, notice the real colors of the light and the objects in the room. Once you train your eyes, it will be easy for you to recognize the true effects of various light sources on colored objects. Until you train your eyes to see what color is assumed by objects under various light sources, you will experience difficulty in getting the objects to appear on film the way you thought they looked in reality.

COLOR MIXING AND BALANCE

Color primaries and secondaries

The complete series of waves that make up the visible part of the electro-magnetic spectrum is important in photography: both color and black and white photography record the visible wavelengths. Within these limits, the human eye sees a change of wavelength as a change of color. Even though the change from one color to another may not be a sharp one, the eye can detect the subtle divisions in the spectrum. See Figure 4-2 for an

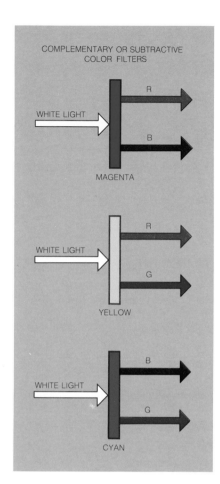
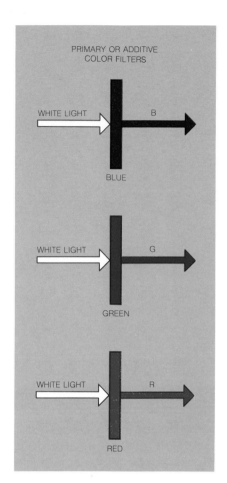

FIGURE 14-4 TRANSMISSION THROUGH PRIMARY AND COMPLEMENTARY FILTERS

illustration of the visible spectrum.

Taken as a whole, we see the colors of the visible spectrum as white light. In photography, this white light is the sum of three primary colors of light: red, blue, and green. Because of this, these colors are referred to as the *primary colors*. Any other color you see is made by mixing various amounts of red, blue, and green. This fact is of great importance to photographers because it makes it possible to reproduce virtually all forms of color on today's films and papers.

You can produce almost any color imaginable by mixing and overlapping the primary colors. Try this yourself by projecting deep blue, deep red, and deep green light onto a white screen. Where all three overlap, you will see a bright white light. You can produce

almost any color by varying the relative brightness of any or all the primary colors projected onto the screen.

When you mix two primary colors, you produce a *secondary color*. Mixing the secondary colors produces interesting results. Try placing filters made from the secondary colors of cyan, magenta, and yellow on a light table. Where all three filters overlap, the area is black. The cyan filter absorbs red light, the yellow absorbs blue light, and the magenta absorbs green light. When all the filters overlap, all the light is absorbed, leaving what we perceive as black: the absence of light. Each subtractive color is said to be "minus" some additive color. Magenta is minus green; yellow is minus blue; and cyan is minus red. (See Figure 14-4.)

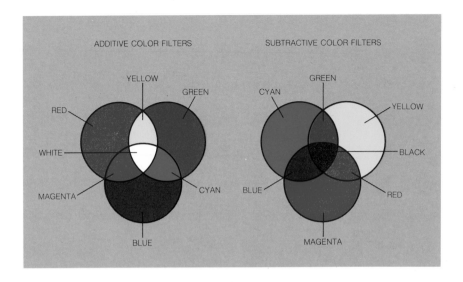

ADDITIVE COLOR FILTERS

SUBTRACTIVE COLOR FILTERS

FIGURE 14-5 COLOR MIXING USING ADDITIVE (PRIMARY) AND SUBTRACTIVE (COMPLEMENTARY) COLOR FILTERS
This is the image seen when light from the three primary color filters is projected onto a screen.
This is the image seen when the three subtractive color filters are placed in this pattern against a luminous background.

Color wheel

When the colors of the visible spectrum are displayed on a color wheel, each of the three *additive colors*—red, green, and blue—is directly opposite its complementary color. These complementary (secondary) colors—cyan, magenta, and yellow—are the three *subtractive* colors. The color wheel, then, provides an easy way to illustrate the relationships of the various primary colors and the results of adding two or more of them together. When all three additive primaries, or all three subtractive primaries, or any two complementary colors are added together, the result is white, black, or shades of gray respectively. The gray tones will vary according to the amount and the intensity of each color in the combination. See Figure 14-5 for information about how to mix the primary and secondary colors in both the additive and subtractive systems. The color wheel is illustrated in Figure 14-6.

Color balance

The balance of different colors in visible light varies from one source of light to another. The mixture of colors in a particular kind of light is referred to in photography as *color tempera-*

ture, which is expressed in degrees Kelvin (K), the international scientific unit of temperature measurement.

Color temperature provides a good way to summarize the different mixtures of color within various kinds of natural or artificial light, but it is *not* the measurement of the amount of heat a light source generates.

The color temperature scale ranges upward from 1,000°K and has no upper limit. Most forms of artificial lighting have a color temperature in the range of 2,000 to 6,000°K; a blue sky measures about 6,000°K. Candles and oil lamps measure about 1,000 K, and a heavily overcast sky measures about 10,000°K. The lower color temperatures occur with wavelengths of red light (candles, tungsten lamps, and studio lamps); the blue wavelengths record the highest temperatures.

COLOR COMPOSITION

The challenge of color photography includes the demands of color composition—the ability to place a variety of visual values together in a pleasing arrangement. Adding color to a photograph does not necessarily increase the picture's statement or elevate its impact. On the contrary, color added the wrong way can actually detract from the picture. A photograph that makes no statement in black and white will usually be just as meaningless in color.

Like black and white composition, color composition is a matter of developing one's personal taste. In addition to following the guidelines for black and white composition in Chapter Three, you must also consider certain problems unique to color composition.

Light and shade

The light and shade recorded in photographs give them a three-dimensional quality. Unless the lighting is flat, the camera will always record combinations of light and shade. In color photography, even the shadow areas will appear in color—either from reflections off nearby surfaces or from nearby sources of direct illumination nearby.

Shadows are invaluable in color photography. They can indicate the weather conditions, the time of day, and the direction of the sunlight, and they can add spectacular drama and mystery to a picture. (See Figure 14-7.)

Dominant color

Black and white photography relies on the elements of tone, texture, balance, shape, and line to set a mood and communicate a message. In color photography, you will find that the color itself can set the mood, express the emotion, or communicate the message. In seeking to set the mood, remember a basic rule: never try to cram too many colors into one photograph. The struggle for dominance will result in confusion.

Decide which color should dominate in the scene. You can make it the dominant (most important) color by photographing either a large area of subdued color or a small glimpse of bright color. The dominant color should relate closely to the center of interest in the picture. If the color itself is not the center of interest, then it should at least support and enhance the center of interest. If a single strong color dominates, pay attention to patterns and textures that accompany it. (See Figure 14-8.)

Contrasting color

In black and white photography, the only way to achieve contrast is through variations between the lightest and darkest areas of a scene. Light and shade are still important in color photography; the additional elements in the composition are the varying

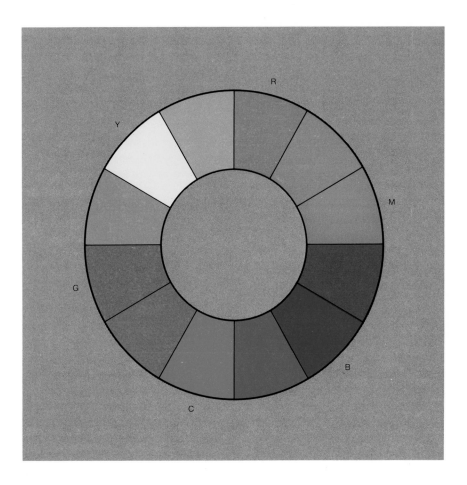

intensities of vibrant colors found in the scene. (See Figure 14-9.)

The colors that contrast most strongly are those opposite each other on the color wheel; large areas of contrasting colors can stimulate the viewer to action, while small areas can create interest and inspire emotion.

Tone and hue

Tone—the range of lightness and darkness in a scene—and hue combine to make up the composition of color photography. The best contrasts of tone and hue depend on the subject you are photographing. Pictures of dark surfaces in dim light convey a somber mood. The white lights near the bright end of the scale help capture the delicate features desired in portraiture. When the picture is monochromatic or is shot in misty or dim light, tone

FIGURE 14-6 COLOR WHEEL

becomes more important than hue. (See Figure 14-10.)

Aggressive and passive color

A color's ability to capture and hold attention is usually determined by the intensity of saturation and the hue of the color. Colors with high saturation values are more *aggressive* than those with low saturation values. Red and colors close to it in hue are considered to be aggressive colors; blue and its neighbors are *passive*. (See Figure 14-11.)

Advancing and receding colors

Some colors are said to *advance* or *recede* in respect to the space they maintain in the print or slide. The reddish colors advance, and the bluish colors recede. Some colors—such as yellow, black, gray, and white—neither advance nor recede.

Saturation also affects whether colors advance or recede—a high-saturation color will advance more than a color with low saturation. A high-saturation blue, for example, may seem to advance, even though blue generally recedes and is passive. (See Figure 14-12.)

Warm and cold colors

Red and its adjacent colors are considered *warm* colors; blue and its neighbors are traditionally *cold* colors. Yellow, gray, black, and white are generally neutral. Any hue can be warmed by adding red or cooled by adding blue.

Other color composition guidelines

Remember: each color is only a part of the total composition, so you need to keep each main color in perspective when arranging a photographic scene.

It is usually better to have a few simple colors than to use a wide variety of colors in a picture. Let one group of hues, expanded with related saturations and hues, dominate the picture.

As leading lines bring the viewer's eye to the center of interest, so do leading colors. Avoid isolating strong colors near the border of the print, because they will lead the eye away from the center of interest and out of the picture.

Skillful color composition can contribute greatly to the impact and statement of a photograph. A certain mood—warm, cool, and so on—can easily be created through proper use of colors in the scene. Subtle psychological undertones can provide depth and interest to the picture. For example, blue usually suggests coolness; but it can also imply dignity, royalty, and wealth when used in certain ways. Red signals danger, but it can also evoke feelings of warmth.

The only way to understand, see, and feel color at a level beyond everyday business is to practice hard at overcoming the repetitious programming of your brain and the standard notion that objects in the environment always remain the same color. Look carefully at a "white" shirt. Almost certainly you will find that it is a very weakly saturated blue, yellow, or green.

COLOR EXPOSURE

Using a light meter

Figuring exposure for color film is much more difficult than for black and white film—there is much less room for error. Only a small area on either side of normal exposure will yield a usable slide or negative. If you are shooting with normal lighting, modern exposure meters will keep you within these limits. But you will run into trouble if you use exposure meters to read in strong backlight or in areas of high contrast, such as sunlit highlights or deep

shadows. In these cases you will have to decide how much detail to record in either the bright highlight or the deep shadow areas.

You will find that the meter reading is influenced most by highlight values, so you will get an underexposure unless you allow for shadows. Underexposure by up to half a stop will help produce a more saturated color in reversal films. Overexposure by up to half a stop has the same result when color negative films are used.

There is a general rule of thumb for shooting color pictures: for normal-looking colors, take pictures in the middle of the day in sunlight or open shade. The first time you use artistic license to deviate from this rule, you will be amazed at the results. Shooting a picture in rain or during early morning or twilight will produce colors that can be dazzling and effective.

Remember that, depending on the time of day and the weather, daylight has different color qualities. Memorable color photographs can be taken in natural light under all kinds of conditions.

Shooting color during the day

Daylight can be divided into five general time periods.

Before sunrise During the time before sunrise, objects are essentially black and white, the light is very cool and shadowless, and the colors are extremely muted. As sunrise draws closer, colors grow in intensity and slowly separate into their hues. Until the sun appears over the horizon, however, the objects appear pearly and flat. (See Figure 14-13.)

Early morning work may require a tripod because of longer-than-normal exposure times. When calculating your exposure time, keep a close eye on your light meter to keep up with rapidly changing conditions.

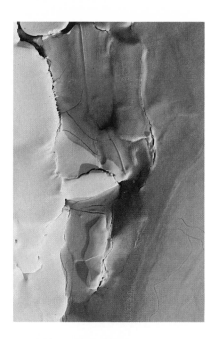

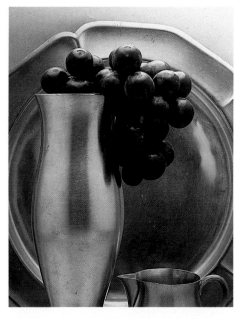

FIGURE 14-7 LIGHT AND SHADE
(Duncan Urquhart)

FIGURE 14-8 DOMINANT COLOR
(Mary Jo Metalonis)

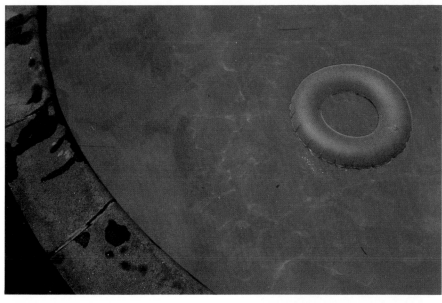

FIGURE 14-9 CONTRASTING COLOR
(Barbara J. Crawford)

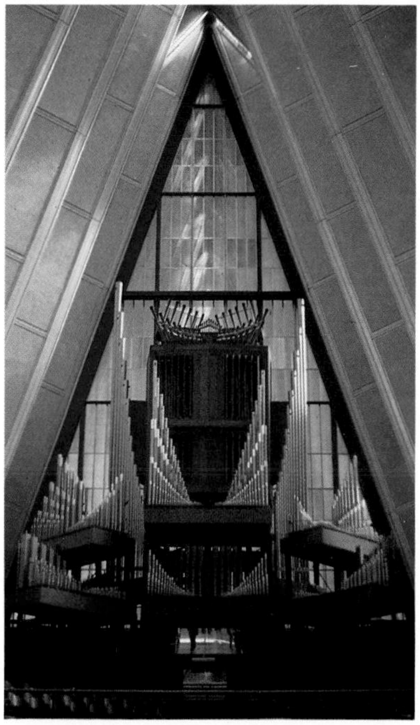

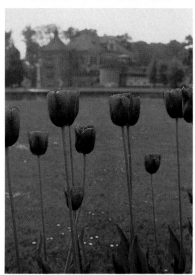

FIGURE 14-10 TONE AND HUE
(R. Colobella)

**FIGURE 14-11 AGGRESSIVE AND PASSIVE
COLOR**
(R. Colobella)

FIGURE 14-12 ADVANCING AND RECEDING COLOR
(Luther Alridge)

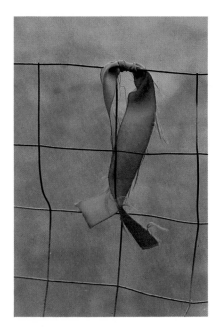

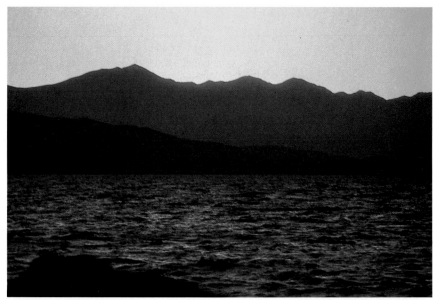

FIGURE 14-13 BEFORE SUNUP (C.R. Katner)

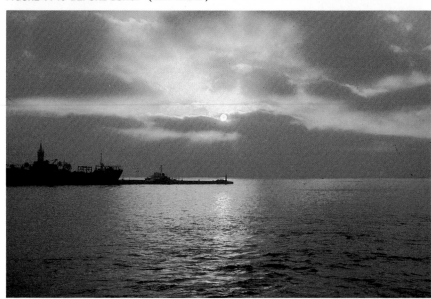

FIGURE 14-15 MIDDAY
(P.W. Hayes)

FIGURE 14-16 LATE AFTERNOON
(Bruce N. Berman)

FIGURE 14-14 EARLY MORNING (P.W. Hayes)

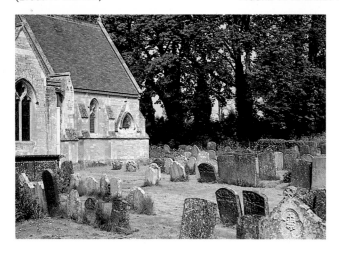

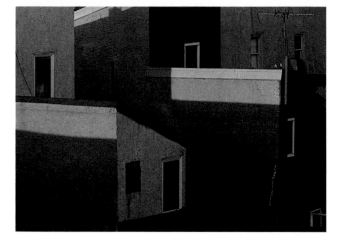

FIGURE 14-18 RAIN AND FOG
(Rose Martin)

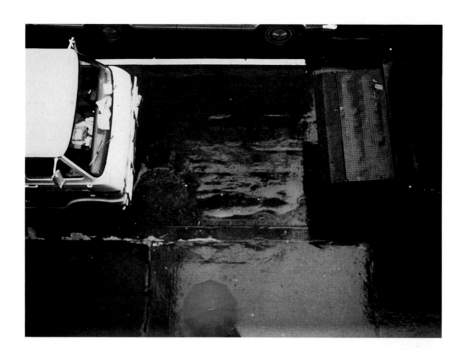

FIGURE 14-17 EVENING
(R. Colobella)

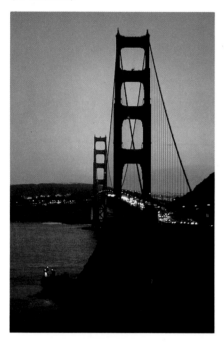

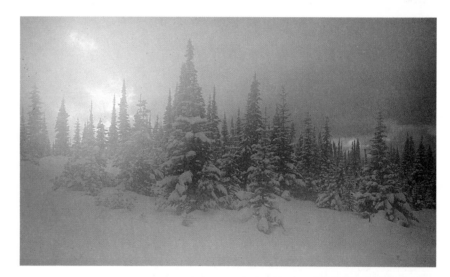

FIGURE 14-19 SNOW SHOT
(R. Colobella)

FIGURE 14-20A&B EFFECT OF USING A POLARIZER ON COLOR INTENSITY

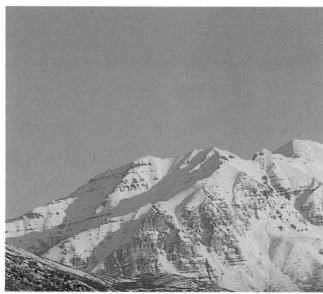

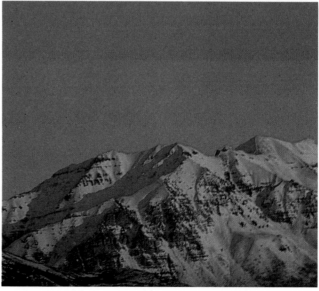

FIGURE 14-20A Without a Polarizing Filter

FIGURE 14-20B Polarizer Adjusted for Maximum Effect

Early morning The moment the sun rises above the horizon, the light quality immediately changes. Light rays reaching the subject are coming through the atmosphere at a very low angle, so the light that gets through is much warmer in color than it will be later in the day. In the early morning, light blue wavelengths are filtered out because they are more easily scattered, so red and orange wavelengths dominate. Shadows, however, take on a bluish tint, because they are illuminated primarily by light reflected from the blue sky. Early morning light lasts from sunrise to approximately 10:00 A.M., and its effects decrease as midday approaches. (See Figure 14-14.)

Midday On a clear day, as the sun climbs toward its high point in the sky, the contrast between colors becomes greater. When the sun is at its zenith, especially in the summer, this contrast is also at its peak. At midday, there is no color distortion in the light coming from the sun, so the rendering of the relationships between colored objects in the scene will be accurate. Each object will stand out strongly in its own true hue, and the shadows at midday will be quite close to black, in comparison to the brightly lighted objects. (See Figure 14-15.) Midday is from approximately 10:00 A.M. to 2:00 P.M.

Late afternoon and early evening When the sun starts to set and the red and orange wavelengths again begin to dominate, the light quality starts to warm again. Because this change happens gradually, you have to train yourself to see it.

On a clear evening, if the setting sun remains visible down to the horizon, objects will almost seem to glow—a phenomenon especially true of gold, yellow, and white objects. Shadows become longer, and bluish-white surfaces become strongly textured and interesting. (See Figure 14-16.) Just as in early morning, conditions change

rapidly, so keep a watchful eye on your light meter. Early evening lasts from about 2:00 P.M. until sundown.

Evening There is still a lot of usable light in the sky—generally reflected by the clouds as reds, yellows, and oranges—after the sun goes down. With increasing exposure, this light can be used until it reaches the point of almost total darkness. Under the right conditions, it can produce a stunning pinkish- or greenish-purple effect. (See Figure 14-17.)

Like pre-sunrise pictures, evening pictures require longer exposure and a steady camera, so you should use a tripod. Since exposure is hard to meter during the evening, you should probably bracket the shot. As night approaches, the contrast between colors lessens and the colors become increasingly muted. Finally, just before night descends, all colors almost disappear, and the world is once again viewed essentially in black and white.

Shooting weather

Most beginning photographers think they cannot shoot pictures outdoors when the weather is bad. If that is what you have always thought, it is time to change your opinion: *there is no such thing as bad weather for shooting color pictures.* Anything in the atmosphere that blocks or filters sunlight can usefully alter the color qualities of the light. All you have to do is learn how to deal with various weather conditions.

Rain and fog Fog produces tones much like those just before sunrise: pearly and muted. Photographing in light mist can yield pictures with soft, delicate qualities. Colors will be subdued, often to the palest of tones, and details may be blurred. Rain will dim some colors and enrich others; objects coated with water have shiny reflective and subdued colors. The light just before and after a storm can

add drama and richness to the hues in any photographic scene. (See Figure 14-18.)

Shooting pictures in rain or fog does create some problems you will need to address. As the light intensity decreases, you will have to increase exposure time, so under some conditions you may need a tripod. Of course, you must keep your film and equipment dry. If your camera or lenses do get wet, dry them off immediately; never touch film with wet hands.

Snow During a snowstorm, color qualities are very subdued and detail is greatly reduced; both the quality of the light and the lack of tones under overcast skies tend to flatten landscapes and allow strong blue hues to dominate. After the storm, when the snow is lit by the sun, the extreme contrast between light and dark is very difficult to handle. When the intensity of reflected light under bright skies is too high for meter readings, underexposed shots usually result. By far the best time to photograph sunlit snow is in the early morning or late afternoon light. (See Figure 14-19.)

FILTERS FOR COLOR PHOTOGRAPHY

Filters are used in color photography for some of the same reasons they are used in black and white. Chapter Ten covers the uses of some of these filters. Table 14-1 summarizes color filters. The kind of filter you use depends on what you are shooting.

Light-balancing filters

Color casts, or shifts along the spectrum so that one color seems to predominate, result when films that are balanced for particular light sources are used with other light sources. Daylight reversal films exposed under artificial light will have a yellow shift; tungsten films exposed outdoors produce a strong blue shift. Color negative films are primarily balanced for daylight. However, if you use these films under tungsten lighting, any resulting color balance problems can usually be corrected during the printing process.

Since color films are balanced for specific light sources, even for specific parts of the country, you do not need a filter to get the correct color rendition, so long as you use a film with its recommended light source. If you cannot use the recommended light source, a conversion filter will allow good color translation by changing the color quality of the light reaching the film to the type of light for which the color film is balanced. For example, you can expose daylight films to a tungsten light source by using an 80A filter; an 85B filter will allow you to expose tungsten films in daylight. Remember, if you are not metering through the lens, to allow for increased exposure time when using a filter. (See Table 14-2.)

Special-purpose filters

Special-purpose filters can be used for color correction or to add drama and impact to a photographic scene. For example, a blue filter used in daylight conveys a feeling of coldness or simulates moonlight. *Split-field* filters have one color on half the filter and a clear side on the other half, allowing you to add color to one part of a scene without affecting the other parts. For instance, with such a filter, you can produce a red sky in a landscape without changing the color of the land.

Neutral-density filters These filters control the overall brightness level of a scene without altering any of the col-

TABLE 14-1 □ COLOR-BALANCING FILTERS AND THEIR USES

LIGHT SOURCE	TYPE OF FILM BALANCED FOR THIS LIGHT SOURCE	FILMS THAT CAN USE THIS LIGHT SOURCE	UNFILTERED COLOR CAST	FILTER TO CORRECT COLOR
100W Tungsten Bulb	None	Daylight	Warms up image	None
		Tungsten Types A and B	Yellow	82C
Studio Lamps	Tungsten Type B	Daylight	Yellow	80A
		Tungsten Type A	Slight Yellow	82A
Photo Floods	Tungsten Type A	Daylight	Yellow	80B
		Tungsten Type B	Slight Blue	81A
Clear Flashbulbs	None	Daylight	Yellow	80C
		Tungsten Types A or B	Slight Blue	81C or 81D
Daylight, Blue Flash, or Electronic Flash	Daylight	Tungsten Types A or B	Strong Blue	85 or 85B
Cloudy or Hazy Sky	Daylight	Daylight	Slight to Moderate Blue	81A

TABLE 14-2 □ SUMMARY OF COLOR FILTERS FOR COLOR PHOTOGRAPHY

FILTER	F/STOP INCREASE	FILTER FACTOR	EFFECT	USE WITH
Amber	$\frac{2}{3}$	1.5×	Corrects color	Tungsten film in daylight or electronic flash
Blue	2	4×	Corrects color	Daylight color film under tungsten light
Magenta	1	2×	Corrects color	Daylight color film in fluorescent light
Neutral density	Varies	Varies	Prevents color shift when using wider aperture or slower shutter speed	Any combination of light source and film
Orange	1	2×	Corrects color	Tungsten color film in fluorescent light
Pale Orange	$\frac{2}{3}$	1.5×	Warms colors not in direct sunlight	Color film in daylight
Polarizing	$1\frac{1}{3}$	2.5×	Reduces glare; darkens sky; strengthens color	Any combination of light source and film
Skylight	None	None	Reduces blue cast in shade and in general light on cloudy days; somewhat reduces UV haze	Color film
Ultraviolet	None	None	Reduces UV haze in landscapes; reduces blue cast in high-altitude and desert scenes	Daylight color film; black and white film

ors; they also prevent overexposure when you are working in high-intensity light.

Polarizing filters These are used in color photography to intensify colors and to eliminate reflections. (See Figure 14-20.) *Ultraviolet and haze filters* can also be used effectively in color photography. Again, remember that some light loss occurs whenever any kind of filter is used, so adjust your exposure accordingly.

SUMMARY

Color photography enables the photographer to record vibrant scenes. Most of the unnatural results and failures in color photography are actually caused by the photographer's lack of color vision. Photographers must force their eyes and brain to look at each scene critically; they must learn to see what is really there, not just what they expect or what memory tells them is there. Remember: *the photographer is the most important factor in photographic work.* It is the photographer's creativity that will produce memorable results, in black and white or in color.

Color is indeed a challenge, and a knowledge of color psychology is essential to producing effective work.

REVIEW QUESTIONS

1 Define the following terms:

Hue

Chroma or Saturation

Value or Brightness

2 What are the receptor cells in the eye called?

3 In reference to color composition, colors can be _____ and _____.

4 Name the parts of a daylight shooting cycle.

5 What is brightness adaptation?

6 What is color adaptation?

7 Name the subtractive primaries.

8 What color is an object with a color temperature of 6000°K?

9 At what end of the spectrum are "aggressive" colors usually found?

10 What time of day produces the most accurate rendition of hue?

FIFTEEN

Color films and processes

Niépce and Daguerre, two of photography's pioneers, both attempted unsuccessfully to create color pictures. After all, nature was in color and since the camera recorded nature, it seemed that the two should be united. But the secret to color photography lay in the correct use and balance of chemicals. Color photography also required a knowledge of physics as well as of advanced chemistry, and few in those days were qualified to make any worthwhile attempts at producing either color film or color prints.

THE FIRST COLOR PHOTOGRAPH

The birth of modern color photography came in 1861, with a lecture on color vision by the Scottish physicist Sir James Clerk Maxwell. The first three-color photographs were prepared as illustrations to support his tri-color theory of color vision.

Maxwell took a series of three photographs of a piece of red tartan ribbon, using black and white film plates. One photograph was shot through a blue filter, the second through a green filter, and the last through a red filter. The film plates were developed to yield three negatives, and positive lantern slides were then produced by printing the negatives. The positive taken through a blue filter was projected through a blue filter; the red and green positives were projected through red and green filters respectively. (See Figure 15-1.) The images were then registered to form a successful color reproduction of the tartan ribbon with a wide range of colors.

ADDITIVE AND SUBTRACTIVE COLOR PROCESSES

Additive process

In Maxwell's process, the choice of colors at the picture-taking stage was limited to the primaries: red, blue, and green, sometimes called *additive primaries*. The amount of each primary color projected onto the screen was controlled by the silver image in the positive slide—a process that became known as the additive color process. When each of the colors was projected on a screen, it formed a color image. The amount of each color was controlled by the silver image in the lantern slide.

Subtractive process

An alternative approach to the selection of colors for reproduction is to utilize the complementary colors. Yellow, magenta, and cyan are used to absorb the three primary colors blue, green, and red respectively, in a process known as the *subtractive system* of color photography. See Chapter Fourteen for more on the subtractive process.

The subtractive system was described by the French pianist Louis Ducos du Hauron. His book, *Les Couleurs en Photographie: Solution du Problème,* published in 1869, laid down all the basic principles of modern color photography and discussed both additive and subtractive color processes.

A primary-color filter (red, blue, or green) can transmit only approximately one-third of the visible spectrum; it absorbs two-thirds of the spectrum while transmitting its own color. For example, a red filter transmits red and absorbs blue and green.

When primary-color filters are placed so that they overlap, the area where any two overlap is black, since the filters have no common bands of transmission. If a red filter and a green filter are placed together, no light can pass through them: the green filter transmits only green and the red filter only red, so no light passes through. Combinations like this cannot be used *together* to control the color of transmitted light.

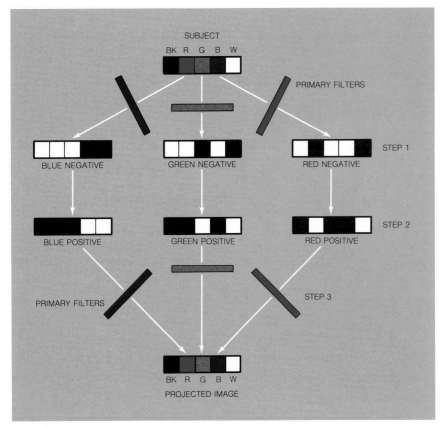

FIGURE 15-1 HOW MAXWELL'S FIRST COLOR PHOTOGRAPH WORKED

Step 1 Three separate exposures of a colored object were made on black and white film, through blue, green, and red filters respectively. The film was processed to give the three separate negatives.

Step 2 The negatives from Step 1 are contact printed onto three new pieces of film. These pieces of film are then developed, to yield black-and-white positives of the negatives.

Step 3 The black-and-white positives from Step 2 are placed in three separate projectors, along with the correct filtration: blue positive with blue filter, etc. The projected images from the three projectors are brought into register, and a color image is seen.

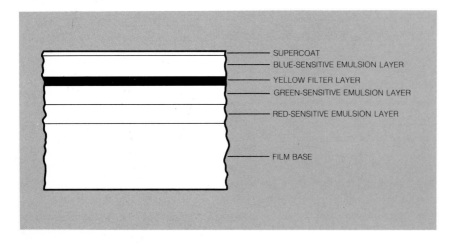

FIGURE 15-2 DIAGRAM OF AN INTEGRAL TRIPAK

Complementary filters (yellow, cyan, and magenta) each absorb only about one-third of the visible spectrum, so such filters *can* be used in combination to control the color of transmitted light. The effects of combining complementary-color filters can be unusual and beautiful. Systems that use yellow, magenta, and cyan dyes or filters to subtract blue, green, and red from the transmitted light are called subtractive processes.

THE DEVELOPMENT OF KODACHROME

As mentioned, the first three-color photograph was made by the additive process in 1861. The viewing system alone required the use of three projectors, so the process was not practical for general use.

By 1910, however, an ingenious use of the additive process had made possible the production of plates yielding color photographs with a single exposure in a conventional camera. The exposure was made through a mosaic grid (or *reseau*) composed of hundreds of very small red, blue, and green squares. The film thus exposed was printed as a transparent black and white positive on glass and was then viewed through a similar grid or mosaic. Unfortunately, the system wasted about 70 percent of the available light, so the pictures were very dim at best. It is interesting that a form of the mosaic method of additive color reproduction survived to flourish in color television.

In 1935, Kodak announced that it had perfected a color reversal (slide) film based on the subtractive process. The only problem was that Kodachrome had to be sent to a Kodak laboratory for processing. A year later, Agfa introduced a color reversal film that could be processed by the user.

Since the introduction of Agfa's film, many other improvements have been made in color films. In 1942, Kodak introduced Kodacolor negative film, based on the subtractive process, for making color prints. Today's color films have the versatility and speed of black and white films.

COLOR FILMS

Most color photographs taken today are made with an emulsion that records blue, green, and red light in distinct layers within the emulsion. The specially designed emulsion assembly is called an integral tripack. (See Figure 15-2.)

Color film consists of three black and white emulsions coated one on top of the other to form a permanent multi-layer structure. The top black and white emulsion layer is sensitized to respond only to blue wavelengths, the middle to green, and the bottom to red. The blue, green, and red parts of an image, then, each record in the properly sensitized emulsion layer. (See Figure 15-3.)

Other colors affect the emulsion layers to varying degrees. Yellow, for example, records in the green- and red-sensitive layers, but not in the blue. A yellow filter is sandwiched between the blue and green emulsions to filter out any blue wavelengths that are not absorbed by the blue emulsion.

There are two types of color film: color negative and color slide. Color negative films produce a negative that is then printed on paper; color slide or reversal film itself forms a color transparency. The transparency is projected to form an image. Common color negative and reversal films are listed in Tables 15-1 and 15-2.

Color film characteristics

Film speed Color slide and color print films now have speeds that match those of black and white films—they range from Kodachrome (ASA 25) to several that have an ASA rating of 400. It is also possible to push pro-

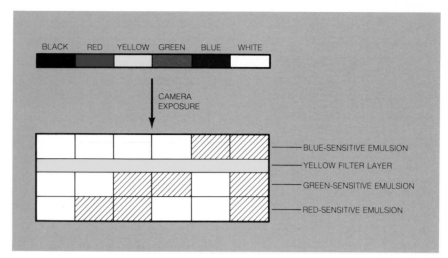

FIGURE 15-3 HOW LIGHT AFFECTS THE TRIPACK
This illustrates where the latent image is recorded in the tripack during exposure.

cess Ektachrome 400 so that it is equivalent to a film with an ASA of 800 or more.

Grain Color slide and print films with standard ASA ratings have grain ranges from very fine to micro fine. As with black and white films, the lower the ASA rating, the finer the grain.

Latitude Traditionally, color slide films have had their exposure range or latitude weighted in favor of underexposure. For example, older, slower Kodachromes could tolerate as much as a full-stop underexposure, but no more than a half-stop overexposure. Today's color slide films have a common latitude of a half-stop underexposure or overexposure, especially films with an ASA rating of 100 or less. As stated in Chapter Fourteen, slight underexposure will produce a more saturated image in the color transparency.

Color negative films have a different exposure range, usually weighted in favor of slight overexposure. Most color negative films can tolerate up to a half stop of overexposure with very few undesirable effects.

Color balance Unlike the human eye, color films are not able to adapt

TABLE 15-1 □ COMMONLY USED COLOR NEGATIVE FILMS

FILM	DAYLIGHT ASA RATING
Agfacolor CNS	80
3M Color Print	80
Fujicolor F11	100
Kodacolor II	100
Sakuracolor II N100	100
Vericolor II Type S	100
Agfacolor CNS 400	400
Fujicolor F II 400	400
Kodacolor 400	400
Sakuracolor 400	400

TABLE 15-2 □ COMMONLY USED COLOR REVERSAL FILMS

FILM	DAYLIGHT ASA RATING
Kodachrome 25	25
Agfachrome 64	64
Ektachrome 64	64
Kodachrome 64	64
3M Color Slide	64
Fujichrome 100	100
3M Color Slide	100
Sakurachrome R100	100
Ektachrome 200	200
Ektachrome 400	400
3M Color Slide	400

Most of these films have a tungsten light version with reduced film speed.

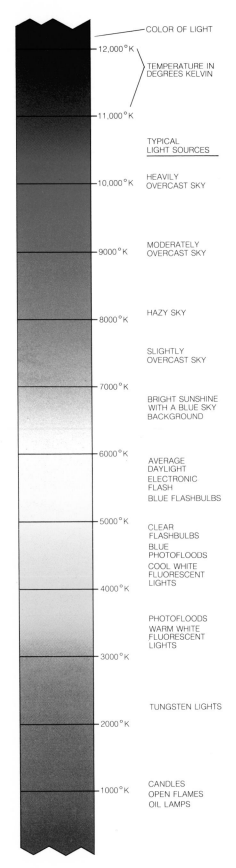

COLOR OF LIGHT

12,000°K

TEMPERATURE IN DEGREES KELVIN

11,000°K

TYPICAL LIGHT SOURCES

HEAVILY OVERCAST SKY

10,000°K

MODERATELY OVERCAST SKY

9000°K

HAZY SKY

8000°K

SLIGHTLY OVERCAST SKY

7000°K

BRIGHT SUNSHINE WITH A BLUE SKY BACKGROUND

6000°K

AVERAGE DAYLIGHT
ELECTRONIC FLASH
BLUE FLASHBULBS

5000°K

CLEAR FLASHBULBS
BLUE PHOTOFLOODS
COOL WHITE FLUORESCENT LIGHTS

4000°K

PHOTOFLOODS
WARM WHITE FLUORESCENT LIGHTS

3000°K

TUNGSTEN LIGHTS

2000°K

1000°K

CANDLES
OPEN FLAMES
OIL LAMPS

FIGURE 15-4 COLOR TEMPERATURES OF SOME PHOTOGRAPHIC LIGHT SOURCES
"Color temperature" describes the color mixtures that exist in different types of normal and artificial light. It is *not* a measure of heat.

to "see" objects as being the same color when they are lit by different light sources. (See Chapter Fourteen for a more detailed explanation.) Multi-layer color emulsions have a fixed, pre-set response, and give truly accurate results only when they are used with the light sources for which they were balanced. For example, someone's face appears to you to be about the same color both in daylight and in the light of a studio lamp. Your eye sees both as being correct, even though the light from the tungsten bulb is more yellow than the sunlight. (See Figure 15-4.)

Color films do not adapt to lighting changes in the same way that our eyes do, so most are balanced for daylight, with tungsten light versions also available. Daylight films can produce good results with tungsten light sources if proper filtration or a flash unit is used. Daylight films exposed in tungsten light without correction will have a pronounced yellow cast; tungsten films exposed in daylight, if not corrected, will have a decidedly blue cast.

COLOR PROCESSING

In color processing, the exact amount of the image dye, each color in its own layer, must be produced in the emulsion; if this does not occur as it should, objectionable color effects result.

The processing conditions under which a tripack gives correct values of speed, contrast, and coloration for all three layers are very limited, so the processing steps—including processing times—are carefully specified by the film manufacturer. Any departure from the processing steps outlined by the manufacturer, which generally include solution temperature, agitation timing, and processing time, will probably cause poor results.

The reversal process

There are two types of color reversal processes. In the Kodachrome process, the color dyes are located in the color developers and the film must be sent to a Kodak lab to be developed. In the Kodak E-6 process, the color couplers are located in the various layers of the tripack, so that the film can be processed by the user. See Figure 15-5 for a diagram of the reversal process of the E-6; Table 15-3 outlines the steps involved.

TABLE 15-3 □ COLOR REVERSAL (SLIDE) PROCESSING STEPS

PROCESSING STEPS	PROCESSING TIME (MINUTES)	TEMPERATURE		AGITATION TIME (SECONDS)		
		°F	°C	BEGIN	REST	CONTINUE
Developer	7	$100 \pm \frac{1}{2}$	37.8 ± 0.3	30	15	5
First Wash	1	92–102	33.5–39	30	15	5
Second Wash	1	92–102	33.5–39	30	15	5
Reversal Bath	2	92–102	33.5–39	30	80	
Color Developer	6	100 ± 2	37.8 ± 1.1	30	25	5
Conditioner	2	92–102	33.5–39	30	80	
Bleach	7	92–102	33.5–39	30	25	5
Fixer	4	92–102	33.5–39	30	25	5
Running-Water Wash	6	92–102	33.5–39	30	25	5
Stabilizer	1	92–102	33.5–39	30	20	
Drying	10–20	75–120	24–49			

Note: Process E-6, for small-tank development.

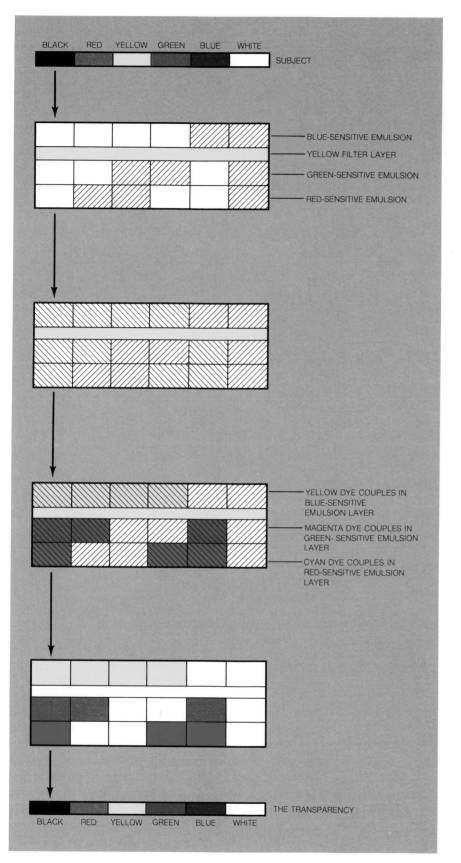

SUBJECT

BLACK RED YELLOW GREEN BLUE WHITE

BLUE-SENSITIVE EMULSION
YELLOW FILTER LAYER
GREEN-SENSITIVE EMULSION
RED-SENSITIVE EMULSION

YELLOW DYE COUPLES IN
BLUE-SENSITIVE
EMULSION LAYER
MAGENTA DYE COUPLES IN
GREEN-SENSITIVE EMULSION
LAYER
CYAN DYE COUPLES IN
RED-SENSITIVE EMULSION
LAYER

THE TRANSPARENCY

BLACK RED YELLOW GREEN BLUE WHITE

FIGURE 15-5 HOW THE REVERSAL PROCESS WORKS

Camera exposure is followed by black-and-white development.

White-light exposure or chemical fogging produces a new latent image.

Color development brings out the latent image from fogging and couples appropriate color dyes to this developing image.

Bleach removes all metallic silver and yellow filter from the emulsion; fix removes any unused silver halides from the emulsion of the transparency.

When the transparency is viewed, this is the resulting image.

Reversal film is first exposed in the camera. Image development begins with the formation of a black and white image in the negative in the first developer stage. After this first developer is rinsed from the film with a water wash, the film is fogged by chemical means in a reversal bath. The fogged silver halide grains are next placed in color developers, where color couplers combine with metallic silver. The manner in which the film and the color developer are manufactured ensures the appropriate location of dye colors. Yellow dyes can only couple with metallic silver in the blue recording layer of the emulsion, magenta dyes only within the green layer, and cyan only within the red layer. The bleaching and fixing steps leave only the image dyes in the gelatin layers. Finally, the film is given a last wash to remove any of the processing chemicals, and it is placed in a stabilizer to increase dye stability and promote spot-free drying.

The Negative—Positive Process

In the color negative–positive process, a negative record is made in the emulsion tripack during exposure, and the film is then processed to yield a negative. As in black and white processing, the negative image is not intended for viewing but is used to produce a positive print.

FIGURE 15-6 HOW THE NEGATIVE–POSITIVE PROCESS WORKS
When the print is viewed, the dyes in the various layers reflect and absorb the rays of white light, so that the image in the print appears like the original scene.

In the negative–positive process, information about the original scene's blue, green, and red light qualities must be available at the printing stage. Color negative film is manufactured so that the blue-, green-, and red-sensitive layers generate yellow, magenta, and cyan image dyes when processed. Metallic silver is also produced in the emulsion at this time, and it is removed by the bleaching and fixing steps. The dye images that remain in the emulsion layers form the color negative. These negative image colors are complements (opposites) to those in the original scene. (See Figure 15-6 and Table 15-4.)

The color negative is then used in the printing stage. In this step, the negative is printed onto a second integral tripack contained in the color paper emulsion. Color paper is processed in a manner similar to that used for color negative film. While color paper is produced in only one contrast grade, it does come in various surface textures for different kinds of photographs. A semi-matte surface is best for landscape shots or portraits, while a glossy finish helps reproduce the highlights in shots of jewelry or water. The textured surfaces, while not as visually brilliant, do not cause a loss of color quality. See Table 15-5 for steps in the production of a positive print.

At the printing stage, color balance is easy to control with subtractive filtration in the enlarger. Because of this, color negative and print materials need not be so closely balanced as reversal materials are.

Color negative and paper processes have been greatly simplified; a modern process may require only two or three

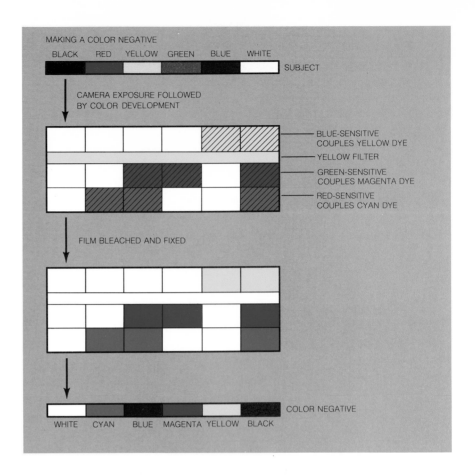

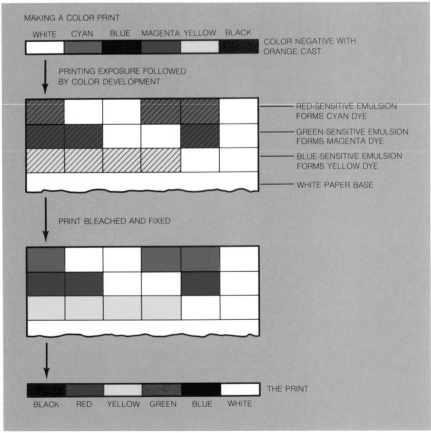

FIGURE 15-7 CROSS-SECTION OF DIRECT POSITIVE OR CIBACHROME PRINTING PAPER

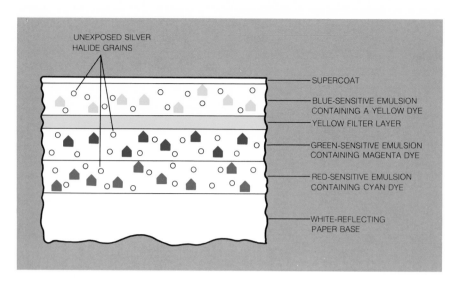

solutions and washing steps. The Kodak C-41 process for film and the Ektaprint 2 process for color paper are typical of today's negative–positive processes.

Positive–positive processes

There are alternatives to forming a color image by having image dyes produced within the emulsion layers during color development. In one of these processes, dyes introduced into the emulsion layers during film manufacture are destroyed. Red light removes cyan dye from the emulsion, green light removes magenta dye, and blue removes yellow.

Ilford's Cibachrome process is a current process that uses this method of image formation to produce positive prints from positive transparencies. The print material is an integral tripack manufactured so that the uppermost blue-sensitive emulsion contains a yellow dye, the green layer contains a magenta dye, and the red layer contains a cyan dye. (See Figure 15-7.) The first step is the black and white development of exposed emulsion grains. The silver image is then used to destroy the corresponding dyes that are present in the emulsion layers. (See Table 15-6.)

By design, fragments from the destruction of the dyes are colorless, soluble, or both. The silver image acts as a pattern for the destruction of the dyes by the bleach bath, after which the unwanted silver salts are removed by fixing. The end result is a positive dye image record left within the gelatin layers. (See Figure 15-8.)

Several manufacturers make starter kits, so you can experiment with any one of the three processes. If you decide to process your own slides, color negatives, or color prints, it is a good idea to begin with the small-volume kits.

TABLE 15-4 □ COLOR NEGATIVE PROCESSING STEPS

PROCESSING STEPS	PROCESSING TIME (MINUTES)	TEMPERATURE		AGITATION (SECONDS)		
		°F	°C	BEGIN	REST	CONTINUE
Developer	3¼	100 ±¼	37.8 ±0.15	30	13	2
Bleach	6½	75–105	24–40.5	30	25	5
Wash	3¼	75–105	24–40.5			
Fixer	6½	75–105	24–40.5	30	25	5
Wash	3¼	75–105	24–40.5			
Stabilizer	1½	75–105	24–40.5	30		
Drying	10–20	75–110	24–43.5			

This is process C-41, for small-tank development. Several manufacturers make processing kits used for color negative film. Each manufacturer's instructions should be carefully followed.

TABLE 15-5 □ COLOR PRINT PROCESSING STEPS

PROCESSING STEPS	PROCESSING TIME (MINUTES)
Prewet (Water)	½
Developer	3½
Stop Bath	½
Wash	½
Bleach–Fix	1
First Wash	½
Second Wash	½
Third Wash	½
Fourth Wash	½

This process is used for Kodak Ektacolor 74 RC and similar papers, with table processors.

TABLE 15-6 □ CIBACHROME PROCESSING STEPS

PROCESSING STEPS	TEMPERATURE (°C)	PROCESSING TIME (MINUTES)	TOTAL ELAPSED TIME (MINUTES)
Developer	30 ±½	3	3
Running-Water Wash	28–30	¾	3¾
Bleach	30 ±1	3	6¾
Running-Water Wash	28–30	¾	7½
Fixer	30 ±1	3	10½
Running-Water Wash (Final)	28–32	4½	15

**FIGURE 15-8 HOW THE POSITIVE–POSITIVE
PROCESS WORKS**

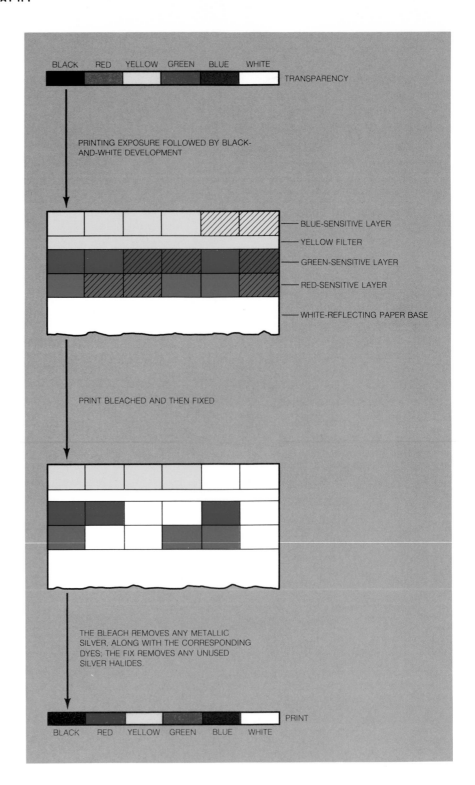

SUMMARY

The field of color photography is as large as and in some ways more complex than the field of black and white photography. Becoming technically competent in either black and white or color photography requires a great deal of time and patience. Both areas can be mastered, though, and the reward will be a great deal of satisfaction. With an investment of time, the photographer can explore the many possibilities inherent in the exciting field of color photography. The important thing to remember is that adding color to a photograph does not mean you can forget about good composition, exposure, visualization, and all the other elements that make up a pleasing photograph. Color is, in the end, just one more tool to test and challenge our creativity.

REVIEW QUESTIONS

1 Who produced the first color photograph?

2 What is the name of James Clerk Maxwell's color process?

3 Who described all the basic principles of color photography in a book published in 1869?

4 What was the first color reversal film to be marketed commercially?

5 What is the emulsion of a color film called?

6 Yellow wavelengths will record in which layer(s) of the tripack?

7 What are the four main characteristics of color film?

8 In what type of film will underexposure by up to half a stop produce a more saturated color?

9 In what type of film will overexposure by up to half a stop produce a more saturated color?

10 In which process are the color couplers located in the emulsion?

11 What process produces both a negative and a print?

12 What process can be used to make a print from a slide?

APPENDIX A

Outline of the history of photography

1400 Glass is discovered.

350 Pinhole images are discussed by Aristotle.

200 B.C. Ptolemy discovers that light bends as it passes from air to water.

c. 1400 A.D. Lenses are first used for optical devices.

Before 1519 Leonardo da Vinci shows a working diagram of a camera obscura and explains how to operate it. *Leonardo's notebooks were not published, however, until 1797.*

1550 Geronimo Cardano suggests use of a biconvex lens to improve the image in the camera obscura.

1558 Giovanni Battista della Porta writes the first published description of the camera obscura and its applications, suggesting that artists could use the camera as a drawing aid. *Della Porta revised his work in 1589, giving a fuller treatment, including improvements since his first edition.*

1568 Daniello Barbaro proposes the use of a diaphragm to improve the sharpness of the camera obscura image.

1573 Ignazio Danti uses a concave mirror behind the camera obscura lens to correct the image.

Before 1580 Friedrich Risner explains how to enlarge and reduce the image and describes the first portable camera obscura.

1600 Georgius Fabricius first reports that silver chloride crystals darken when exposed to light.

1604—11 Johannes Kepler suggests using a concave lens in addition to the convex, to get larger images. *This is the basic principle used in modern telephoto lenses.*

1685—86 Johann Zahn describes a portable camera obscura with several lenses, a ground-glass image screen, and light shields.

1725 Johann Schulze establishes the light sensitivity of a solution of chalk, aqua regia, and silver nitrate: the mixture turned purple when exposed to light.

1763—77 W. Lewis, J. Priestley, and C.W. Scheele carry Schulze's experiments further. ·

1802 Thomas Wedgwood and Sir Humphry Davy publish their experiments in producing images on paper and leather sensitized with silver nitrate. *In other experiments, they used silver chloride as the sensitizer. The sensitized material was too slow for use in the camera obscura.*

1819 Sir J.F.W. Herschel discovers that silver salts can be dissolved with thiosulfates (hypo).

1822 J.N. Niépce makes printing plates by exposing plates sensitized with asphault, which is normally soluble in lavender oil but becomes insoluble upon exposure to light. *The plates were then etched in a weak acid to form the printing plates.*

1827 J.N. Niépce produces the first permanent photograph, the result of a bitumen process on a pewter plate.

1835 W.H. Fox Talbot produces the first paper negatives. *Talbot used several different combinations of chemicals; his negatives were sensitized with silver chloride, silver iodide, and silver nitrate in various combinations, and fixed with solutions including potassium iodide, common salt, and sodium thiosulfate. Positive prints were produced by contact printing the negative onto a new sheet of sensitized paper.*

1837 L.J.M. Daguerre, in partnership with Niépce, produces the first successful daguerreotype, employing a silver-coated plate sensitized with iodine vapor just before exposure. *The result was a light-sensitive layer of silver iodide. Mercury vapor was used for development, and common table salt was the fixative.*

J.B. Reade produces photomicrographs using a solar microscope on paper sensitized with common salt and silver nitrate, developed by washing immediately before and during exposure with gallic acid, then fixed with hypo. *Without realizing it at the time, Reade was developing a latent image.*

1839 Sir J.F.W. Herschel suggests the use of hypo as a fixing agent to Fox Talbot; Herschel takes a photograph on a glass plate coated with silver carbonate.

1840 W.H. Fox Talbot discovers that a latent image can be developed using gallic acid.

1841 W.H. Fox Talbot works out the positive–negative process, which he calls the calotype process. *Negatives were made on silver iodide paper, developed by bathing the paper in a solution of silver nitrate and gallic acid, and fixed with hypo. Positives were made by contact printing the negative image onto silver chloride paper.*

J. Petzval designs the first fast camera lens—a lens ten times faster than that used in daguerreotype photography.

1847 A. Niépce de Saint-Victor produces negatives on glass plates, yielding faster printing and clearer prints than paper negatives.

1848 A.N. de Saint-Victor proposes albumen as the vehicle for the silver iodide emulsion.

D.O. Hill and R. Adamson complete their collaboration on some of the finest calotypes ever made.

1850 L.D. Blanquart-Evrard produces the first albumen-coated paper, capable of recording more detail than Fox Talbot's. *The new paper was used almost exclusively as the printing papers of choice until the end of the century.*

1851 F.S. Archer develops the wet collodion process. *A glass plate was coated with an alcohol-ether solution of cellulose nitrate in which potassium iodide had been dissolved. The glass plate was then dipped in silver nitrate and exposed while still wet. The emulsion could be developed with pyrogallic acid or ferrous sulfate and fixed with hypo or with potassium cyanide. The wet collodion process rapidly replaced the daguerreotype process and dominated the field for almost thirty years. Inconvenient at best, the process nonetheless produced excellent results.*

1860 J.M. Cameron, one of the most remarkable amateurs of all time, takes up photography at the age of forty-eight. *Her pioneering efforts greatly improved the field of portrait photography.*

1860–65 M.B. Brady drags photographic equipment to the American Civil War battles, risking personal injury to become one of the first photographers of combat in action.

1861 Sir James Clerk Maxwell demonstrates the three-color separation and the additive system color processes.

The focal plane shutter is introduced.

1864 B.J. Sayce and W.B. Bolton prepare a silver bromide collodion emulsion.

1868 D. du Hauron develops the theoretical methods of three-color photography and proposes the subtractive system of color mixing.

1871 R.L. Maddox makes the first gelatin dry plates, the forerunners of modern-day emulsions, by substituting gelatin for collodion.

Mechanical shutters are introduced, making faster speed films practical.

1873 W. Willis patents platinum (nonsilver) printing process.

1874 W.B. Bolton discovers how to wash the silver bromide emulsion to remove the soluble salts formed in its precipitation.

1875 W.H. Jackson sets out to photograph the Rocky Mountains and the Southwest. *His stunning photographs inspired the United States Congress to establish Yellowstone as the first National Park in the country.*

L. Warnerke introduces roll film, each spool containing enough film for 100 exposures.

1877 Wratten & Wainwright of London commercially produce gelatin dry plates.

1880 Sir W. de W. Abney uses hydroquinine as a developer.

1882 J. Clayton and P.A. Attout develop the first isochromatic color-sensitive plates.

1884 George Eastman patents continuous-coating system for photographic paper.

1885 G. Eastman and W.H. Walker manufacture commercial roll film.

1887 H. Goodwin applies for a patent for the manufacture of sensitive material on a celluloid base, granted in 1898.

The leaf shutter is introduced.

1888 G. Eastman produces the first roll film camera, the No. 1 Kodak.

When all the pictures had been taken, the owner sent the camera back to the company; there, the film was developed, the prints made, and the camera loaded with new film.

1890 F. Hurter and V.C. Driffield, pioneers in the field of photographic sensitometry, develop the characteristic curve.

1891 A. Bogisch is the first to use metol as a developing agent.

First daylight loading film is introduced.

1901 The work of A. Stieglitz, an early advocate of straight photography, begins to earn recognition.

1902 P. Rudolph designs the most popular lens of all time, the Zeiss Tessar.

1906 Wratten & Wainwright introduce commercial panchromatic plates.

1914 Eastman Kodak produces first panchromatic film.

1925 The 35 mm Leica is marketed in Germany.

1927 The twin lens Rolleiflex is introduced.

1928 Panchromatic film makes its debut.

1931 H.E. Edgerton invents the electronic flash.

J.T. Rhamstine introduces the first photoelectric exposure meter, the Electrophot.

1935 The Eastman Kodak company introduces Kodachrome film, the first practical color film to be marketed commercially. *The film was the result of research headed by L. Mannes and L. Godowsky.*

1937 The Exacta single lens reflex camera is placed on the market.

1941 The Eastman Kodak Company introduces Kodacolor film.

1942 Both Agfa (Ansco-Color) and Kodak (Ektachrome) introduce slide film that the photographer could process.

1947 The birth of the instant picture era comes with the Polaroid Land Camera, named for its developer, Edwin Land. *The camera that could produce a black and white print in sixty seconds.*

1963   The Polaroid Corporation markets the first instant color print film.

1976   The first electronic computer-controlled cameras are introduced. *The camera was equipped with miniaturized circuitry, i.e., an IC chip, that automatically set the f/stop and shutter speed.*

1978   The Polaroid Corporation introduces the first practical auto-focus camera.

1979   Ilford introduces black and white film system in which all the silver used is recoverable. Film is developed much like color print film.

1982   Sony introduces digitized camera, the Mavika, which uses no film. Pictures are played back on a television screen; permanent prints can also be made from the camera's record of the image.

Kodak introduces first practical disk camera, with fifteen frames per disk. Compactness of film disk makes sophisticated electronic flash, automatic film advance, exposure control, and other features feasible.

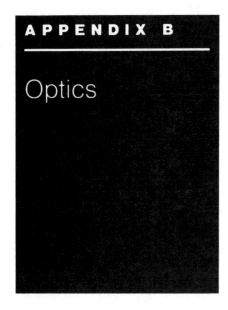

APPENDIX B

Optics

An acquaintance with the principles of how light forms images is necessary for the photographer. After all, optical images are what we are trying to record on film. Collectively, these principles are known as the *geometrical laws of optics*. These ''laws'' are simply descriptions of how light behaves. In fact, it is our understanding of these optical laws that enables us to manipulate light—with lenses, film, and the other tools of photography—in order to capture a permanent image of that light.

THE LAWS OF GEOMETRIC OPTICS

Rectilinear propagation

Generally, light rays travel in straight lines. This rule holds true so long as the ray is traveling in a single medium, such as air, water, or glass. Once it passes from one medium to another (from air to water, for example), its direction of travel is changed. (See Figure B-1.)

Reflection

Depending on the nature of the surface, the reflection of light may be direct or diffused.

Direct reflection Also often called *specular reflection,* direct reflection takes place without scattering of the light rays. A example of direct reflection is reflection of light from a mirror. In direct reflection, the angle of incidence is always equal to the angle of reflection. The angle of incidence is the angle between the surface and the light that hits it; the angle of reflection is the angle between the surface and the reflected light. (See Figure B-2.)

Diffuse reflection Reflection from a matte surface, scattering the light in many directions, is called *diffuse reflection.* (See Figure B-3.) Diffusely reflected light enables us to see detail and texture, qualities that are absent from a direct reflecting surface, such as a mirror.

The reflected light that we see combines both direct and diffuse reflection and is called *mixed reflection.*

Absorption

When light is absorbed, it disappears as light and reappears in another form of energy. In most cases, this new form of energy is heat. Photochemical and photoelectrical effects may also occur. Certain materials, such as filters, can selectively absorb and transmit specific wavelengths of light.

Refraction

When a ray of light traveling in one medium passes into another medium

FIGURE B-1 RECTILINEAR PROPAGATION
The light beam from a flashlight illustrates rectilinear propagation of light. The light rays all travel in straight lines in the same direction.

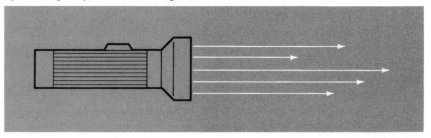

with different optical properties, its direction is changed. This change of direction, or bending, is called refraction. The bending results from a change in the speed of light as it passes from one medium into another. It should be noted that, unlike sound waves, light does not need a medium to carry it; it travels through empty space as well as through air and other transparent media.

Lenses utilize the refractive properties of various types of materials to form images. The light is bent from its straight-line path, so that it is focused on the film.

Another example of refraction is the prism effect. Figure B-4 illustrates what happens when a ray of white light strikes a prism. As the light ray passes from air to glass, it slows down, causing the ray to be bent, or refracted. Since each wavelength is bent to a different degree, the light ray is separated or dispersed into its component colors. Red wavelengths are bent the least, and blue-violet the most.

Polarization

Polarization is the production of orderly vibrations from the random vibrations of ordinary light. Plane polarization occurs when the waves

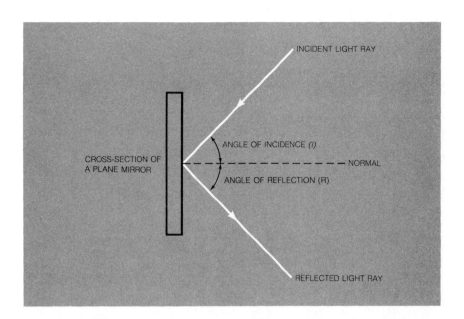

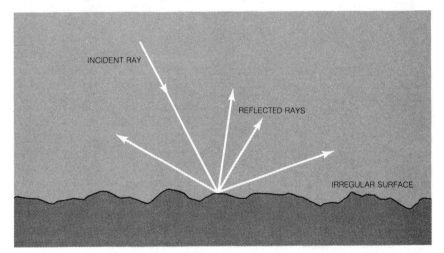

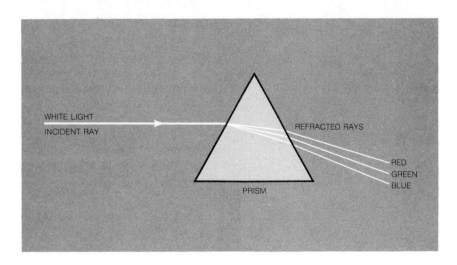

FIGURE B-2 DIRECT REFLECTION
In the case of direct reflection, angle *i* is always equal to angle *r*.

FIGURE B-3 DIFFUSE REFLECTION
Diffuse reflection means there are reflections in many directions. There is no way of knowing what the angle of reflection will be.

FIGURE B-4 PRISM EFFECT
A beam of white light enters the prism and is refracted. Upon exiting the prism, the beam is divided into the various colors that compose white light.

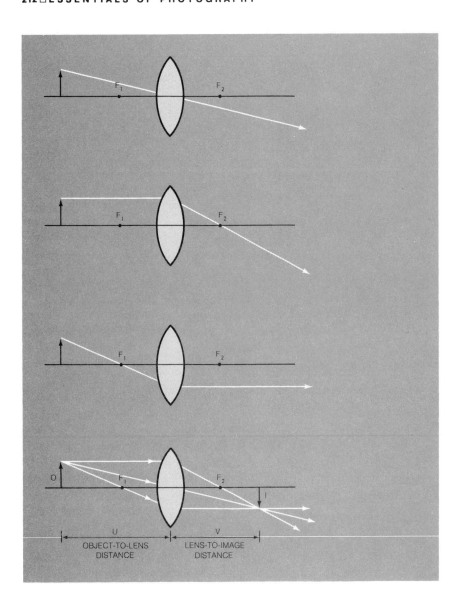

FIGURE B-5 RAY TRACING: POSITIVE LENS
Ray 1 travels through the center of the lens.
Ray 2 travels parallel to the axis and then passes through the rear focal point.
Ray 3 passes through the front focal point and then travels parallel to the axis.
All three rays are needed to locate the image position. The image of the object is located where the three rays intersect.

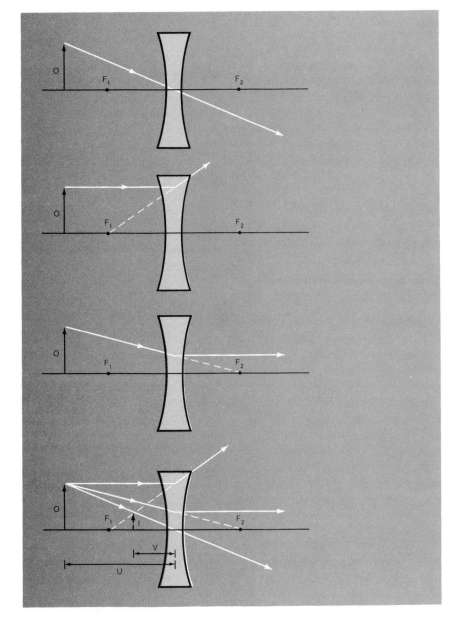

FIGURE B-6 RAY TRACING: NEGATIVE LENS
Ray 1 passes through the center of the lens.
Ray 2 runs parallel to the axis. It is also connected to the front point by an imaginary line.
Ray 3 passes through the lens and is connected to the rear focal point by an imaginary line. Because of refraction this ray emerges and travels parallel to the axis.
The imaginary image for a negative lens is located at the intersection of rays 1 and 2.

vibrate in a single direction. The polarization effect can be obtained in three ways: with special filters, by reflection from nonmetallic glossy surfaces at specific angles, or by scattering from small particles, as in the atmosphere.

RAY TRACING FOR A SIMPLE POSITIVE LENS

Camera lenses, irrespective of their construction details, can be considered similar to simple positive or negative lenses in their image-forming abilities. In particular, they always form a real image by refracting light rays to a point of focus. You can get a better idea of how an image will be formed if you apply the five laws of geometric optics. These laws can also tell you what the image will look like once it is formed. One way to visualize where and how an image will be formed is to use ray tracing.

The action of a lens is more easily understood if the paths of some of the image-forming rays are traced. For a positive lens, a few simple rules can be given, based on definitions of lens properties.

1 A ray passing through the center of the lens is undeviated.

2 A ray traveling parallel to the optical axis, after refraction, passes through the far focal point of the lens.

3 After refraction, a ray passing through the near focal point of the lens emerges from the lens parallel to the axis.

4 The intersection of these three rays indicates where the image is formed.

The distance an object is from the lens is termed the object distance; in the illustrations, it is denoted by the letter u.

The image distance is the distance from the lens to the point where the image is focused; it is denoted in the illustrations with the letter v. (See Figures B-5 and B-6.)

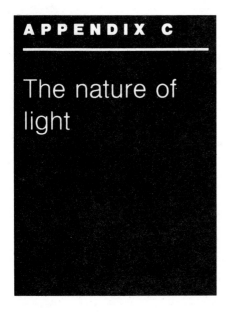

APPENDIX C

The nature of light

The nature of light, or what it is composed of, has been the subject of a great deal of speculation through the years. The essential problem is that light acts as if it is made up of particles under some conditions and as if it is waves under other conditions. The various early theories of light, none of which really explained the "double nature" of light, have been discussed briefly in the text. This appendix will treat only what is known—and still not fully understood—in the twentieth century.

WHAT LIGHT IS

In 1900 German physicist Max Planck advanced a theory that developed into the *quantum theory* of light. He reasoned that light was always emitted in discrete amounts, or *quanta*; each quantum of light was called a *photon*. With some modifications in the years since Planck's work, the quantum theory is accepted today as the best explanation for light's seemingly contradictory behavior. That is, light is believed to be composed of photons, which sometimes act like particles, but travel in wave form. The study of how light behaves is called *optics*. Modern optics has three main branches that apply to photography: physical, geometrical, and quantum optics.

Physical optics

Physical optics assumes that light behaves strictly as a wave. The field of physical optics includes the study of how light moves through space. Physical optics explains how light gets to the subject and then from the subject to the camera.

Geometrical optics

Geometrical optics assumes that light travels in straight lines, or *light rays*. The concept of light rays is important for understanding how an image is formed by the camera lens.

Quantum optics

Quantum optics assumes that light consists of individual quanta of energy, or photons. It is used to study the effects that take place when light is absorbed by matter. For example, quantum optics explains what happens when light is absorbed by a photographic emulsion.

LIGHT WAVES

It is easy to explain many of the properties of light if we assume that light takes the form of a wave. Although sound waves require air or some other medium and ocean waves require water, light waves can travel freely in a vacuum. In free space, light travels at 3×10^8 meters per second (186,000 miles per second); in air, light's velocity is approximately the same. The speed of light is reduced by up to 30 percent when it travels through water or glass; it travels 2.25 $\times 10^8$ meters per second through water and about 2×10^8 meters per second through glass. In other words, the denser the medium through which light must pass, the slower its speed.

There are many other waves that travel through space at the same speed as light; the entire group of waves, including light waves, are called *electromagnetic waves* or *electromagnetic radiation*. Waves composed of two parts are called *transverse waves*; waves composed of only one part are called *longitudinal waves*. (See Figure C-1.) While sound waves have only one part, electromagnetic waves have two parts—one along the direction of travel, and the other at right angles to the direction of travel. (See Figure C-2.)

The distance from a point on one wave to the corresponding point on the next wave is called the *wave-*

length, usually denoted by the Greek letter lambda (λ). The number of waves passing a given point in one second's time is called the *frequency of vibration*. Different electromagnetic waves are distinguished by their wavelengths and by their frequencies. The distance the wave moves above and below the axis of travel is called its *amplitude*. (Amplitude is a measure of the intensity of the light, but it is rarely used in photography.)

The speed of an electromagnetic wave is the product of the wavelength and the frequency. Suppose your favorite radio station broadcasts at 1100 KHz, which is equal to 1,100,000 cycles per second. The length of one wave is 272.7 meters. By multiplying 1,100,000 cycles per second by 272.7 meters, you get 3.0 × 108 meters per second. This shows that radio waves travel at the same speed as light waves.

THE ELECTROMAGNETIC SPECTRUM

As mentioned earlier, other waves besides light travel in space; their wavelengths may be longer or shorter than those of light. The complete series of electromagnetic waves, arranged in order of their wavelengths, is called the *electromagnetic spectrum*. (See Figure 4-1.) The electromagnetic spectrum is continuous from the shortest to the longest wavelengths; there is no sharp, clear-cut line between one wave and another or between one group of waves and another.

The different types of electromagnetic waves vary widely in what they do. Waves with very long wavelengths, such as radio and television waves, have no effect on the body. Even though they cannot be seen or felt, they can be readily detected with a proper receiver, i.e., with a radio or television set. Microwaves and infrared waves can be felt as heat. The human

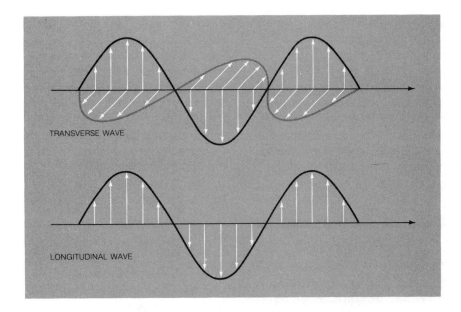

FIGURE C-1 COMPARISON OF TRANSVERSE AND LONGITUDINAL WAVES

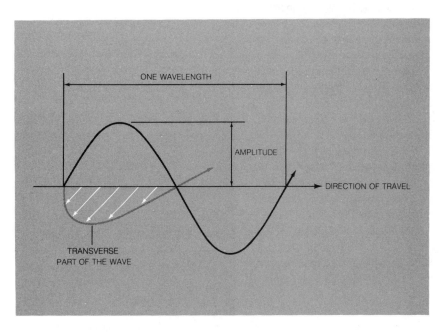

FIGURE C-2 PARTS OF A TRANSVERSE WAVE

eye is sensitive to only a very narrow band of wavelengths—the *visible spectrum,* what we call light. Much shorter wavelengths are the source of radiation—X rays, which can penetrate the human body, and gamma rays, which can penetrate several inches of steel. Unless they are properly controlled, both X rays and gamma rays can pose a threat to human health.

THE VISIBLE SPECTRUM

The waves in the visible spectrum are those most important to photography. The visible spectrum is composed of electromagnetic radiation with wavelengths from approximately 400 to 700 nanometers. (One nanometer, abbreviated *nm,* is equal to 10^{-9} meters.) Within these limits, the human eye sees a change of wavelength as a change of color. Although the change from one color to another is not clear-cut, the approximate color ranges can be indicated on the visible spectrum. (See Figure 4-2.)

The eye has a very slight sensitivity beyond this region; it is sensitive from about 390 nm on the short end to about 760 nm on the long end of the visible spectrum. The useful range for most photographic purposes, however, is from 400 to 700 nm. In photography, the visible spectrum consists of only three bands: blue-violet, from 400 to 500 nm; green, from 500 to 600 nm; and red, from 600 to 700 nm. (See Figure C-3.) While this division is an approximation, it helps solve many practical problems associated with light and photography.

Photographs make use of reflected light that travels from the subject to the camera. The other essential part of the picture-recording process is a light-sensitive material, called film, that records the image when it is exposed to the reflected light.

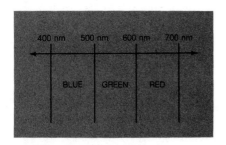

FIGURE C-3 DIVIDING THE VISIBLE SPECTRUM INTO THREE COLORS

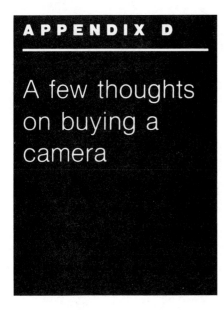

APPENDIX D

A few thoughts on buying a camera

You have probably wondered which camera is the best one to purchase. Maybe you have even made inquiries.

Unfortunately, there is no single camera that will suit the needs of every photographer. The best camera for you is the one that is tailored to meet your individual needs and desires. There are seven simple steps that can help you determine which one is best for you.

Step 1

Try to determine exactly what you are going to need the camera for. Will you be taking pictures of family members and friends, or will you concentrate on scenic and architectural shots? Is the size of the camera an important factor for you? Would a larger or smaller camera allow you greater flexibility? Which format would be best for you? Will you be using your camera every day, or will you be likely to dust it off once a month (or less often)? Be realistic in evaluating what you want and need in a camera.

Step 2

Have a good idea about the features you will want and need. Do you need such features as interchangeable lenses, electronic modes of operation, instant print capability, power winder, synchronized flash, or varied shutter speeds?

Step 3

Decide how much you can pay or how much you want to pay for your camera equipment. Camera features and ruggedness generally increase with the price. Do you want to invest in new equipment, or would you rather buy used camera equipment? (More on used equipment in Step 7.)

Step 4

Consult the equipment reviews in monthly photography magazines and in the various consumers' guides to help you narrow down your choice to a few prime candidates.

Step 5

Once you have narrowed your choice to a few cameras that feature the extras you want at a price you can afford, visit several local camera shops and handle the cameras that fall within your price range. Do a little comparison shopping: the price on any one camera may fluctuate widely from store to store. Generally, you can expect better prices in an area where there is some competition.

Step 6

Decide whether you want to purchase the camera from a store or whether you want to go the mail-order route. Mail order has some distinct advantages; chief among them is lower price. But it carries with it some disadvantages, too—it is difficult to get personalized service from a mail-order company, whereas a camera dealer down the street is available if you have problems with your equipment or need instruction on how to use it.

If you are a first-time camera buyer, you should probably stick with a local dealer who can offer individualized service. If you do decide to order camera equipment through the mail, check with friends and the Better Business Bureau for information about the reputation of the firm.

Step 7

Before you make the final selection, consider the used market. Many camera stores accept trade-ins. You can also check the classified ads in your local newspaper. There is a big advantage to buying used equipment: you can get much more for your money. Before you hesitate because you have been burned on other "used" items, consider the fact that many photography hobbyists trade in perfectly good cameras because their needs change or because they want the latest model with the extra options.

If you do decide to buy used equipment, inspect it carefully. Check for signs of abuse—dents, damaged screw heads, and so on. Look at both sides of the lens for scratches, fungus, chips, and other deformities; carefully shake it to determine whether or not the glass elements have separated. Examine all moving parts; work the shutter, the dials, and any knobs. Steer clear of any camera that appears to have been abused; also stay away from cameras that are so old that parts and repairs will be difficult to obtain.

Many places let you take a used camera for a trial period before you decide whether or not to buy it. Run at least one entire roll of film through the camera during the trial period, develop it, and assess the camera's performance.

APPENDIX E

Characteristic curves

There are many useful tools to help a photographer understand the relationship between exposure and development; one of the most important of these is the characteristic curve.

Sensitometry, an area of science that deals with photography, is the study of how photographic emulsion reacts to changes in exposure and development. The word *sensitometry* comes from the Latin words for *sensitivity* and *measurement.* The results of sensitometric experiments are plotted on graphs called *characteristic curves.* Characteristic curves demonstrate how the silver grains in the negative increase or decrease when exposure or development is increased or decreased.

SENSITOMETRY

Sensitometry is easy to understand if you first examine what happens in the emulsion layer. A thin slice from a negative placed under a microscope reveals the emulsion layer; higher magnifications reveal the individual silver deposits. The individual silver deposits in the negative are called *silver grains.* The light is blocked from passing through the negative where the silver grains are tightly packed; light passes through areas where the silver grains are sparse.

A normally exposed and developed negative has a wide range of silver grain deposits. Both exposure and development affect the silver grains. An increase or decrease in exposure will change the total *number* of silver grains in the emulsion; an increase or decrease in development will change the *size* of each grain. A black negative can have either a large number of individual silver grains or a smaller number of larger grains.

Sensitometry, then, is the study of how exposure and development change the light-passing ability of a negative. A two-step system is used to make sensitometric measurements. A *sensitometer* is first used to make a precise exposure on the emulsion being tested, and the emulsion is carefully processed to give the desired development. The resulting negative is then placed in a *densitometer,* which measures the number of silver grains in a given area of the emulsion. Densitometer readings are called *density values.* Density values represent the number of silver grains in the measured section of the exposed emulsion.

THE CHARACTERISTIC CURVE GRAPH

The characteristic curve is plotted on a graph with horizontal and vertical axes. Exposure values, representing the amount of light necessary to activate a given number of silver grains, are plotted on the horizontal axis; density values, indicating the number of silver grains in the emulsion, are plotted on the vertical axis. Both exposure and density values increase with movement away from the zero point on the graph. Figure E-1 gives a layout of the characteristic curve; the S-shaped line indicates what happens to the number of silver grains when there is a change in exposure or development.

Originally produced during the late 1890s, the characteristic curve graph was first called the H and D curve after Hurter and Driffield, the British photographers who developed the graph. Today it is called the characteristic curve graph, because it always maintains its characteristic "lazy S" shape over a wide range of conditions.

Each kind of film and printing paper has a unique characteristic curve. Some film and paper emulsions have a long straight-line region and a condensed shoulder region; others have a long toe region and a comparatively short straight-line region. You can obtain information about your film and printing paper from the manufacturer.

Parts of the characteristic curve

The characteristic curve includes four main areas.

Toe area The toe-area density values do not increase at the same rate as the exposure values. Density readings taken from the shadow areas of the negative fall in this area of the curve. The bottom limit of the curve is formed by the *fog density,* produced by the film base and the unexposed but developed emulsion, and the *threshold density,* the first density that can be measured above the fog density.

Straight-line area The density and exposure values increase at the same rate in the straight-line area of the curve, called the *area of correct exposure.* Density readings taken from the

moderate shadows and highlights in the negative fall in the straight-line area of the curve.

Shoulder area Like the toe, the shoulder area has density values that do not increase at the same rate as the exposure values. Readings taken from the highlight areas of the negative fall in the shoulder area. *Maximum density*—the maximum number of silver grains that this combination of emulsion, exposure, and development can produce—indicates the upper limit of the curve and is reached at the top of the shoulder.

Region of solarization In the region of solarization—usually used only in special-effects photography—an increase in exposure actually results in a decrease in density. The exposure time necessary to produce solarization is about one thousand times greater than normal exposure time. However, different materials vary widely in the degree of solarization they show.

Characteristic curve terminology

To use the characteristic curve successfully, you must learn to read the six signals linked to the information the curve generates.

Exposure Exposure equals the intensity of the light multiplied by the time it shines on the emulsion; these values are measured with a light meter. When exposure values are plotted on a charcteristic curve, they are generally converted to logarithmic values. Exposure values are always located on the horizontal axis of the graph.

Transmittance Transmittance is the measure of how much light is allowed to pass through a negative. *Transmitted light* passes through a given part of a negative; *incident light* falls on the surface of the negative. Transmittance values are the numerical expressions for the transmitted light divided by the incident light; they are always equal to or less than 1. and are usually reported as a percentage of light transmitted. For example, suppose 6 units of light fell on some part of a negative, and the negative only allowed 3 units of light to pass through. The transmittance value is $\frac{3}{6} = 0.5 = 50$ percent.

Opacity The inverse of the transmittance, opacity measures the amount of light that is *not* allowed to pass through a negative. Opacity is figured by taking the incident light from a given area and dividing it by the transmitted light; opacity values are always greater than or equal to 1. Increasing opacity means that there are increasing numbers of silver deposits in the negative. If 6 units of light are incident and 3 units are transmitted, the opacity is $\frac{6}{3} = 2$.

Density Density is the unit most often used in sensitometric measurements, because it is a more meaningful measurement than either

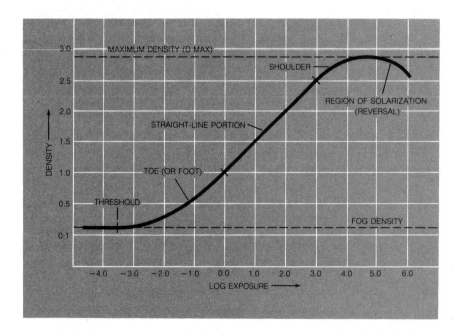

FIGURE E-1 PARTS OF THE CHARACTERISTIC CURVE

transmittance or opacity. Density measures the increasing blackening in a negative because of increased silver deposits. By taking the logarithm of the opacity, we arrive at the density value. If the opacity equals 2, then the density is log 2, or about 0.3.

Over a wide range of viewing conditions, the response of the eye to changes in blackness is approximately logarithmic. Logarithmic density values closely correspond to values that the eye sees as increasing degrees of blackness.

See Figure E-2 for a characteristic curve that shows the relationship among transmittance, opacity, and density; if one of these values is known, it is easy to determine the other two. Exposure values are also represented in log form on the graph. Figure E-3 gives the characteristic curve for normal exposure.

Gamma A term used to indicate the measurement of contrast in a negative, gamma is limited to the straight-line area of the characteristic curve. The value for gamma is found by determining the slope of the straight-line part of the curve. To determine the slope, or *rise,* mark the ends of the straight-line part of the graph. Measure the vertical difference between these points and the horizontal difference. The slope is the vertical difference divided by the horizontal difference. For example, in Figure E-2, if *y* is 4 and *x* is 7, then the slope, or gamma, is $\frac{4}{7}$ = 0.57.

Further information on logarithms and how to determining slopes can be found in any good mathematics text.

Film speed An emulsion's sensitivity to light, or its film speed, can also be determined from its characteristic curve. While the calculations necessary to determine the film speed are complex and of little consequence to a practicing photographer, it is important to know that all film-speed rating systems are based on the characteristic curve.

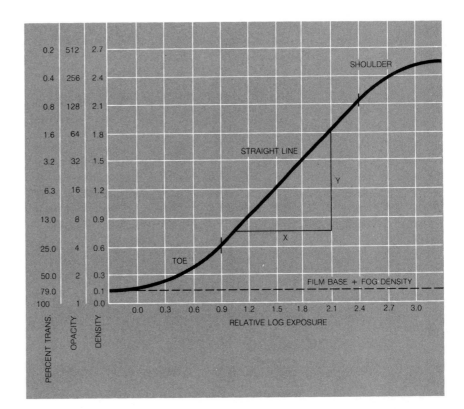

FIGURE E-2 GRAPHING THE CHARACTERISTIC CURVE

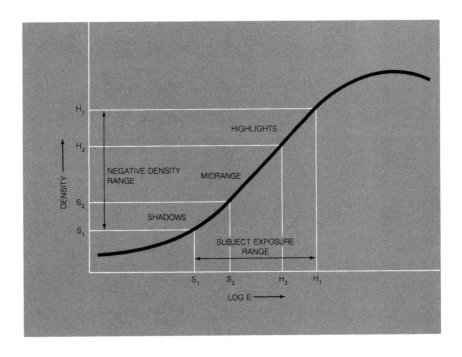

FIGURE E-3 CHARACTERISTIC CURVE FOR NORMAL EXPOSURE

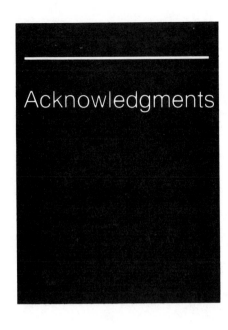

Acknowledgments

The authors gratefully acknowledge the contribution of their Editorial Consultant, C. Geoffrey Berken of the Community College of Philadelphia, who first suggested the use of the many student photographs in this text. He was tireless in selecting, printing, and supplying these illustrations and in securing permission from the photographers. His unselfish efforts have helped make *Essentials of Photography* what it was intended to be: a practical and useful book.

It is our hope that those who use this text will derive inspiration from seeing what excellent results students can achieve with the right combination of knowledge and practice. The Community College of Philadelphia students who contributed their work to *Essentials of Photography* are

Luther Alridge (p. 192)
Patricia M. Artis (p. 166)
Terry Ashe (p. 151)
Joseph T. Baiocco (pp. 50 and 61)
Robert L. Bentley (p. 62)
Bruce N. Berman (p. 192)
Diane Biondi (p. 157)
Michael Cathey (p. 66)
John W. Clifton (p. 169)
Barbara J. Crawford (p. 191)
Paul E. DeWalt (p. 59)
Arnold H. DiBlasi Jr. (p. 54)
Mike Fasone (p. 165)
Janet Fornia (p. 165)
Charles D. Hatcher (p. 60)
David Hering (p. 53)
Rogers C. Horsey Jr. (p. 65)
Michael J. Huffert (p. 59)
Debra M. Jacob (p. 157)
Kenneth C. Jennings Jr. (p. 156)
Joseph C. Lawless (p. 151)
Rose Martin (p. 193)
John J. McGurk (p. 58)
Mary Jo Metalonis (p. 191)
Linda P. Montague (p. 159)
W. F. Mruk (p. 57)
Richard Osborn Jr. (p. 167)
Nathan Pierson (p. 50)
Eileen Polsenberg (p. 51)
Monica Rohn-Turner (p. 166)

Kurtd Schmick (p. 61)
Randi Lyn Schor (pp. 60 and 173)
Lois B. Sharkey (p. 60)
Duncan Urquhart (p. 191)
Karin F. Wheeler (p. 51)
Patrice Williams (p. 59)

In putting together a book of this kind, many difficult decisions must be made. Among the hardest for us was which pieces to include and which to omit. Several people were generous in giving us permission to reproduce photos, yet will not find their work shown here. In making so many fine photographs available to us, Geoff Berken and other friends have made our task both more pleasant and more difficult. There were many excellent examples of student work to choose from, but because of the physical and financial limitations of any such publishing project, we inevitably had to do without some beautiful photographs. Omissions are certainly not meant as criticism of the photographers' work: we wish we could have used them all.

Paul W. Hayes
Scott M. Worton
October 1982

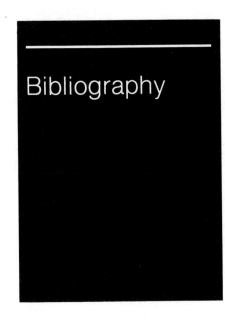

Bibliography

Adams, A. *Basic Photo Series* (5 volumes). Dobbs-Ferry, New York: Morgan and Morgan.

Book I, *Camera and Lens,* revised edition. 1976

Book II, *The Negative,* fourth edition. 1968

Book III, *The Print,* revised edition. 1968

Book IV, *Natural Light Photography,* fifth edition. 1965

Book V, *Artificial Light Photography,* revised edition. 1968

_____ . *Natural Light Photography.* New York: New York Graphic Society, 1977.

Andre, J., *William H. Fox Talbot.* New York: Macmillan Publishing Company, 1975.

Avon, D., and A. Hawkins. *Photography: A Complete Guide to Technique.* New York: Amphoto, 1973.

Blaker, A. *Photography: Art and Technique.* San Francisco: W.H. Freeman, 1980.

Cole, S. *Amphoto Guide to Basic Photography.* Garden City, New York: Amphoto, 1978.

Davis, P. *Photography,* third edition. Dubuque: Wm. C. Brown Company, 1979.

Dixon, D.R. and P.B., *Photography Experiments and Projects.* New York: Macmillan Publishing Company, 1976.

Dowdell, J.J. and R.D. Zakia. *Zone Systemizer.* Dobbs Ferry, New York: Morgan and Morgan, 1973.

Eastman Kodak (ed.). *Adventures in Existing-Light Photography, AC44.* Rochester, New York: Eastman Kodak Company, 1973.

_____ . *Applied Infrared Photography, M-28.* Rochester, New York: Eastman Kodak Company, 1972.

_____ . *Basic Developing, Print, and Enlarging, AJ-2.* Rochester, New York: Eastman Kodak Company, 1977.

_____ . *Basic Photographic Sensitometry Workbook, Z-22-ED.* Rochester, New York: Eastman Kodak Company, 1977.

_____ . *Composition, AC-11.* Rochester, New York: Eastman Kodak Company, 1976.

_____ . *Contrast Index, F-14.* Rochester, New York: Eastman Kodak Company, 1976.

_____ . *Creative Darkroom Techniques, AG-18.* Rochester, New York: Eastman Kodak Company, 1973.

_____ . *Darkroom Data Guide, R-20.* Rochester, New York: Eastman Kodak Company, 1974.

_____ . *Filters for Scientific and Technical Use, B-3.* Rochester, New York: Eastman Kodak Company, 1978.

_____ . *Filters and Lens Attachments, AB-1.* Rochester, New York: Eastman Kodak Company, 1975.

_____ . *Kodak Color Films, E-77.* Rochester, New York: Eastman Kodak Company, 1977.

_____ . *Kodak Infrared Films, N-17.* Rochester, New York: Eastman Kodak Company, 1976.

_____ . *Photography with Large Format Cameras, O-18.* Rochester, New York: Eastman Kodak Company, 1973.

_____ . *Practical Densitometry, E-59.* Rochester, New York: Eastman Kodak Company, 1975.

_____ . *Processing Chemicals and Formulas for Black and White Photography, J-1.* Rochester, New York: Eastman Kodak Company, 1977.

_____ . *Professional Photoguide, R-28.* Rochester, New York: Eastman Kodak Company, 1975.

_____ . *Professional Portrait Techniques, O-4.* Rochester, New York: Eastman Kodak Company, 1973.

_____ . *Reversal Color Processing, E-63.* Rochester, New York: Eastman Kodak Company, 1977.

_____ . *Some Questions and Answers about Camera Lenses, AA-3.* Rochester, New York: Eastman Kodak Company, 1976.

_____ . *Understanding Graininess and Granularity, F-20.* Rochester, New York: Eastman Kodak Company, 1973.

_____ . *What Is Black and White Quality? G4.* Rochester, New York: Eastman Kodak Company, 1977.

Eisenstadt, A. *Eisenstadt's Guide to Photography.* New York: Viking Press, 1978.

Feininger, A. *Light and Lighting in Photography.* Garden City, New York: Amphoto, 1976.

Freeman, M. *The 35mm Handbook.* New York: Ziff-Davis, 1980.

Gernsheim, H. *A Concise History of Photography.* London: Thymes and Hudson, 1965.

_____ . *The History of Photography to 1914.* Oxford: Oxford University Press, 1955.

Hattersley, R. *Photographic Lighting.* Englewood Cliffs, New Jersey: Prentice-Hall, 1979.

Hedgecoe, J. *The Art of Color Photography.* London: Mitchell Beazley Publishers Ltd., 1978.

_____ . *The Book of Photography.* London: Ebury Press, 1976.

_____ . *The Photographer's Handbook.* New York: Alfred A. Knopf, 1977.

Jacobs, L. *Basic Guide to Photography,* second edition. Los Angeles: Petersen Publishing, 1977.

Jacobson, R.E. *The Manual of Photography,* seventh edition. London: Focal Press, 1978.

Langford, M. *Better Photography.* New York: Focal Press, 1978.

Morgan and Morgan (ed.). *The Morgan and Morgan Darkroom Book.* Dobbs Ferry, New York: Morgan and Morgan, 1977.

Osman, C., and P. Turner (ed.). *Creative Camera Collection.* New York: Coo Press/ Two Continents, 1978.

Patterson, F. *Photography for the Joy of It.* New York: Van Nostrand Reinhold, 1978.

Pittard, E.M. *The Compact Photo Lab Index.* Dobbs Ferry, New York: Morgan and Morgan, 1977.

Rehm, K. *Basic Black and White Photography.* Garden City, New York: Amphoto, 1976.

Rhode, R.B., and F.H. McCall. *Introduction to Photography,* third edition. New York: Macmillan Publishing Company, 1976.

Rosen, M.J. *Introduction to Photography.* Boston: Houghton Mifflin Company, 1976.

Sanders, N. *Photographic Tone Control.* Dobbs Ferry, New York: Morgan and Morgan, 1977.

Smith, R.C. *Antique Cameras.* North Vancouver, B.C.: David and Charles Ltd., 1975.

Strobel, L. and H. Todd. *Dictionary of Contemporary Photography.* Dobbs Ferry, New York: Morgan and Morgan, 1977.

Swedlund, C. *Photography: A Handbook of History, Materials, and Processes.* New York: Holt, Rinehart, and Winston, 1974.

Time-Life (ed.) *Time-Life Library of Photography.* New York: Time-Life Books.

> *The Art of Photography.* 1971.
>
> *The Camera.* 1970.
>
> *Color.* 1970.
>
> *The Print.* 1970.

Upton, B. and J. *Photography.* Boston: Little, Brown and Company, 1976.

Vestal, D. *The Craft of Photography.* New York: Harper and Row, 1975.

White, M., R. Zakia, and P. Lorenz. *The New Zone System Manual.* Dobbs Ferry, New York: Morgan and Morgan, 1976.

Yulsman, J. *The Complete Book of 35mm Photography.* New York: Coward, McCann, and Geoghegan, Inc., 1976.

Zakia, R. and H. Todd. *101 Experiments in Photography.* Dobbs Ferry, New York: Morgan and Morgan, 1969.

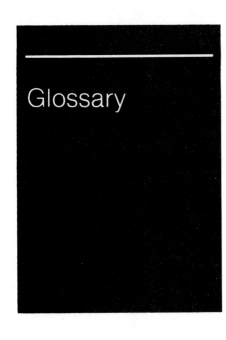

Glossary

A

Aberration
Blurring or distortion caused by a defect in a lens.

Absolute zero
Zero on the Kelvin temperature scale, equal to approximately −273°C. The Kelvin scale is divided into degrees equal in magnitude to those of the Celsius scale.

Absorption
The assimilation of material or energy by an object. Absorbed radiant energy is converted by the absorbing object into another form of energy, generally heat.

Accelerator
One of the parts of a developing solution, which causes an increase in the rate of development. It is usually an alkaline solution.

Acetic acid
The acid in vinegar, used in the development process of film and paper. Acetic acid is diluted with water to produce a solution which stops the developer activity.

Additive mixing
A process of reproducing various colors with combinations of the primary wavelengths of red, green, and blue. Color television depends on the additive process.

Aerial perspective
The effect of atmospheric haze, dust, or smoke on objects at a distance, making them appear lighter. Haze tends to decrease contrast and give an illusion of depth to the picture.

Agitation
The movement or action used to circulate the developer, the stop bath, and the fixer evenly over the emulsion of film and paper, to replace exhausted solution with fresh and ensure uniform chemical activity.

Air bells
Small bubbles of air that form on the emulsion of photographic film and paper during processing. Air bells prevent the developer and other solutions from working at that site, causing uneven development and spots of lighter density.

Ammonium thiosulfate
Main ingredient of rapid fixers, used in place of sodium thiosulfate.

Amplitude
In a wave form, the maximum height of the wave, measured from the base or zero level.

Antihalation backing
Light-absorbing layer applied to the film base to prevent light from being reflected back onto the emulsion after it has passed through.

Aperture
A circular opening in a lens system that controls the amount of light that strikes the film. An aperture may be fixed or adjustable.

Artificial light
A light source, whether man-made or naturally occurring, that is contrived, controlled, or otherwise manipulated.

Atom
The smallest division of a chemical element retaining the distinctive properties of the element.

Available light
Natural light.

B

Background merger
A distracting element of the background that appears to become a part of the main subject, e.g., a tree that seems to be growing from a person's head.

Balance
A factor of composition, the even distribution of objects and light and dark areas in a photographic print.

Barrel distortion
A lens defect that causes straight lines to appear bowed outward at the center. Barrel distortion is a characteristic of fisheye lenses and is the opposite of pincushion distortion.

Bellows
A flexible light-tight enclosure used to connect the film plane to the lens in some cameras and enlargers.

Bitumen of Judea
Asphaltum, the material used by

Niépce to serve as the emulsion for his photograph on a pewter plate. The image is developed in lavender oil.

Blocked highlights
Highlight areas with less than normal detail or contrast because of various factors, such as overexposure and overdevelopment.

Blue
Electromagnetic radiation of 400–500 nm in wavelength on the visible spectrum. One of the additive primaries.

Border merger
An important element of the photograph that is cut off by one of the edges or borders of the print or negative.

Bounce flash
A flash aimed at a wall, ceiling, or other reflective surface, rather than directly at the subject. Bounce flash helps create the illusion of existing or natural light.

Bracketing
Making several exposure variations of the subject to ensure accuracy. For example, if the best estimate of correct exposure is $\frac{1}{125}$ at f/16, a bracket exposure would be one stop under the estimate ($\frac{1}{125}$ at f/22) and one stop over ($\frac{1}{125}$ at f/11).

Brightener
A fluorescent material added to photographic papers to intensify the whites.

Brightness adaptation
Automatic adjustments made by the eye for various levels of illumination, producing high sensitivity in low illumination and low sensitivity in high illumination.

Bromide paper
A fast photographic printing paper with silver bromide as the light-sensitive emulsion, used for projection printing.

Burning-in
Giving selected areas of an enlargement additional exposure to increase density and detail. The opposite of dodging.

Butterfly light
One type of portrait lighting. The main or key light is positioned directly in front of and above the subject. The shadow from the nose is projected directly down onto the upper lip.

C

Calotype
A photographic process developed by William Henry Fox Talbot. Calotype was the first reliable negative process, the forerunner of modern negative processes.

Camera obscura
A small light-tight room or box with a lens or aperture in one wall that forms images on the opposite wall. The images formed can be traced to make a permanent record of the scene.

Catalyst
A substance that, although it does not itself have a direct effect on the process, is used to start or speed up a chemical reaction.

Center of interest
The object or area of the image that attracts and holds the attention of the eye most strongly.

Characteristic curve
A graph drawn for any combination of film and developer. A characteristic curve is obtained by plotting the logarithm of various exposures and the resulting densities after development. Also known as *H & D (Hurter and Drifield) curve* and *sensitometric curve.*

Chemical development
The reduction of silver ions in the silver halide grain to metallic silver by a developer, forming the visible silver image from the latent image.

Chemical sensitization
Increasing the response sensitivity of a silver halide during the manufacturing process, generally by adding sulfur to the emulsion.

Chloride paper
A relatively slow photographic paper with a silver chloride emulsion, used mostly for contact printing.

Chlorobromide paper
Photographic printing paper with a mixture of silver chloride and silver bromide as the emulsion; speed and tone characteristics are between those of chloride and bromide papers.

Chroma
An attribute of color that describes the saturation or intensity of the hue.

Chromatic aberration
A lens defect that causes various wavelengths (colors) to image differently. Modern lenses are coated to correct for chromatic aberration.

Circle of confusion
The measure of to what degree an image point is out of focus. The larger the circle of confusion, the more out of focus the image is. Circles of confusion are used in making acceptable depth-of-field determinations.

Clear time
The time required for cloudiness to disappear from film placed in fixer. Doubling the clear time is a good rule of thumb for fix time.

Cold light
A fluorescent light source of high voltage and low temperature, used as an enlarger light source.

Color
Light is composed of separate wavelengths, perceived visually as color. Light is described in terms of hue, chroma, and value. *Hue* defines a specific wavelength; *chroma,* the saturation or amount of the hue present, and *value,* the lightness or darkness of the hue.

Color balance
The apparent realism of the colors, especially the neutral colors, in a photographic image. For example, if the whites of a print appear bluish or pinkish, the color balance is said to be blue or red.

Color constancy
The degree to which the color of an object appears unchanged when viewed under various sources of illumination. A white shirt, for example, may appear white whether viewed under sunlight or tungsten light.

Color reversal
A color film process whereby positive color images are produced directly from the source rather than by a negative process.

Color temperature
A scale for rating the color of any illu-

mination. Color temperature is measured in degrees Kelvin (°K).

Compaction
A zone system term based on exposure readings. By decreasing the film development, negative density ranges are compressed.

Composition
The arrangement of the physical elements of a photograph and the relationship of these elements to each other and to the whole arrangement.

Concave
A lens surface that curves inward; opposite of *convex*.

Condenser enlarger
A projection printer that uses directed light, as opposed to a diffusion system, using scattered light.

Condenser lens
A lens or lens system for concentrating illumination at a specific point.

Contact print
A photographic print exactly the same size as the negative. It is made by placing the negative and the printing paper emulsion in contact with each other and exposing through the negative.

Contact sheet
A number of contact prints on the same sheet of photosensitive paper.

Contrast
The difference in density from one portion of the negative to another and from highlight to shadow in the print.

Contrast filter
Transparent filters of yellow, blue, green, red, etc., that absorb certain wavelengths. They are used to lighten or darken certain colors in black and white photography.

Converging lens
A lens that bends parallel light rays toward the center of the lens.

Correction filter
A filter used on the camera in black and white photography to correct the tonal rendition of certain colors.

Cropping
Eliminating a part of a negative or slide by trimming or masking, then reproducing only the desired part of the original exposure.

Cross light
Illumination of the subject from the side.

Curvature of field
A lens defect preventing the image from being focused on a single plane.

Curvilinear distortion
A lens defect that causes image lines to bend outward (barrel) or inward (pincushion).

Cyan
Wavelength in the region of 485 nm; may be produced by removing red from white light or by mixing blue and green.

D

Daylight
Light composed of sunlight and skylight. Daylight quality and color temperature depend on the time of day, atmospheric conditions, etc.

Densitometer
An instrument used to measure the light-stopping ability of a photographic image, as in finding the various densities of a negative.

Density
The measure of the light-absorbing characteristics of a photographic image.

Depth of field
The range of distances from the camera that are within acceptable focus. Depth of field depends on f/number, lens focal length, object distance, and personal preference.

Developer
A chemical solution containing a reducing agent, used to change the latent image into a visible image on photosensitive material.

Diaphragm
In photography, synonomous with *aperture*: a usually adjustable hole for controlling light quantity.

Diffuse light
Light that has been scattered or reflected in various directions.

Diffusion enlarger
A printing projection system that scatters the light source so that the negative is evenly illuminated; the opposite of condenser enlargers.

Dispersion
The separation of white light into individual colors (frequencies), e.g., barrel and pincushion distortion.

Dodging
A method for reducing exposure in selected portions of a print, usually by placing an object between the lens and the easel of the enlarger. During exposure, the object casts a shadow on the portion of the print where reduced exposure is required.

Dry mounting
Using a usually heat-sensitive tissue-paper adhesive between a photographic print and the mounting medium. By applying pressure (and sometimes pressure), the print is permanently attached to the mount.

Drying aid
A chemical solution used in film and paper to retard curling and stop water spots.

E

Edge burning
Giving more exposure to the edges of a photographic print, which directs the eye towards the center.

Eighteen-percent gray
A standard gray value that reflects eighteen percent of the light that strikes it. Eighteen percent gray is the medium value that photoelectric meters are adjusted to and upon which black and white exposure is based.

Electromagnetic spectrum
The range of radiant energy wavelengths from gamma rays to radio waves that includes visible light.

Electronic flash
Illumination produced by passing electrical current through a tube of inert gas (usually xenon); the light produced approaches the color of sunlight.

Element
(1) A single glass part of a lens sys-

tem. (2) A substance composed of atoms having the same number of protons in their nuclei, e.g., silver, bromine, oxygen, hydrogen.

Emulsion
The light-sensitive coating on photographic film or paper, usually suspended in a gelatin base.

Enlarger
Device used to project photographic images at sizes larger than the negative.

Enlargement
A print made from a projection printer in which the print is larger than the negative.

Enlarger head
The part of the enlarger that houses the light source, the negative carrier, and the lens.

Exposure
The amount of light allowed to strike the photographic material. It is expressed by the equation $E = I \times T$, or exposure equals intensity multiplied by time.

Exposure–development matrix
A 3×3 matrix of 9 prints or negatives, illustrating the effects of various exposure and development combinations. also called *E–D matrix*.

Exposure latitude
The maximum amount exposure can change, either increasing or decreasing, without a significant effect on the image.

F

f/number
A numerical designation assigned to aperture openings. The f/number is equal to the focal length of the lens divided by the diameter of the lens opening. Also known as f/stop.

f/stop
Another name for *f/number*.

Fiber paper
Photographic printing paper whose paper base is composed entirely of cellulose fiber.

Fill light
A light source of less intensity than the key or main light, used to fill in the shadow created by the main light.

Film
A flexible plastic, usually acetate, coated with a light-sensitive material.

Film plane
The plane within the camera body where the image is focused on the emulsion during exposure.

Film speed
The ASA or DIN number associated with each film identifies the relative sensitivity of the emulsion to light; the number is referred to as the speed of the film.

Filter
Any of various kinds of materials used to change the quality or quantity of light from any given source, e.g., color filters, polarizing filters, neutral density filters; usually glass or acetate.

Filter factor
A series of numbers used to increase exposure and compensate for the different amounts of light absorbed by various filters.

Fixer
A chemical solution that dissolves silver halides but will not dissolve metallic silver, to fix or stop the material's sensitivity to light.

Flashbulb
A sealed glass bulb containing oxygen and a combustible material that produces a short burst of light when ignited by an electric current.

Flood light
A light that spreads illumination over a broad area.

Focal-plane shutter
A flexible curtain shutter close to the focal plane, with a window of varying size that moves across the film during exposure.

Fog
Densities on film that result from extraneous light striking the film. Fog can also be caused by chemical action.

Foreground merger
Something in the foreground of the picture that interferes with the subject and becomes distracting to the composition.

Format
A term describing cameras that is essentially determined by the size of the negative. For example, a $2\frac{1}{4} \times 2\frac{1}{4}$ format camera has a $2\frac{1}{4}$- × -$2\frac{1}{4}$-inch negative.

Forty-five-degree light
Common portrait light.

Framing
(1) The area within the borders of the camera viewfinder. (2) Using natural frames to isolate and emphasize the subject, e.g., framing a shot with tree limbs in the borders.

Front lighting
Light directed from the camera position toward the subject.

G

Glossy
Smooth, shiny photographic printing paper. Glossy prints are used for reproduction.

Graded
Photographic prints have a certain amount of contrast which is expressed as a number on a scale from one through five, five being the highest contrast.

Grain
Clumps of silver halide crystals in the emulsion, so-called because they give the image a granular texture when viewed under high magnification.

Gray scale
A series of ten neutral gray tones ranging from black to white. Each step in the scale represents one f/stop difference in exposure.

H

Halation
Light that passes through the emulsion, strikes the film base, and is reflected back into the emulsion, causing a halo around the original image. Most modern films are coated with an antihalation backing to prevent halation.

Halogen
A group of elements which contains bromine, chlorine, iodine, and fluorine.

Hardening fixer
Fixer to which an agent has been added to harden the gelatin in the film emulsion, helping to reduce the chance of scratches and other damage.

Haze
The optical effect caused by the scattering of light by particles in the atmosphere. Haze appears bluish because short wavelengths of light are scattered more than long wavelengths.

Highlight
Generally, the lightest tonal area of a print or the most dense areas of the negative.

Hydroquinine
A developing agent associated with high-contrast developers or combined with other developers (metol) in general developers.

Hyperfocal distance
The distance from the camera to the nearest object that is in focus when the lens is focused on infinity.

Hypo
General term for a fixing agent.

I

Incident light
Light that is falling on a subject, as opposed to light that is reflected or emitted by the subject.

Ion
An atom that is charged either positively or negatively, by losing or gaining an electron, respectively.

Ionic bond
The sharing of electrons by two ions to form a stable configuration of atoms.

Integral tripack
A type of color photographic film with several different layers of emulsions. Each emulsion is sensitive to a different color of light.

Inverted
Upside down. An image passing through a single positive lens element is inverted.

K

Key light
The main light source on the subject when more than one flood or flash is used.

Kelvin
In physics and chemistry, a temperature scale sometimes referred to as the *absolute scale*. The Kelvin scale increments are equal to those of the Celsius scale. Zero on the Kelvin scale is equal to $-273°C$. The Kelvin scale is used in photography to specify color temperature.

L

Latent image
The invisible image formed on photosensitive material when it is exposed. Development is necessary to make the image visible.

Latitude
Exposure range: the amount of exposure change possible without affecting the image quality. Latitude is usually measured in f/stops.

Lens
A curved piece of glass or transparent material capable of focusing light to form an image.

Leading lines
Lines within a composition that tend to lead the eye in a certain direction.

Leaf shutter
A shutter, made of interleaving blades, usually positioned between the elements of a camera lens.

Lens flare
Re-reflected or "loose" light from lens surfaces that reaches the film or paper. It causes a lowering of contrast. Flare is controlled by coating the lens.

Light
Electromagnetic radiation between 400–700 nanometers that is visible to the human eye. The visible part of the spectrum.

Lightness constancy
Brightness constancy, the phenomenon of seeing what one "knows" is there, with respect to the lightness of a surface under varying illumination. For example, if a white shirt is seen under bright light and then under much dimmer light, the viewer perceives the shirt as "white," even though the light that reaches the eye is in fact gray rather than white.

Linear perspective
A feeling of depth produced by the apparent convergence of parallel lines and/or by diminishing image size with increasing distance of the object from the viewer.

Liter
A metric unit of measure equal to 1000 milliliters or about 1.06 quarts.

Logarithm
An exponent or power applied to a constant base. For example, if the base is 10, the logarithm of 100 is 2, because $10^2 = 100$; the log of 1000 is 3, because $10^3 = 1000$.

Loop lighting
A type of portrait light, so-called because of the looping shadow cast by the subject's nose.

Luminance range
The range in f/numbers or other increments between the textured highlight luminance and the detailed shadow luminance of a scene.

Luster
A photographic paper surface between glossy and matte.

M

Macro
Photography of items that are visible to the naked eye but are reproduced by the camera with an image ratio of one to one or greater.

Magenta
Visible wavelength of 500–600 nm. One of the subtractive primaries. It is equal to minus green by the additive process. Magenta is a combination of red and blue.

Matte
A flat, dull-surfaced printing paper.

Medium format
Refers to camera forms in the range of $2\frac{1}{4} \times 2\frac{1}{4}$ inches to 6×7 centimeters.

Meniscus lens
A lens in which both lens surfaces curve in the same direction, i.e., a concave-convex or convex-concave lens.

Mergers
Term for composition errors in which the subject of the print blends in with the scene itself.

Metol
A developing agent (p-methylaminophenol) for general-purpose use. It is often mixed with hydroquinine.

Midtones
Values of gray in a print between black and white.

Molecule
The smallest particle of a substance that has all the characteristics of that substance. A molecule contains one or more atoms of the same or different elements, e.g., gaseous hydrogen (H_2), water (H_2O), and silver bromide ($AgBr$).

N

Natural light
Light that exists at the scene and is used in its natural state, without manipulation by the photographer.

Negative
Photographic opposite of the original scene or final print. Light tones of the original scene are rendered dark, and dark tones are rendered light.

Negative carrier
The part of the enlarger that holds the negative flat and in position during printing.

Neutral black
The black part of the image on the photographic printing paper. A black without any noticeable blue or brown tinting.

Neutral-density filter
A light decreasing filter that absorbs all wavelengths equally.

O

Object merger
Object which interferes with the main subject.

Opacity
The light-stopping ability of the negative. Opacity is the opposite of transmittance. As opacity increases, transmittance decreases. For example, if the incident light is 100 and the transmitted light through the negative is 5, the opacity is 20.

Optical axis
A line through the centers of curvature of a lens or lens system.

Optics
The study of light, its creation and propagation, and how it changes and is changed.

Orthonon
Black and white film emulsions sensitive only to blue and ultraviolet frequencies, also termed *color-blind emulsions.*

Orthochromatic
Black and white emulsions sensitive to blue, ultraviolet, and green frequencies. The green sensitivity is obtained by adding a dye to the orthonon emulsion.

Overdevelopment
Overprocessing of photographic material by developing it too long or at too high a temperature or by agitating the tank too vigorously. Overdevelopment results in high density, high contrast, increased grain size, and increased fog.

Overexposure
The problem of having too much light on the photographic material, characterized by high-density negatives which lose detail in the highlights.

P

Panning
Movement of the camera during exposure, usually to follow a moving subject.

Panchromatic
Black and white emulsions sensitive to the entire visible spectrum.

Parallax
Differences in image position that are especially noticeable at close range. If the viewfinder on the camera is in a different position than the lens, the image seen through the viewfinder is different from the image seen through the lens. To illustrate this, try looking at an object approximately 15 inches away, first with one eye, then with the other. Because your two eyes see the object from two different positions that are not in line with the object, the images are slightly different. If you perform the same experiment with an object farther away, the shift in image position will be less, the greater the object's distance from your eyes.

Paramount light
Portrait light that is distinguished by a characteristic shadow directly under the nose, which generally resembles the shape of a butterfly.

Pattern
Visual elements that are orderly and usually repeated several times over a given space.

Perspective
The creation of depth as a third dimension in a two-dimensional photograph. Several types of perspective may be involved in developing this illusion. See *Linear perspective, Aerial perspective, Leading lines.*

Photochemical reaction
A chemical reaction that changes electromagnetic radiation, usually light, into chemical energy.

Photon
A quantum of light; the fundamental unit of radiant energy.

Pincushion distortion
A lens distortion displacing image points, causing straight lines to appear bowed; the opposite of barrel distortion.

Pinhole
A small aperture that can be used to form an image without a lens.

Polarization
The process of causing random light vibrations to vibrate in a single direction, for example, by passing the unpolarized light through a sheet of diffraction grating.

Positive
A photographic image that has approximately the same tone as the original scene: light tones are light and dark tones are dark.

Previsualization
A zone-system term, the mental rendering of a scene or subject by the photographer, who then adjusts exposure and development to produce the previsualized result.

Printing frame
A device for making contact prints, usually under a projection enlarger. A printing frame holds the negative(s) tightly against the printing paper.

Processing
Any of a number of procedures that follow exposure of a photographic material.

Push processing
Increasing effective film speed by increasing development. Push processing usually results in higher contrast and increased grain size.

Q

Quantum
In light theory, a discrete amount, or packet, of light energy: associated with the photon.

R

Radiator
A source of electromagnetic energy.

Rangefinder
A type of camera featuring a device for estimating distance. A rangefinder uses mirrors or prisms and the parallax effect to bring images into alignment.

RC
Resin coated. RC photographic printing paper is coated with a plastic so it will absorb less liquid during processing, allowing shorter processing times.

Reciprocal
The number obtained by dividing any (nonzero) number into 1. The reciprocal of 4 is $\frac{1}{4}$ or .25; the reciprocal of 5 is $\frac{1}{5}$ or .2; etc.

Reciprocity failure
Failure of the reciprocity laws, which usually occurs at low light levels or with long exposure times.

Red
One of the three additive primaries. Red lies in the visible spectrum at approximately 650 nm and longer.

Reflection
A change in the direction of energy at the intersection of two materials. For example, light traveling through the air strikes a mirror and is reflected back into the air, in a different direction. Reflection is responsible for the distortion of the image seen when you look into the curved mirror formed by the bowl of a spoon. Not only are the proportions of your face changed when you look at the convex side; when you look into the concave side, your image is upside down. Some energy is always lost in reflection, i.e., some of the energy is not reflected but rather remains in the reflecting material.

Refraction
A change in the speed and direction of energy at the intersection of two transparent media. For example, light traveling through the air strikes a glass lens and continues to travel through the glass, but in a different direction and at a different speed. Another familiar example is a glass of water with a spoon in it. The spoon handle appears to be bent, because the light from the lower part of the spoon is refracted as it passes through the water, then through the glass, then through the air; the light from the upper part passes only through the air.

Region of solarization
The area above the shoulder of the H & D characteristic curve where density begins to decrease with increased exposure.

Rembrandt light
Light that produces a diamond-shaped highlight on the shadow side of the subject's face.

Restrainer
A chemical that reduces the rate of development and the rate of fog formation.

Reticulation
Wrinkling of the film emulsion caused by abrupt changes in processing temperature. Reticulation is rare in modern films except when intentionally produced.

Rule of thirds
A principle of composition. According to the rule, the most effective proportion for composition is a one-to-two relationship, that is, a subject is best placed in the lower or upper third of the print, rather than centered in the frame.

S

Safelight
A light source, usually filtered, for use with photographic materials that has little or no exposure effect on the materials. Different materials require different safelight filters.

Selective focus
An effect obtained by selecting a shallow depth of field and focusing on the subject. The subject remains in sharp focus but the foreground and background of the scene are blurred and out of focus.

Semi-gloss
A photographic printing paper surface that is smooth and slightly glossy.

Semi-matte
A photographic printing paper surface that is flat but not as dull as matte.

Sensitivity speck
A small spot believed to be on or within a silver halide grain that acts as the site for the beginning of latent-image formation.

Sensitometry
The study of how photographic materials react to light energy.

Sepia
A yellowish brown color. Sepia toning is a process for producing such color in black and white prints.

Shadow
An area of the scene not directly illuminated by the light source.

Shoulder
Portion of the characteristic curve

relating to high density and exposure above the working area. Contrast in exposure following the shoulder begins to decrease.

Shutter
A device within the camera which controls the time of exposure.

Shutter speed
The time of exposure, usually the time from when the shutter is half-open to when it is half-closed.

Side light
A light source that illuminates the subject at approximately 90 degrees from the imaginary line between the camera and the subject.

Silhouette light
Light producing only a dark outline against a lighter background.

Silver halide
A compound of silver with iodine, chlorine, or bromine. Silver halides are the light-sensitive components of most photographic materials.

Simple lens
A single lens element, which may be concave, convex, etc.

Single lens reflex
A camera that uses a mirror between the lens and the film. Subject composition is done through the lens just prior to exposure. The mirror moves up out of the way and the film is exposed.

Skylight
Light reflected from the atmosphere; generally bluish in color. Skylight and sunlight together make daylight.

Slide
A transparency, usually 35 mm, made for projection viewing.

Sodium thiosulfate
The most common fixing agent, or hypo.

Soft focus
A special lens or lens attachment to produce a slightly diffused or blurred image.

Solarization
A reversal of image tones caused by drastic overexposure of the photographic materials.

Specular reflection
A mirror-like reflection.

Split lighting
Lighting placed to illuminate exactly one side of the subject's face and create a strong shadow on the other side.

Spotting
Covering small print defects, dust spots, small scratches, etc., with dye and blending the defective spot into the rest of the print.

Spot meter
Type of reflection exposure meter with a very narrow angle of view, which can be as small as one degree.

Squeegee
Soft, flexible blade used to remove excess water from the photographic material.

Stop bath
A diluted solution of acetic acid used to stop the action of the developer.

Straight line portion
The middle area of the characteristic curve between the toe and shoulder, where an increase in exposure produces an equal increase in density.

Subject contrast
The ratio of luminance from highlight to shadow. On an average day, outdoor luminance ratio is approximately 160:1.

Sunlight
One of the components of daylight. Sunlight is radiation of approximately 5500°K.

Surface textures
The look, feel, or both of a photographic printing paper surface. Such surfaces may be described as smooth, fine grained, rough, tweed, silk, and tapestry.

Swing
An adaptation on a view camera that allows the lens to rotate around a vertical axis. This adjustment will correct certain distortions of the image.

Synchronization
Matching of the flash or strobe unit to the timing of the camera shutter.

T

Telephoto lens
A lens with a long focal length.

Test strip
A series of different exposures on the same piece of photographic materials in order to determine the correct exposure.

Texture
A surface characteristic of photographic paper: rough or smooth; also used to describe a small-scale visible pattern.

Thin
Term describing a negative that has too little silver deposits because of underexposure, underdevelopment, or both.

Threshold
A level in photographic material where response just begins to produce a density.

Tint
A characteristic of photographic paper, specifically the color of the paper stock that the emulsion is coated on, such as white or grey.

Toe
A part of the characteristic curve associated with short exposure times and low densities. The toe is the portion between the fog density and the straight-line portion.

Tone
A photographic paper characteristic. Cold-toned prints are bluish; warm-toned prints are brownish.

Toning
Changing the hue of the photographic image by chemical means, such as sepia or selinium toning.

Tone control
A system for altering image density to produce a desired effect; a similar technique to the zone system.

Twin lens reflex
A camera equipped with two lenses of

equal focal length, one for viewing and one for making the photograph.

U

Ultraviolet
Electromagnetic radiation in the range of 400 to 10 nm, which is invisible to the human eye. Most photographic materials, however, are sensitive to ultraviolet. Sometimes referred to as *black light.*

Underdevelopment
Insufficient development, caused by low developer temperature, not enough agitation, or too short a time in development. Underdevelopment causes lower than normal contrast.

Underexposure
Not enough light for desired film response. Underexposure causes low density and loss of contrast.

V

Value
One of the terms in the Munsell system of color designation: the lightness or darkness of the color. White has a high value; black has a low value.

Variable contrast
Printing paper, either paper or RC, that is coated with two emulsions of different contrasts. Variable contrast is obtained by coloring the exposure light with filters that cause one of the emulsions to respond more than the other.

View camera
Usually a large-format camera with the ability to adjust for distortion by adjusting the lens tilt or camera back.

Vignette
Darkening or lightening the background, usually during printing, to cause the subject to merge gradually into the background toward the edges.

Violet
Visible light near 400 nm, at the short end of the visible spectrum.

W

Warm
Refers to the tone of a photographic print; warm tones are brownish in hue.

Washing
Putting film and paper in water to remove unwanted chemical residue.

Washing aid
A bath that chemically speeds up the washing process; usually an alkaline solution.

Wavelength
The distance between two corresponding points of a wave or other form of radiation. The larger the wavelength, the smaller the frequency. Wavelength and frequency distinguish light from other forms of electromagnetic radiation.

Wet collodion process
An early photographic process using a silver chloride emulsion coated on glass plates that had to be exposed and developed before the emulsion dried.

Wetting agent
A chemical substance used in the processing of film to prevent water from beading on the film surface and to promote more even drying.

Whitener
A fluorescent substance used to brighten the paper base and thus make brighter highlights.

X

Xenon
An inert gas used in electronic flash lamps.

Y

Yellow
Light of approximately 580 nm, located between green and red. Yellow is one of the subtractive primaries and is minus blue.

Z

Zone system
A method for controlling exposure and development to produce a preconceived image rendition. A visual change of one zone of exposure is equal to one stop.

Zoom lens
A lens with movable elements capable of several different focal lengths.

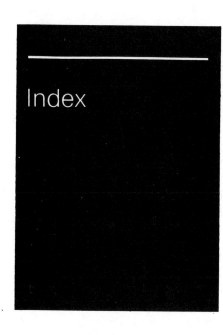

Index